Spine Disorders

Spine Disorders

Medical and Surgical Management

J. D. Bartleson, M. D.
Mayo Clinic

H. Gordon Deen, M. D.
Mayo Clinic

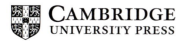
CAMBRIDGE
UNIVERSITY PRESS

CAMBRIDGE UNIVERSITY PRESS

Cambridge, New York, Melbourne, Madrid, Cape Town, Singapore, São Paulo, Delhi

Cambridge University Press
The Edinburgh Building, Cambridge CB2 8RU, UK

Published in the United States of America
by Cambridge University Press, New York

www.cambridge.org
Information on this title: www.cambridge.org/9780521889414

First published 2009

Printed in the United Kingdom at the University Press, Cambridge

A catalog record for this publication is available from the British Library

Library of Congress Cataloging-in-Publication Data

Spine disorders : medical and surgical management / edited by
J. D. Bartleson, H. Gordon Deen.
    p. ; cm.
  Includes bibliographical references and index.
  ISBN 978-0-521-88941-4 (hardback)
1. Spine–Diseases. 2. Spine–Surgery. I. Bartleson, J. D. II. Deen,
H. Gordon.
  [DNLM: 1. Spinal Cord Diseases–surgery. 2. Spinal Diseases–
surgery. 3. Spinal Cord Diseases–diagnosis. 4. Spinal Diseases–
diagnosis. WE 725 S7594 2009]
  RD768.S6743 2009
  617.5′6059–dc22

                                                        2009012561

ISBN 978-0-521-88941-4 hardback

To my wife Ruth, for her steadfast love and support. To my children Joseph and Ruthie, who continually inspire me to look at the world in new ways.

H. Gordon Deen, M. D.

To past, present, and future patients with spine disorders.

J. D. Bartleson, M. D.

Contents

Preface

It is fair to ask why another spine textbook is needed, especially one authored by a neurologist and a neurosurgeon. There are several reasons.

First, spine disorders are very common, cause considerable morbidity, and have a tremendous economic impact.

Second, the evaluation of a patient with back and limb pain can be challenging. While a clear-cut diagnosis is often possible, in many cases the diagnosis is uncertain. Even if a diagnosis can be established, there are typically multiple treatment options available. Experts disagree about the best course of treatment for an individual patient, and many therapies are only partially helpful. The uncertainties and frustrations associated with the diagnosis and treatment of spine conditions are felt by providers, patients, their families, employers, and payers.

Third, many healthcare providers have limited training in spine disorders. As a result, many providers are ill prepared to manage spine patients who often comprise a significant segment of their practice.

Fourth, we believe that the optimal management of the patient with spine pain, limb pain, or both involves a multidisciplinary approach. Neurologists and neurosurgeons have a long tradition of working together as a team in the evaluation and treatment of many neurologic conditions including tumors, cerebrovascular disease, and spine disorders. A neurologic and neurosurgical perspective is important because most of the spine problems that require surgery involve compression of nervous tissue (the spinal cord, individual nerve roots, or the cauda equina). Fifth, while most spine textbooks now available are written by and for surgeons, the bulk of spine care is provided by non-surgeons. We believe a concise book targeted at the full range of providers who care for spine patients is needed.

This book grew out of a course that we have given for several years at the Annual Meeting of the American Academy of Neurology. The book describes the anatomy, physiology, and pathophysiology of the spine. It describes how to evaluate clinically and with laboratory and imaging studies the patient with disease affecting the cervical, thoracic, and lumbar levels of the spine. We describe available medical and surgical treatment options for the patient with various spine disorders. The book can be read from cover to cover or piecemeal as one encounters specific spine symptoms or considers potential surgical procedures. The goal of the book is not to teach the nonsurgeon how to do spine surgery but to inform the reader when surgery should be considered, what surgical interventions can be offered, and the risks and benefits that are involved. We hope and believe that this book will benefit all healthcare providers who see patients with spine disorders.

Acknowledgments

I am very grateful to Dr. Timothy P. Maus for his help with the neuroradiology testing section and many of the images and to Dr. W. Neath Folger for his review of the electrophysiology testing section. I am deeply indebted to Ms. Linda A. Schmidt for her steadfast assistance and countless hours of work.

J. D. B.

I am deeply indebted to my neurosurgical mentors, David F. Dean, M. D., Thoralf M. Sundt Jr., M. D., and Sidney Tolchin, M. D. These individuals were outstanding surgeons, teachers, and role models who did so much to stimulate my interest in neurosurgery during the early years of my career.

I am also grateful to my neurosurgical colleagues at Mayo Clinic Florida, Robert E. Wharen Jr., M. D., Ronald Reimer, M. D., Eric W. Nottmeier, M. D., and Ricardo A. Hanel, M. D., Ph. D., for their advice, encouragement, and support during the writing of this text.

H. G. D.

Introduction

Spine-related disease is, both literally and figuratively, a painful proposition. Pain in the neck, mid back, and low back is one of the most common medical conditions in adults. Other conditions affecting the spine do not cause pain (e.g., myelopathy) but contribute to cost and disability. Low back pain alone is said to be the most common cause of disability for persons under the age of 45 in the United States; at any one time, 1% of the U.S. population is chronically disabled and another 1% temporarily disabled by their back pain. In any given 3-month period, about 25% of U.S. adults report low back pain, and nearly 15% report neck pain. About 2% of all physician office visits relate to low back pain alone. Low back problems are reported to be the second-most common cause for absenteeism from work (after upper respiratory tract infections) and the most common cause for office visits to orthopedic surgeons, neurosurgeons, and occupational medicine physicians. Low back operations are said to rank third among all surgical procedures in the United States. A recent study of estimated healthcare expenditure for spine problems among U.S. adults when adjusted for inflation showed a 65% increase from 1997 to 2005; the total expenditure in 2005 was about $85 billion. The estimates do not include indirect costs such as lost wages, disability payments, or "suffering." Despite the increase in expenditures, self-reported measures of mental health, physical functioning, and limitations at work, school, and in social situations were worse in 2005 than in 1997. It is discouraging that we are spending more on spine problems in the United States but helping people less over time.

Scope of the problem

The scope of spine-related problems is reflected by the great number of different kinds of healthcare providers who treat patients with cervical, thoracic, and lumbar spine conditions (see Table 1.1). In addition, there is a very long list of different treatments that are given to patients for their spine conditions (see Table 1.2).

Why do so many different kinds of providers treat spine patients with so many different therapies? There are four chief reasons. The first is that spine-related conditions, especially those due to spondylosis and those associated with pain, are very common. The second reason is that there are many different causes for the same clinical presentation. Because of the many potential causes for the same complaint and the lack of accurate diagnostic tests for the different conditions, the third reason is that providers have great difficulty making an accurate diagnosis. For example, healthcare providers can accurately diagnose only about 15% of patients with acute low back pain. The fourth and last reason is that whether or not we can diagnose the patient's problem, we have great difficulty effectively treating their symptoms, in particular their pain, especially if it is chronic, and pain is often the spine patient's chief complaint. Our inability to provide an accurate diagnosis and specific, promptly effective treatment spawns confusion and a multitude of potential therapies. The natural history for many patients is one of gradual improvement or, at the least, stability with fluctuation. As a result, any and all treatments may seem to be effective. The spine patient is not certain if they need a chiropractic manipulation or an operation on their back, and providers have honest disagreements about which course of treatment has the best outcome. The commonness of spine problems and their chronicity attract large numbers of practitioners who typically favor one avenue of treatment which may be of substantial help to a minority of patients or very modest benefit to a large number of patients. Patients desperately want to get better and often look for an easy answer and quick treatment and sometimes benefit from a very genuine placebo effect. In truth, for many patients, the goal of treatment of their back condition is to keep their symptoms under control rather than to cure them. For many patients with chronic spine problems, especially those

Table 1.1. Healthcare providers who treat spine-related problems

Anesthesiologists

Chiropractors

Homeopaths

Internal medicine specialists

Massage therapists

Naprapaths

Neurologists

Neurosurgeons

Occupational medicine specialists

Occupational therapists

Orthopedic surgeons

Pain medicine specialists

Physical medicine and rehabilitation specialists

Physical therapists

Primary care providers (MDs, osteopaths, physician assistants, nurse practitioners)

Radiologists

Others

Table 1.2. Treatment options for back pain

Medications

  Botulinum toxin injections

  Disk injections

  Epidural injections

  Facet blocks

  Herbal medicines

  Homeopathy

  Medications, both prescription and over-the-counter given by various routes and including analgesics, muscle relaxants, local anesthetics, and centrally acting drugs such as tricyclic agents and serotonin-norepinephrine reuptake inhibitors

  Nerve blocks

  Trigger point injections

Surgical

  Anterior discectomy and fusion with instrumentation

  Anterior discectomy and fusion without instrumentation

  Anterior fusion without discectomy

  Anterior and posterior fusion

  Discectomy with placement of artificial disk

  Intrathecal pump placement for purposes of medication administration

  Laminectomy with discectomy

  Laminectomy without discectomy

  Microdiscectomy

  Posterior fusion with instrumentation

  Posterior fusion without instrumentation

  Radiofrequency lesioning of nerves especially the medial branches of dorsal rami

  Spinal cord stimulator placement

Physical treatments

  Acupuncture

  Bed rest

  Connective tissue massage

  Corsets

  Crutches

  Electrotherapy

  Exercises

  Magnet therapy

  Massage

  Multimodal rehabilitation

  Stretching

  Traction and distraction

  Transcutaneous electrical nerve stimulation, high and low frequency

  Ultrasound

Cognitive and behavioral

  Back school

  Behavioral therapy

  Biofeedback

  Holistic therapy

  Meditation

  Relaxation techniques

involving pain, a combination of different therapies is more likely to be helpful than searching for a single magic bullet.

Epidemiology

Accurate assessment of the incidence (the rate at which people develop a new symptom or disease over a specified time period) and prevalence (measure of the number of people in a population who have a symptom or disease at a particular time) for spine pain is difficult to ascertain because of different definitions, collection methods, and populations studied. The following discussion relates mostly to spine and limb pain due to spondylosis. By spondylosis we mean the degenerative wear and tear changes that affect the intervertebral disks and facet joints and the associated pain arising from these structures and the adjacent bones, ligaments, and muscles of the spinal column.

Cervical level

Neck pain is less common than low back pain and less studied. The lifetime prevalence of significant neck pain is about two-thirds to three-fourths of all individuals, and about 20% of adults experience neck pain over a 1-year period. About 5% of patients report significant disability from their neck pain. Neck pain occurs in about 15%–30% of adolescents. The incidence and prevalence of neck pain increase from adolescence until around the age of 50 and are slightly more frequent in women than men. After the age of 70, neck pain is about two-thirds as common as low back pain. Although not as common as lumbar radiculopathy, the annual incidence of cervical radiculopathy is about 1 in 1000 per year. About 18% of the population visits a healthcare provider each year for neck pain. The frequency of neck pain decreases somewhat after the age of 50.

Risk factors for neck pain include certain occupations (e.g., dentists). Risk factors in the workplace include time pressure demands, low co-worker support, working in a seated position with the neck flexed, and working with arms above the shoulders. Degenerative joint and disk changes on cervical spine imaging are also probably associated with increased risk of neck pain and cervical radiculopathy.

One of the main risk factors for persisting neck pain is a whiplash-type injury. Lighter individuals may be more susceptible to acute neck injury than heavier people, and there is a positive correlation with height where taller individuals are more susceptible to neck injury. Age does not seem to be a significant factor in injury-provoked neck pain. Litigation and emotional issues may complicate neck pain following injury. Neck pain is relatively less common in children and adolescents.

Thoracic level

Thoracic spine disease is less common than cervical, which in turn is less common than lumbar spine disease. It is estimated that only 1% of all disk herniations affect the thoracic spine. While there are fewer data, it is likely that many of the risk factors that lead to neck and low back pain are also associated with mid back pain. Thoracic pain commonly follows trauma from sports, leisure activities, and accidents.

Thoracic pain is relatively common in childhood and fairly common in adolescence. Osteoporosis is a major risk factor for vertebral compression fracture in the thoracic and lumbar spine.

Lumbar level

Two-thirds to three-fourths of people will experience low back pain during their lifetime; half of Americans report at least 1 day of low back pain in the past year; and many international surveys report a point prevalence of low back pain of between 15% and 30% of the studied population. Sciatica is less common with a lifetime prevalence of 14%–40%, and lower yet for significant sciatica secondary to disk herniation (4%–5% lifetime prevalence, higher in men than women). Low back pain begins in adolescence as a rule and gradually increases in frequency, then levels off, and may decline in the very elderly, over the age of 85.

In children and adolescents, the following factors have been linked with a possible increase in the risk of low back pain: genetic predisposition, lower socioeconomic status, athletic activities, presence of scoliosis, rapid growth, and increased height.

Risk factors for low back pain in adults include a history of low back pain in adolescence, lower socioeconomic status, lower level of education, poor physical conditioning, certain physical activities usually experienced in work (heavy lifting, bending and twisting, static work positions such as prolonged sitting or standing, exposure to whole body vibration), certain psychological and psychosocial work factors (monotony at work, job dissatisfaction, and poor relations with co-workers), depression, obesity, cigarette smoking, some congenital spine abnormalities (scoliosis, transitional vertebra), and prior episodes of low back pain as an adult. Low back pain is very common even in people without any of these risk factors.

Spinal anatomy

The vertebral column

The vertebral column consists of seven cervical vertebrae, twelve thoracic vertebrae, five lumbar vertebrae, the sacrum which consists of five fused segments, and the coccyx which is a small triangular bone consisting of three to five fused, rudimentary vertebrae (see Figure 1.1). The mature vertebral column has several curves. The cervical spine from the first cervical through the second thoracic vertebra is convex forward, the thoracic curve from the second to the twelfth vertebra is convex backward, the lumbar

3

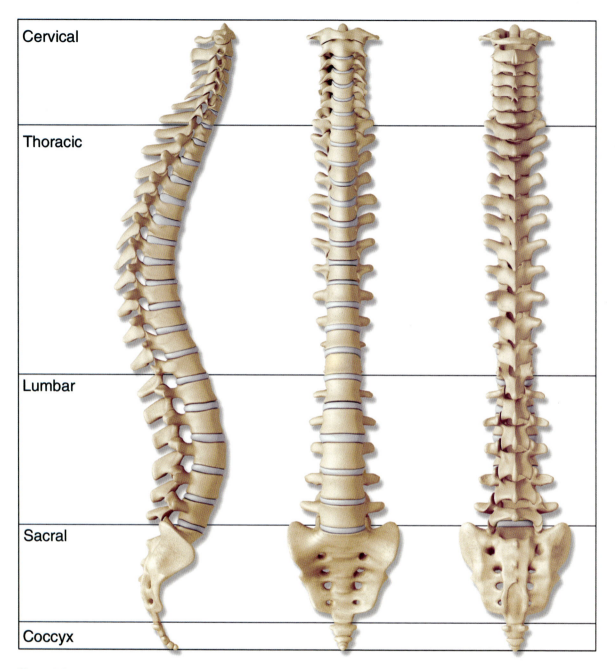

Cervical

Thoracic

Lumbar

Sacral

Coccyx

Figure 1.1. Anterior, posterior, and lateral views of the vertebral column showing the cervical, thoracic, and lumbar levels and the sacrum and coccyx.

curve from T12 to the lumbosacral junction is convex forward, and the sacrum and coccyx are concave forward (and convex backward) and help to form the posterior wall of the pelvis. The twelve paired ribs articulate with the thoracic vertebrae, and the sacrum is wedged between the ilium of the innominate bone on each side.

The typical vertebra consists of an anterior part, the vertebral body, and a posterior arch enclosing the vertebral (or spinal) foramen. The foramina of the individual vertebrae line up to form a vertebral (or spinal) canal which contains the spinal cord from the upper border of the atlas (the first cervical vertebra) usually to the lower end of the first lumbar vertebral body in adults, and below that level, the vertebral canal contains the bundle of lumbosacral nerve roots termed the cauda equina (see Figure 1.2). In adults, the end of the spinal cord may be as high as the twelfth thoracic vertebra or as low as the interspace between the second and third lumbar vertebrae. In the newborn, the spinal cord ends at the level of the upper border of the third lumbar vertebra. As we grow, the spine grows more rapidly than the spinal cord and, as a result, the spinal cord is at a higher level within the spine in the adult compared to the infant and child. The usual vertebral body is roughly cylindrical but flattened posteriorly. The vertebral bodies change in shape and size at different levels. From the second cervical to the first sacral level, each vertebra is connected to the next by fibrocartilaginous complexes termed intervertebral disks between the vertebral bodies, synovial joints between the posterior arches, and various ligaments. The intervertebral disks lack synovium, are termed symphyses, and do permit limited motion.

The intervertebral disks are about the same size as the apposing vertebral bodies and vary in thickness at different spinal levels, being thicker at levels where the vertebral bodies are taller. The disks are thicker in the front than in the back in the cervical and lumbar regions and thus contribute to the spinal curvatures at these levels. Conversely, in the thoracic region, the intervertebral disks are fairly uniform in thickness, and the posterior convexity is due to the shape of the vertebral bodies, which are narrower in the front than in the back. When compared to their associated vertebral bodies, the cervical and lumbar disks are relatively thicker than the thoracic disks.

The intervertebral disks consist of an outer annulus fibrosus, which does receive some blood supply from adjacent vessels, and an inner nucleus pulposus which is avascular. The annulus fibrosus is outwardly convex and heavily laminated. Within each lamina, the majority of the collagenous fibers run in parallel, but fibers in adjacent laminae run in different directions such that overlapping fibers are at oblique angles to one another (see Figure 1.3). The disks are contained superiorly and inferiorly by cartilaginous plates which are firmly fixed to the bony end plates of the adjacent vertebral bodies.

The vertebral arch is composed of two short, round, rod-like bones called pedicles which project backward from the upper, dorsal surface of the vertebral body. Each pedicle meets a broad, vertical lamina. The two laminae are angled posteriorly and medially and meet in the midline behind the vertebral foramen where they fuse with the posteriorly projecting spinous process. The spinous processes vary considerably in size, shape, and direction throughout the spine. In the cervical spine, the spinous processes are rather short and nearly horizontal, and usually have bifid tips. In the thoracic region, they are directed obliquely downward, and in the lumbar region are nearly horizontal. At the junctions of the pedicles and laminae, there are paired superior and inferior articular processes termed zygapophyses. The superior articular process projects upward, and the inferior process downward. Each process has a synovium-covered articular surface, and the superior process of one vertebra articulates with the inferior process of the vertebra above, forming a zygapophyseal or facet joint (see Figure 1.4). These paired facet joints permit a limited amount of movement while restricting excessive motion.

There are variably sized transverse processes which project laterally from the junction of each pedicle and lamina. They are rather diminutive in the cervical region and larger in the thoracolumbar spine. In the region of the transverse process of the cervical vertebrae is a foramen transversarium on each side through which passes a vertebral artery. In the thoracic spine, these transverse processes articulate with the ribs. The transverse processes and posteriorly projecting spinous processes serve as attachment sites for the strong paraspinal muscles.

Each pedicle has concave notches on its inferior and superior surfaces. The inferior notch is larger and deeper than the superior notch. The inferior notch of the pedicle of the vertebra above, the superior notch of the pedicle of the vertebra below, the intervertebral disk and vertebral body anteriorly, and the zygapophyseal joint posteriorly form the intervertebral foramen. The intervertebral foramina, also called neural foramina, are paired structures at each spinal level through which the spinal nerves and blood vessels travel (see Figure 1.4).

The anterior longitudinal ligament extends along the anterior surfaces of the vertebral bodies and intervertebral disks; the posterior longitudinal ligament is within the vertebral canal and runs along the posterior aspect of the vertebral bodies and intervertebral disks. Running along the posterior aspect of the vertebral canal and connecting the laminae of adjacent vertebrae are the ligamenta flava. The ligamentum nuchae in the neck, the supraspinous ligament in the thoracolumbar spine, and the interspinous

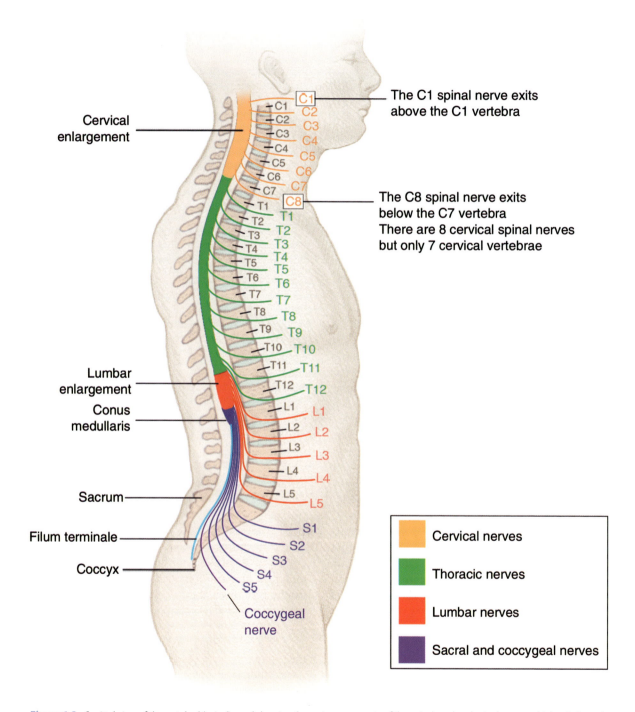

Cervical enlargement

The C1 spinal nerve exits above the C1 vertebra

C1
C2
C3
C4
C5
C6
C7

The C8 spinal nerve exits below the C7 vertebra
There are 8 cervical spinal nerves but only 7 cervical vertebrae

Lumbar enlargement

Conus medullaris

Sacrum

Filum terminale

Coccyx

Coccygeal nerve

	Cervical nerves
	Thoracic nerves
	Lumbar nerves
	Sacral and coccygeal nerves

Figure 1.2. Sagittal view of the vertebral (spinal) canal showing the various segments of the spinal cord and spinal nerves which exit through the intervertebral foramina. The spinal cord ends at about the level of the L1 vertebral body, and below that is a bundle of nerve roots called the cauda equina which leave the vertebral canal in pairs at the appropriate level.

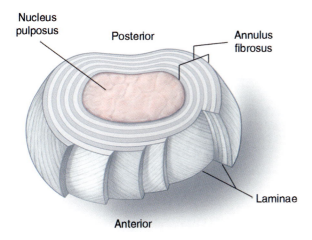

Nucleus
pulposus

Posterior

Annulus
fibrosus

Laminae

Anterior

Figure 1.3. Diagram of intervertebral disk showing the outer annulus fibrosus and the inner nucleus pulposus. The annulus fibrosus has multiple layers or laminae. Within each lamina, the fibers run in parallel and usually at an oblique angle. Fibers in adjacent laminae run in different directions, helping to limit movement and strengthen the attachment between adjacent vertebrae. Individual laminae are much smaller than is shown in this diagram.

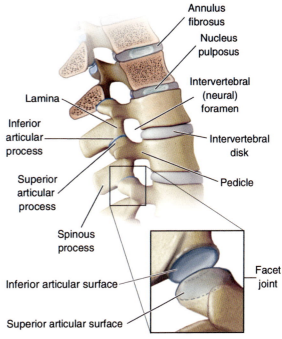

Annulus
fibrosus

Nucleus
pulposus

Intervertebral
(neural)
foramen

Lamina

Inferior
articular
process

Intervertebral
disk

Superior
articular
process

Pedicle

Spinous
process

Facet
joint

Inferior articular surface

Superior articular surface

Figure 1.4. Lateral (lower) and mid sagittal (upper) views of the vertebral column show the component parts and relationships. The apposition of the synovium-covered articular surfaces of the inferior and superior articular processes form the paired facet (zygapophyseal) joints found at each spinal level. The intervertebral (neural) foramina through which the spinal nerves exit the vertebral foramen are formed by the undersurface of the pedicle above, the vertebra and intervertebral disk in front, the facet joint posteriorly, and the upper surface of the pedicle of the next lower vertebra below.

ligaments connect adjacent spinous processes. These ligaments also connect with deep paraspinal muscles.

The first and second cervical vertebrae, the atlas and axis respectively, merit special mention. The atlas lacks a typical vertebral body and consists of a ring-type structure. It supports the skull. Interlocking with the anterior aspect of the vertebral foramen at the level of the atlas is a small, hard cylindrical bony process, called the dens or odontoid process, which projects upward from the axis (the second cervical vertebra). The front of the dens forms a small joint with the back of the anterior arch of the atlas. The dens is kept in place by a transverse ligament. The atlas has two rather large lateral masses, and the upper aspect has a superior articular facet on each side which articulates with an occipital condyle on the bottom of the skull on each side. The articulations between the skull and atlas and between the atlas and axis facilitate rotational and nodding movements of the head and upper neck (see Figure 1.5). There is no intervertebral disk between the atlas and axis.

The lower five cervical vertebrae (C3–C7) have a unique lateral connection to the vertebra above. The upper surface of each of these vertebrae is concave from side to side, and this concavity is formed in large part by lateral uncinate processes on each side of the upper surface of C3–C7 (see Figure 1.6). The bony protuberance which extends upward along the lateral aspect of the upper surface of each of these vertebrae

interfaces with a beveled edge of the cervical vertebra above and helps to prevent posterolateral disk protrusions. It is unclear whether this cleft is a fibrocartilaginous connection or a true synovial joint, but these articulations are termed uncovertebral joints or the joints of Luschka. Whether or not there is a true joint present, these "joints" can degenerate and hypertrophy and, given their posterolateral location, they are in a position to compress exiting cervical nerve roots (see Figure 1.6).

The combination of the intervertebral disk system, the ligaments which attach the vertebrae to one another, the facet joints, and the muscles which attach the vertebrae and adjacent structures permits a modest amount of movement between any two adjoining vertebrae. The intervertebral disks which bind the vertebrae together allow movement between adjoining vertebrae by virtue of their compressibility and slight ability to rotate. The summation of multiple small movements at multiple spinal levels gives

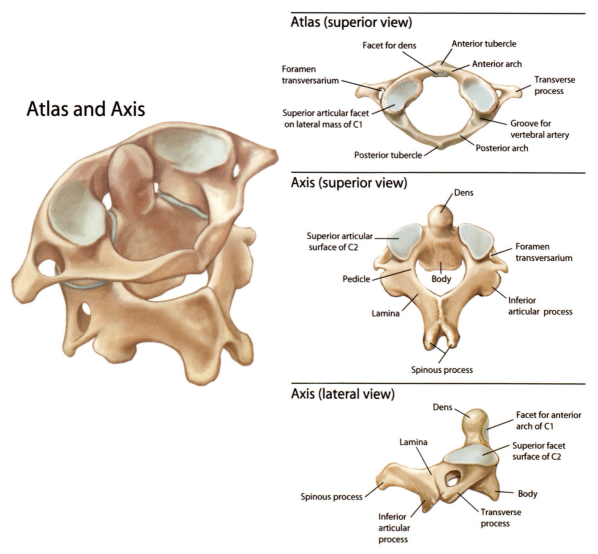

Atlas and Axis

Atlas (superior view)

Facet for dens
Anterior tubercle
Foramen transversarium
Anterior arch
Transverse process
Superior articular facet on lateral mass of C1
Groove for vertebral artery
Posterior arch
Posterior tubercle

Axis (superior view)

Dens
Superior articular surface of C2
Foramen transversarium
Pedicle
Body
Inferior articular process
Lamina
Spinous process

Axis (lateral view)

Dens
Facet for anterior arch of C1
Lamina
Superior facet surface of C2
Spinous process
Body
Inferior articular process
Transverse process

Figure 1.5. The image on the left shows the relationship between the atlas (the first cervical vertebra or C1) and the axis (the second cervical vertebra or C2) from above and behind. The three images on the right show separate views of the atlas and axis. The atlas articulates with the base of the skull above and with the axis below. The dens (odontoid process) is a peg which extends up from the axis and articulates with the back of the anterior arch of the atlas. A ligament behind the dens helps to keep it in place. There is no intervertebral disk between the atlas and axis.

rise to a fairly substantial range of motion for the vertebral column as a whole. Greater movement is possible in the cervical and lumbar regions because the disks are thicker at these levels.

The spinal cord is not round but oval, being wider than it is deep, more so in the cervical levels than elsewhere. The spinal cord and exiting nerve roots are covered by three membranes or meninges which are, from outside in, the dura mater, the arachnoid mater, and the pia mater (see Figure 1.7). The dura mater extends from the foramen magnum to the

second sacral vertebral level and has tubular prolongations along the nerve roots and spinal nerves as they pass through the intervertebral foramina to leave the spine. The space between the dura and the periosteum and ligaments within the vertebral canal contains a plexus of veins, loose fat, and areolar tissue. Local anesthetics, infection, and tumors can spread through this epidural space. Beneath the dura mater is the arachnoid, a delicate membrane that is loosely attached to the dura and envelops entering and exiting nerves and blood vessels. Between the dura

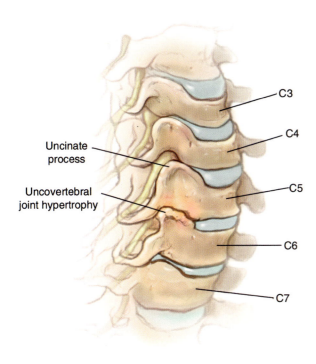

Uncinate
process

Uncovertebral
joint hypertrophy

C3

C4

C5

C6

C7

Figure 1.6. The C3–C7 vertebrae have uncinate processes which are upward projections of the lateral edges of the vertebral body on each side. Each uncinate process contacts the disk and beveled inferolateral surface of the vertebra immediately above. These so-called uncovertebral joints (joints of Luschka) can degenerate and hypertrophy. Such hypertrophy can cause cervical nerve root impingement, especially if it occurs posteriorly.

and the arachnoid mater is a potential subdural space which also ends at the second sacral level. The pia mater covers the spinal cord and also invests the nerve roots. Between the arachnoid and pia mater is the subarachnoid space which contains spinal fluid. The arachnoid and dura can expand such as when spinal fluid pressure is increased. The ability to expand can dampen transmitted spikes in spinal fluid pressure such as accompany the pulse-driven production of cerebrospinal fluid in the choroid plexus within the ventricles intracranially.

There are two areas of enlargement of the spinal cord: the cervical enlargement which extends from about the third cervical to the second thoracic spinal cord segment, and the somewhat smaller lumbar enlargement from the first lumbar to the third sacral spinal cord segment. The cervical and lumbar enlargements relate to the increased number of nerve cells and nerve fibers required for innervation of the

upper and lower limbs respectively. The cervical nerve roots travel downward only slightly before leaving the spinal canal and never more than one vertebral level from the corresponding spinal segment. Thus, the cervical spinal cord enlargement is only slightly higher than the corresponding vertebral levels. However, because the spinal cord typically ends at about the level of the first lumbar vertebral body, the lumbar enlargement lies at the ninth through twelfth thoracic vertebral levels, and, as a result, the lumbosacral nerve roots descend for some distance within the vertebral canal before exiting. As noted above, the spinal cord usually ends at the lower end of the first vertebral body but can be as high as the twelfth thoracic vertebra or as low as the disk below the second lumbar vertebra (see Figure 1.2).

The termination of the spinal cord is called the conus medullaris. Below the conus medullaris is a bundle of nerve roots termed the cauda equina (horse's tail) which descend within the lumbosacral spinal canal to exit in pairs through the appropriate intervertebral foramina. Within the cauda equina the sacral segments are located most medially and the first exiting, upper lumbar segments are located more laterally. From the bottom of the conus medullaris there is a connective tissue filament, the filum terminale, which extends all the way to the bottom of the vertebral canal into the sacrum and attaches to the coccyx.

Detailed spinal cord anatomy

Superimposing an H over an oval can separate a generic spinal cord level into the following sections (see Figure 1.8). The upper (posterior or dorsal) arms of the H surround paired funiculi or white columns which transmit ascending first-order sensory information dealing mostly with proprioception (vibration, joint precision sense, pressure, and touch). The ascending fibers in these columns are uncrossed and most have their cell bodies in the ipsilateral spinal (dorsal root) ganglia. Each of the paired dorsal funiculi is further divided into a lateral fasciculus cuneatus and a medial fasciculus gracilis. The fasciculus cuneatus carries fibers from the upper thoracic and cervical nerves, and the fasciculus gracilis carries nerve fibers from the lumbosacral and lower thoracic segments. Sacral level nerve fibers are medial to lumbar, which are medial to thoracic, which are medial to cervical level fibers. The ascending sensory nerves in the two fasciculi synapse in the nucleus cuneatus and the nucleus gracilis in the medulla oblongata after which the second-order neurons

9

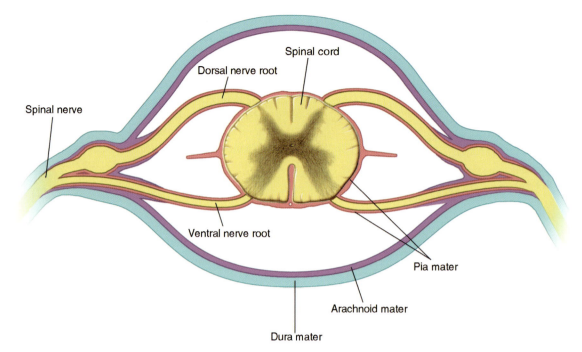

Figure 1.7. The meninges are shown covering the spinal cord, nerve roots, and spinal nerves. The pia mater (red) is closely attached to the spinal cord and nerve roots. The pia is separated from the arachnoid mater (purple) by spinal fluid. The arachnoid layer is loosely attached to the dura mater. The dura mater (teal) has tubular extensions or sleeves lined with arachnoid which cover the nerve roots and spinal nerves as they pass through the intervertebral foramina. The dura becomes continuous with the epineurium of the spinal nerves.

decussate and ascend to the thalamus in the medial lemniscus. Lateral to the uprights of the H are two large lateral funiculi or white columns (one on each side) which include both ascending and descending tracts. The ascending tracts include anterior and posterior spinocerebellar tracts, the lateral spinothalamic tract which is the predominant pathway for pain and temperature sensation, and several other lesser tracts. The most important descending tract is the lateral corticospinal tract which carries motor signals to the spinal cord. The lateral corticospinal tract contains mostly fibers from the contralateral hemisphere which have crossed in the lower ventral medulla oblongata (pyramidal decussation). The lateral corticospinal and lateral spinothalamic tracts are organized such that fibers serving the lower limbs are more peripheral within the spinal cord than those serving the upper extremities. Between the two legs of the H are small anterior funiculi or white columns which contain a small but variable descending anterior corticospinal tract which has motor function and is uncrossed, and an ascending anterior spinothalamic tract which is close to the lateral spinothalamic tract.

The H itself has thick lower (anterior or ventral) legs and somewhat thinner (posterior or dorsal) arms

which contain mostly gray matter. These are termed anterior or ventral and posterior or dorsal gray columns or horns. In the thoracic spinal cord, there is a lateral gray column which projects from each side of the H at the level of the crossbar of the H. The anterior gray columns contain important motor neurons which control movement and muscle tone. They are comparatively broad and short and do not reach the anterior surface of the spinal cord. The lateral gray columns in the thoracic and upper lumbar spinal cord segments contain preganglionic sympathetic nerve cells. In the sacral cord there are similar parasympathetic gray columns that do not have a clear lateral projection. The posterior gray columns consist of several layers of nerve cells chiefly related to sensory function. Nerve cells in the posterior gray columns receive input from neurons in the ipsilateral dorsal root ganglia and elsewhere within the spinal cord. After ascending one or two segments ipsilaterally, much of the output from the posterior gray columns crosses to the opposite side through a white commissure in the crossbar of the H. These second-order sensory fibers ascend in the contralateral anterior spinothalamic tract (touch and pressure more than pain sensation) and the contralateral lateral

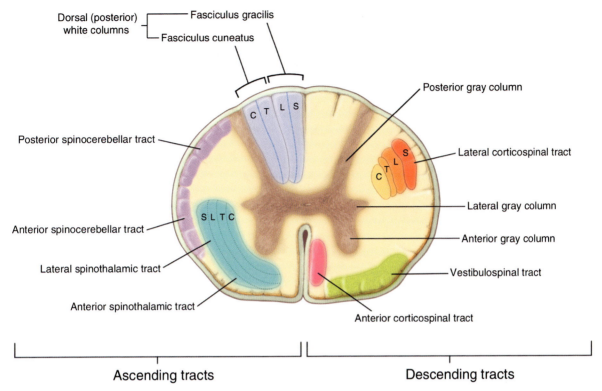

Dorsal (posterior) white columns
— Fasciculus gracilis
— Fasciculus cuneatus

Posterior gray column

C T L S

Posterior spinocerebellar tract

S
L
C T

Lateral corticospinal tract

Anterior spinocerebellar tract

S L T C

Lateral gray column

Anterior gray column

Lateral spinothalamic tract

Anterior spinothalamic tract

Vestibulospinal tract

Anterior corticospinal tract

Ascending tracts

Descending tracts

Figure 1.8. Transverse section of a typical spinal cord segment. The "H" within the spinal cord consists largely of gray matter, while the remainder of the spinal cord is largely white matter. The "arms" of the H and the dorsal white columns between the arms of the H deal mostly with sensory function. The legs of the H relate mostly to motor function. The lateral white columns (lateral to the arms and legs of the H) and the anterior white columns (between the legs of the H) contain motor and sensory nerve tracts. Ascending tracts are on the left and descending on the right. Nerve fibers are somatotopically organized within tracts as shown: C = cervical, T = thoracic, L = lumbar, and S = sacral level of origin or termination of sensory and motor nerve fibers respectively. When describing structures within the spinal cord the terms anterior and ventral are used interchangeably as are the terms posterior and dorsal.

spinothalamic tract (pain and temperature sensation) to synapse in the thalamus contralateral to their side of origin.

Finally, the crossbar of the H contains the small central canal and crossing chiefly spinothalamic tract nerve fibers. The small central canal is a remnant of the ventricular system, contains spinal fluid, and is surrounded by ependyma and a few nerve cells. The central canal or a separate central fluid-filled channel can enlarge and create hydromyelia or syringomyelia respectively.

The spinal nerves

There are a total of thirty-one paired spinal nerves: eight cervical, twelve thoracic, five lumbar, five sacral, and one coccygeal. Each spinal nerve is formed by the joining of ventral (anterior) and dorsal (posterior) spinal nerve roots. The first cervical nerve exits between the occipital bone and atlas and is called the

suboccipital nerve. The second cervical nerve exits between the atlas and the axis (C1 and C2) and, thus, the numbered root (C2) is one higher than the intervertebral level (C1–C2). This is true for the remaining cervical levels with the eighth cervical nerve root exiting between the seventh cervical and first thoracic vertebrae. In the thoracic and lumbar spine, the nerve roots exit at the same level as the vertebral level (i.e., T7 exits at T7–T8, and L3 exits at L3–L4).

The ventral nerve roots emerge from the anterolateral aspect of the spinal cord as rootlets and contain axons of neurons located in the anterior and lateral gray columns. The dorsal nerve roots house spinal or dorsal root ganglia which contain unipolar sensory nerve cells. The spinal ganglia usually lie within the intervertebral foramina. The peripheral processes of the spinal ganglia neurons convey sensory information of all kinds which is passed on to the spinal cord through the dorsal nerve roots. The central processes

11

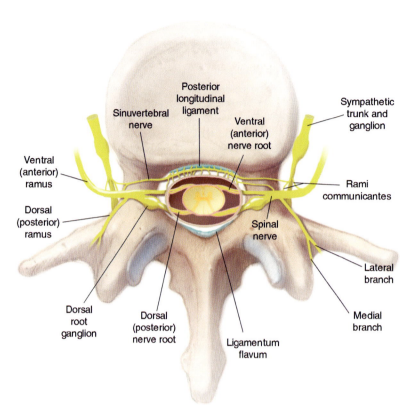

Figure 1.9. This figure shows the formation of a typical spinal nerve. Dorsal and ventral nerve roots join just distal to the dorsal root ganglion to form a spinal nerve. Soon thereafter, the spinal nerve divides into a smaller dorsal ramus and a larger ventral ramus. The ventral rami supply the limbs and anterolateral aspects of the torso, while the dorsal rami supply paraspinal muscles, posterior midline cutaneous sensation, and the facet joints. At each spinal level, sinuvertebral (recurrent meningeal) nerves are formed by the union of a branch from the spinal nerve or its ventral ramus and a branch from a gray ramus communicans. Sometimes the two branches do not meet. The sinuvertebral nerves pass back through the intervertebral foramina to enter the spinal canal where they divide into ascending, descending, and transverse branches. They innervate structures in the anterolateral vertebral canal (posterior longitudinal ligament, superficial annulus fibrosus, periosteum, and the anterolateral dura) and may play a significant role in transmitting pain from degenerated intervertebral disks.

of the spinal ganglia enter the spinal cord dorsolaterally in small fascicles where they divide into a group of more lateral fibers that ascend or descend a short distance and synapse on neurons in the posterior gray column, and a group of medial fibers that ascend ipsilaterally in the posterior white columns to synapse in the lower brain stem. The ventral and dorsal nerve roots receive a covering of dura and arachnoid and join and form a spinal nerve. The spinal nerve promptly divides into a large ventral or anterior ramus and a smaller dorsal or posterior ramus usually just before exiting the intervertebral foramen (see Figure 1.9). The term nerve root is loosely applied to the ventral and dorsal nerve roots and spinal nerve just before and after they merge.

The ventral ramus of each spinal nerve receives a gray ramus communicans from the sympathetic trunk and ganglia, while the ventral rami of the thoracic and upper lumbar nerves each send a white ramus communicans to the sympathetic trunk and ganglia. The ventral rami of the spinal nerves supply the limbs and anterolateral aspects of the chest and abdomen with motor and sensory nerves. In the cervical and lumbosacral regions, the spinal nerves unite

and intermix near their origins in so-called plexi. The smaller dorsal rami do not intermingle, and supply posterior paraspinal structures with motor and sensory functions. Each dorsal ramus divides into lateral and medial branches. The lateral branches of the dorsal rami supply larger, more lateral paraspinal muscles and cutaneous sensation near the midline posteriorly. The medial branches innervate the multifidus, other medial paraspinal muscles, the interspinous ligament, the zygapophyseal (facet) joints at the level of the corresponding spinal nerve and the one below, medial cutaneous sensation in the cervical and thoracic levels, and likely some periosteum. Because the facet joints are a possible source of spine pain, treatment is often directed at the medial branches which supply them with sensation. The dorsal rami of the first three cervical spinal nerves supply the occiput and suboccipital region with sensation.

The sinuvertebral or recurrent meningeal nerves are small but important structures that are present at all vertebral levels. One or more sinuvertebral nerves arise at each spinal level on each side. A branch from the spinal nerve or ventral ramus joins with a branch from a gray ramus communicans (or directly from a sympathetic ganglion) to form a sinuvertebral nerve (see Figure 1.9). Sometimes the somatic and sympathetic nerve filaments do not join. The sinuvertebral nerves immediately course back through the intervertebral foramen passing in front of the dorsal root ganglion where they divide into ascending, descending, and transverse branches which interconnect with similar branches of sinuvertebral nerves from adjacent spinal levels and the opposite side. These nerves supply sensory and autonomic sympathetic innervation to the posterior longitudinal ligament, the posterolateral intervertebral disk (normally only the superficial layers of the annulus fibrosus), periosteum, anterolateral dura mater, and blood vessels. The sinuvertebral nerves are thought to play a significant role in transmitting axial spine pain including that due to disk degeneration.

Muscles directly influencing the spine
There are three major muscle groups which affect the spine: those that are along the posterior aspect of the torso; those along the anterior aspect of the torso; and the psoas and iliacus muscles which are joined to each other laterally and sometimes called the iliopsoas muscle. The posterior aspect of the torso has multiple layers of muscles which are thickest adjacent to the midline. The more superficial muscles, such as the trapezius and latissimus dorsi, connect the upper limb to the trunk. The deep, intrinsic back muscles are all innervated by dorsal rami of the spinal nerves. These deep dorsal muscles attach to the back of the skull, the transverse and spinous processes of the vertebrae, various ligaments, the iliac crests, and the sacrum, and extend from the back of the head to the back of the pelvis. The more superficial muscles span more vertebrae than the deeper muscles. The dorsal muscles extend and laterally bend the spine, contribute to torsional movements, and help maintain posture. On the anterior aspect of the torso, the abdominal wall muscles help with flexion of the spine, lateral bending, and torsional movements. These include the rectus abdominis and external and internal oblique muscles. The psoas muscle originates from the anterolateral aspect of all five lumbar vertebrae and their transverse processes and inserts via a tendon to the lesser trochanter of the femur. The iliacus muscle originates from the anterior aspect of the ilium and lateral sacrum and also inserts on the lesser trochanter. The psoas and iliacus muscles work in concert, are frequently grouped together and called the iliopsoas, and are innervated by the L1–L3 spinal

nerves. The right and left iliopsoas groups powerfully flex the thigh on the pelvis and, when the thigh is fixed, bend the pelvis and trunk forward which helps to maintain an erect posture.

Vascular supply of the spinal cord and cauda equina
The spinal cord is supplied by a single anterior spinal artery that runs longitudinally along the anterior surface of the spinal cord in the midline and two smaller posterior spinal arteries that run longitudinally just medial to each dorsal root entry zone (see Figure 1.10). The anterior spinal artery is formed rostrally by the union of arterial branches from the two vertebral arteries. Deep arteries along the vertebral column supply small spinal branches at virtually every segmental level. These spinal branches pass through the intervertebral foramina and divide into anterior and posterior radicular arteries which supply the ventral nerve root and the dorsal nerve root with its associated ganglion respectively. The radicular arteries are asymmetric and can be absent. Most do not contribute to the anterior spinal artery but a handful, perhaps four to nine, do contribute. The larger anterior radicular arteries are usually situated in the lower cervical, lower thoracic, and upper lumbar levels. Typically, one of the anterior radicular arteries is substantially larger than the others. This vessel, often called the great radicular artery of Adamkiewicz, usually arises from a segmental branch of the descending aorta at the level of the upper lumbar or lower thoracic spine. In two-thirds of individuals, this vessel is on the left side and accompanies the spinal nerve through the intervertebral foramen usually from T9 to L1 but ranging from T5 to L3. The posterior radicular arteries contribute blood flow to the posterior spinal arteries.

Through surface and sulcal branches, the anterior spinal artery supplies the anterolateral two-thirds of the spinal cord while each posterior spinal artery supplies the ipsilateral posteromedial one-sixth of the spinal cord including the dorsal funiculi and the posterior horn. The blood supply to each level of the spinal cord is proportionate to the amount of gray matter it contains, and is thus greatest at the levels of the cervical and lumbar spinal cord enlargements which contain the nerve cells and fibers that supply the upper and lower limbs respectively.

Flow through the anterior spinal artery is more tenuous than through the paired posterior spinal

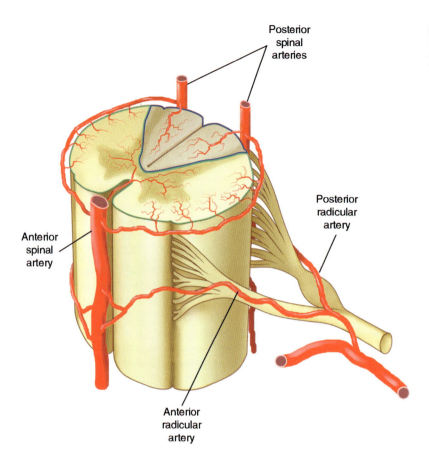

Posterior
spinal
arteries

Posterior
radicular
artery

Anterior
spinal
artery

Anterior
radicular
artery

Figure 1.10. Vascular supply of spinal cord showing the single anterior spinal artery which supplies the anterolateral two-thirds of the spinal cord and two posterior spinal arteries, each of which supplies one-sixth of the spinal cord.

arteries. This is in part because the anterior spinal artery has a larger area of spinal cord to supply and in part because the posterior spinal arteries receive more contributions from radicular arteries than does the anterior spinal artery. Between the vertebral artery contributions to the origin of the anterior spinal artery rostrally and the substantial supply at the lower end from the artery of Adamkiewicz along with the effect of gravity, there is a watershed area in the thoracic spinal cord so that when blood flow is disrupted, especially from the caudal end, spinal cord infarction can occur. The lower thoracic spinal cord is most often affected. Because of two posterior spinal arteries and better anastomotic flow between these two vessels, which often form collateral channels, the spinal cord infarction typically affects the antero-lateral two-thirds of the cord. This results in a characteristic syndrome of severe paraplegia, pain and temperature sensation loss below a thoracic spinal level, bowel and bladder dysfunction, and preservation of posterior column function (touch, joint position, and vibration sense).

Pathophysiology – extrinsic and secondary conditions

Trauma

Trauma to the spinal cord, nerve roots, and cauda equina can result from direct injury to the nervous tissue; compression by bone fragments, blood clot, or intervertebral disk material; or ischemic damage related to the effects of the injury on spinal cord and nerve root circulation. Significant injuries almost always present acutely; lingering or delayed effects of trauma will be included under spondylotic and other musculoskeletal categories later in this chapter.

Until proven otherwise, a patient with any of the following should be assumed to have a spinal cord injury and immobilized until appropriately imaged: anyone with a significant head injury, who is unconscious, who has multiple serious injuries, has been in a motor vehicle accident, has had a severe sports or recreational injury, has had a serious fall, has severe acute spine pain, who is unable to move, or who has lost sphincter control. Patients with underlying

Table 1.3. American Spinal Cord Injury Association (ASIA) Impairment Scale

A = **Complete**: no motor or sensory function is preserved in the sacral segments S4–S5

B = **Incomplete**: sensory but not motor function is preserved below the neurologic level and includes the sacral segments S4–S5

C = **Incomplete**: motor function is preserved below the neurologic level, and more than half of key muscles below the neurologic level have a muscle grade less than 3 (out of 5)

D = **Incomplete**: motor function is preserved below the neurologic level, and at least half of key muscles below the neurologic level have a muscle grade of 3 (out of 5) or more

E = **Normal**: motor and sensory function are normal

Source: Reproduced with permission from *International Standards for Neurological Classifications of Spinal Cord Injury*, revised edition. Chicago, IL: American Spinal Injury Association; 2000, pp. 1–23.

instability, osteoporosis, or occult malignancy may sustain a fracture with less severe trauma. Given the same degree of injury, patients with pre-existing spinal stenosis (congenital or acquired) sustain more spinal cord and/or nerve root damage than patients who do not have underlying narrowing of their spinal canal. Patients with acute spinal cord injury often have spinal shock with complete loss of function below the level of their cord injury, transient hypertension followed by hypotension, and sometimes priapism. Neurologic impairment can take the form of paraplegia, quadriplegia, paralysis of the upper limbs only or upper limbs more than the lower limbs, or a Brown–Séquard syndrome. Patients may have a spinal level below which sweating is impaired or absent, a Horner syndrome, or hypothermia. The American Spinal Injury Association (ASIA) Impairment Scale is listed in Table 1.3 and includes grades A (complete loss of function without sacral sparing) through E (normal sensory and motor function). Sacral sparing (sensory or motor function preserved in the sacral segments) reflects preserved function of long-tract nerves serving these distal segments which are peripherally located within the spinal cord.

One should be aware of the central cord syndrome, the most common incomplete spinal cord injury syndrome. The central cord syndrome is an acute cervical spinal cord injury that typically affects the lower cervical cord. Central cord syndrome usually follows a hyperextension injury, often in the patient with congenital or acquired narrowing of the spinal canal. The damage is greatest in the central spinal cord as a result of contusion or, sometimes,

bleeding. The central long tracts and cervical cord gray matter sustain the brunt of the damage, helping to explain why patients present with upper-limb greater than lower-limb sensory and motor deficits. The syndrome can also occur with fracture dislocations and compression fractures. Most patients improve, and many are left with only upper limb deficits which frequently affect the hands.

Patients with suspected traumatic spinal injuries require emergent imaging, possibly followed by surgical stabilization. About 3%–4% of patients with traumatic spinal cord injury go on to develop symptomatic post-traumatic syringomyelia.

Bacterial infections

Bacterial vertebral osteomyelitis and intervertebral disk space infection share similarities. Both present with spine pain, may or may not have constitutional symptoms initially, are typically accompanied by spine tenderness, and often occur together. Most vertebral body bacterial infections (osteomyelitis) occur in the lumbar spine, and the vast majority of pyogenic spinal infections involve the vertebral body rather than the posterior elements of the spine. Bacteria usually reach the lumbar vertebrae through an arterial route, but can spread through the venous plexus that surrounds the thecal sac in the lumbosacral spine. In perhaps half of patients, an origin for the vertebral osteomyelitis can be found such as a urinary tract infection, skin infection, respiratory tract infection, or previous spinal intervention such as surgery or discography. Immunosuppression of any mechanism, diabetes mellitus, intravenous drug use, underlying cancer, and advancing age may predispose to vertebral osteomyelitis. *Staphylococcus aureus* is the most common bacterium identified followed by streptococcus species but Gram-negative species can occur. It is rare to have more than two adjacent vertebral bodies affected. Disk space infection and psoas or epidural abscess may occur in association with vertebral osteomyelitis. Intervertebral disk space infection has a similar pathogenesis to osteomyelitis, but is more likely to occur after operative intervention (e.g., fusion, discectomy) and, rarely, after needle procedures such as discography and therapeutic injections. Disk space infection also most commonly affects the lumbar spine. Disk space infection frequently involves the adjacent vertebral end plates and can also result in the development of epidural abscess.

The clinical presentation of pyogenic vertebral osteomyelitis is similar to that of disk space infection.

Both typically present with localized, progressive, severe spine pain that is aggravated by movement and often wakes the patient from sleep. Both conditions may be associated with constitutional symptoms such as fever and are accompanied by localized spine tenderness. Cervical vertebral osteomyelitis is more likely to be associated with neurologic deficits. Both osteomyelitis and discitis are associated with increased erythrocyte sedimentation rates and elevated C-reactive protein levels. Blood cultures are more likely to be positive with vertebral osteomyelitis than with disk space infection. Bone loss, gas formation, swelling, disk space narrowing, and adjacent edema and uptake with gadolinium on magnetic resonance imaging (MRI) and on radionuclide scans including technetium-99 m (^{99m}Tc) and gallium-67 (^{67}Ga) are characteristic of pyogenic vertebral osteomyelitis. Intervertebral disk space infection is characterized by loss of disk space height, then irregularity and loss of definition of the adjacent vertebral end plates with subsequent vertebral body destruction. In both disk space infection and vertebral osteomyelitis, radionuclide imaging is usually positive well before plain X-rays show characteristic changes. MRI with and without enhancement is probably better than computed tomography (CT) in diagnosing these vertebral infections.

The diagnosis of bacterial vertebral osteomyelitis and disk space infection is confirmed, and antibiotic treatment planned through culture of the infected site, typically achieved through CT-guided needle aspiration. Occasionally, open biopsy for culture is necessary. Blood cultures and cultures of a suspected primary infection source are also helpful. An associated epidural abscess may require surgical drainage.

Mycobacterial (TB) osteomyelitis is most likely to occur in the thoracic spine and also is more likely to affect those who are immunosuppressed. The onset is indolent with localized spine pain with or without radicular pain, and sometimes accompanied by the development of a sharp forward angulation of the spine (gibbus). Tuberculous osteomyelitis has a predilection for the anterior aspect of the vertebral body, accounting for the tendency to form a gibbus. Tuberculous vertebral osteomyelitis is always associated with a focus elsewhere in the body. On imaging, TB osteomyelitis may affect several vertebral bodies, there can be scalloping of the anterior surface of the vertebral bodies by tuberculous abscesses, the disk space is typically spared, and vertebral body collapse tends to occur anteriorly. In contrast to bacterial

vertebral osteomyelitis, TB osteomyelitis may require surgical intervention to reduce deformity and prevent or treat neurologic impairment.

Spinal epidural abscess is a life-threatening condition that requires prompt diagnosis and treatment. The pain can be quite severe. Meningismus may be present. Patients typically present with focal spine pain, radicular pain, motor weakness, sensory loss, sphincter disturbance, and constitutional signs and symptoms. The thoracolumbar spine is more commonly affected. Patients are commonly immunosuppressed or have had previous spinal intervention. *Staphylococcus aureus* is the most common bacterium. Blood-borne spread from a distant infection is more common than direct extension from a nearby source, which is more common than cases arising from spinal interventions. Elevated white blood cell count and erythrocyte sedimentation rate are usual. Blood cultures are often positive. Lumbar puncture is inadvisable at the level of the abscess and, in general, should not be performed below the level of the abscess for fear of causing neurologic worsening. MRI is the diagnostic procedure of choice. Treatment consists of appropriate antibiotic therapy and typically surgical intervention with drainage of the abscess except in patients without neurologic deficits and/or whose medical condition will not allow surgery.

Lyme disease can cause an infectious radiculitis. Tertiary syphilis (tabes dorsalis) causes a myelopathy characterized by posterior column dysfunction and brief, focal, migratory pains chiefly in the lower extremities (lightning pains).

Viral infections

Many viruses can infect the spinal cord and nerve roots. The most common is infection of the dorsal root ganglia due to varicella-zoster virus (VZV). So-called shingles causes severe radicular pain along with a vesicular rash in the dermatome of the infected dorsal root ganglion. Less commonly but especially in immunosuppressed patients, the VZV can spread to involve the spinal cord and cause myelitis. Other herpes viruses such as herpes simplex type 2 (genital herpes), and cytomegalovirus can also infect the spinal cord. A number of enteroviruses have been associated with transverse myelitis, often as a post-infectious phenomenon. Poliovirus is an enterovirus which can spread to the central nervous system where it has a predilection for the brain stem and anterior column motor neurons. Poliovirus can cause typically asymmetric flaccid paralysis followed by improvement which is often incomplete (paralytic poliomyelitis). Nonparalytic poliovirus infections are often asymptomatic or cause a mild febrile illness or apparent aseptic meningitis. West Nile virus, a flavivirus transmitted to humans by mosquito bite, can cause aseptic meningitis, encephalitis, or myelitis in less than 1% of persons infected with this virus. A very small percentage of infected patients develop acute flaccid paralysis.

Human immunodeficiency virus (HIV) can cause a vacuolar myelopathy which causes symptoms in about 5%–10% of patients with acquired immuno-deficiency syndrome (AIDS). Manifestations include painless spastic paraparesis with impaired proprio-ception more than pain and temperature sense.

Human T-cell lymphotrophic virus, types I and II (HTLV-I and II), are retroviruses which are much less common than HIV and can cause a chronic progressive myelopathy sometimes known as tropical spastic paraparesis.

Most of these viral spinal infections can be diagnosed with blood and/or cerebrospinal fluid (CSF) analysis for antibodies and/or polymerase chain reaction study for virus-specific target nucleic acids. Some, such as VZV, herpes simplex, and cytomegalovirus, can be treated with antiviral drugs such as acyclovir, valacyclovir, or famciclovir. Immunization is, of course, available for poliomyelitis. In 2006, a live attenuated herpes zoster virus vaccine was approved for use in adults, and time will tell whether or not the incidence of shingles will decline as a result.

Fungal and parasitic infections

Fungal myelopathies are rare and are more likely to cause meningitis or extradural disease than an infectious myelitis. Specific infectious agents include *Aspergillus*, *Blastomyces*, *Coccidioides*, and *Cryptococcus* and are more likely to infect patients with a compromised immune system.

In the United States, parasitic infections of the spinal cord are uncommon but should be suspected in natives of or travelers from areas where certain parasitic infections are commonplace. Cysticercosis, echinococcosis, and schistosomiasis can affect the spinal cord. Toxoplasmosis of the spinal cord can be seen in any immunosuppressed patient, such as those with AIDS.

Inflammatory demyelinating myelopathies

There is a large overlapping group of noninfectious, non-compressive, inflammatory, and often demyelinating myelopathies. Imaging and blood and spinal fluid testing aid in diagnosis. The most common condition within this group is multiple sclerosis (MS). In recent years, a group of patients previously thought to have a form of MS called neuromyelitis optica (NMO) or Devic disease has been found to have a distinct condition. Neuromyelitis optica is characterized by "longitudinally extensive transverse myelitis" (LETM) in which the demonstrable spinal cord lesion extends over three or more spinal cord segments usually centrally within the spinal cord, optic neuritis, and humoral NMO immune globulin G (lgG) antibodies which target the water channel aquaporin-4. MS is more common in White populations, and NMO is more common in non-White groups. Patients with NMO frequently have recurrent LETM or develop optic neuritis. MS is characterized by the frequent presence of oligoclonal bands, an increased IgG index, and modest CSF pleocytosis. MRI in MS affecting the spinal cord reveals short segment abnormalities which may show gadolinium enhancement, are often peripheral rather than central, and may be multifocal. Typically, MRI also reveals intracranial demyelinating lesions in MS.

Acute transverse myelitis is a distinct condition that can be confused with MS or NMO. This acute inflammatory myelitis reaches peak worsening somewhere between 4 hours and 21 days after onset. There is evidence of inflammation on CSF examination and/or MRI, which shows a gadolinium enhancing intrinsic spinal cord abnormality with few or no intracranial imaging lesions. Acute transverse myelitis is often a one-time illness that can leave behind significant residual neurologic impairment, but some patients may go on to develop MS, NMO, or another identifiable form of myelitis.

Transverse myelitis can also occur after vaccination or after an infectious illness, usually viral in nature. Post-vaccinal or post-infectious myelitis occurring within 3 weeks of vaccination or infection is more common in children and adolescents. Immunizations linked to myelitis include hepatitis B, influenza, measles, pertussis, rabies, rubella, and smallpox. The antecedent infectious illness or immunization may have served as a nonspecific trigger for the development of myelitis.

Acute disseminated encephalomyelitis (ADEM) encompasses multifocal brain and spinal cord symptoms and signs and can occur after vaccination or systemic illness. It is more common in children. The patient may present with predominant brain or spinal cord symptomatology. As with the other inflammatory myelopathies, there is often CSF pleocytosis, but oligoclonal bands are generally not present. ADEM is often considered a one-time illness but could represent an initial manifestation of MS or NMO.

Noninfectious inflammatory myelopathies can be seen in systemic autoimmune diseases such as systemic lupus erythematosus, Sjögren syndrome, Behçet disease, and mixed connective tissue disease. The association is much more likely to be valid if the patient presents with myelitis after the diagnosis of their systemic autoimmune disease rather than when the myelitis is the first manifestation, in which case associated serologic markers may be falsely positive or unrelated to the neurologic condition.

Sarcoidosis with or without systemic manifestations can present with granulomatous involvement of the spinal cord and/or nerve roots usually seen on MRI. Inflammation is evident on CSF examination, serum angiotensin-converting enzyme may be elevated, and other organs are often involved.

Myelitis can occur as a remote effect of an underlying malignancy such as breast, ovarian, and non-small cell lung cancer. The presence of serum paraneoplastic antibodies is suggestive of a paraneoplastic myelopathy. In the appropriate setting and presence of a positive paraneoplastic antibody, a search for an underlying malignancy including imaging of the chest, abdomen, and pelvis with CT or MRI and possibly positron emission tomography (PET) scanning should be pursued.

Many of these noninfectious inflammatory myelopathies are treated acutely with immunosuppressant therapy. Intravenous methylprednisolone, 1000 mg per day for five consecutive days, is often given for acute myelitis. For patients with established relapsing remitting MS, preventive therapy with a medication such as interferon beta is commonly used. Patients with NMO are at risk for relapse and are often treated with immunosuppressive therapy such as azathioprine and prednisone. Neurosarcoidosis is often treated with systemic corticosteroids, other immunosuppressive treatments, and sometimes infliximab. For patients with a paraneoplastic myelopathy, treatment of the associated malignancy is sometimes associated with improvement in or stabilization of their myelopathy.

Toxic, metabolic, and hereditary myelopathies

Noncompressive, noninflammatory myelopathies can be due to metabolic disturbances (typically deficiency of a key substrate), toxins (typically ingested), and hereditary causes.

A common myelopathy occurs with vitamin B_{12} deficiency. MRI shows increased T_2 signal in the posterior and lateral columns as well as the subcortical white matter. Visual loss and cognitive impairment can occur. Vitamin B_{12} (cobalamin) can be measured in the serum; elevated serum methylmalonic acid and homocysteine levels aid in diagnosis of patients with low–normal B_{12} levels. B_{12} deficiency can be due to pernicious anemia, an autoimmune condition which is associated with elevated serum gastrin and anti-intrinsic factor antibodies, gastrointestinal surgery, gastrointestinal disease, fish tapeworm infestation, nitrous oxide (laughing gas) toxicity, and dietary deficiency. Treatment consists of parenteral or very large doses of oral vitamin B_{12}.

Folic acid deficiency rarely causes neurologic manifestations similar to those due to B_{12} deficiency and can be seen in nutritional deficiency such as with alcoholism, gastrointestinal disease, treatment with folic acid antagonists such as methotrexate, and inborn errors of folic acid metabolism.

Nitrous oxide (N_2O or laughing gas) causes irreversible inactivation of vitamin B_{12} and can be seen in medical personnel working in poorly ventilated surgical suites, in individuals who abuse nitrous oxide, and in rare patients who have a single exposure and have concomitant unsuspected vitamin B_{12} deficiency.

Copper deficiency can cause a myelopathy similar to "swayback" disease seen in animals. Intrinsic spinal cord abnormalities may be seen on T_2-weighted MRI. Copper deficiency can result from malabsorption such as that secondary to prior gastric surgery and excess consumption of zinc. Low serum copper, ceruloplasmin, and urinary copper excretion aid in diagnosis, and oral or parenteral copper supplementation can be helpful. In patients with zinc-induced copper-deficiency-related myelopathy, stopping the zinc supplementation may be all that is needed.

Vitamin E deficiency can be due to gastrointestinal, pancreatic, or hepatic conditions, genetic defects especially those related to serum lipids, or nutritional factors. The presentation is often that of a progressive spinocerebellar syndrome combined with a peripheral neuropathy. Low serum vitamin E levels are helpful diagnostically, and treatment consists of vitamin E supplementation.

Konzo is an abrupt, symmetric, nonprogressive spastic paraparesis seen in central and east Africa due to regular consumption of large amounts of insufficiently processed cassava which results in cyanide toxicity. Lathyrism is due to excess consumption of the legume *Lathyrus sativus* (grass pea) and causes a progressive spastic paraparesis. This condition is seen in India, Bangladesh, and Ethiopia. Consumption of large amounts of fluoride, present in large quantities in the soil in certain geographic areas, can be deposited in bones and result in bony overgrowth. The vertebral column can be affected, causing spinal cord or nerve root impingement.

Superficial siderosis of the central nervous system is associated with hearing loss, progressive ataxia, and myelopathy. MRI shows hemosiderin deposition in the nervous system. The pathogenesis is thought to be related to recurrent bleeding into the cerebrospinal fluid, the cause of which may be difficult to determine. If a source of hemorrhage can be found and eliminated, progression of the superficial siderosis may be prevented.

Radiation therapy can cause a transient, reversible myelopathy within months of treatment which is characterized by tingling often with a positive Lhermitte sign and is thought to be due to demyelination. Radiation can also cause a delayed, progressive, irreversible myelopathy 1 to 2 years after treatment. MRI can be normal or show spinal cord edema with or without enhancement and late in the course shows cord atrophy. Corticosteroids may provide temporary benefit only. Intrathecal chemotherapy can cause a transient or persistent myelopathy. Myelopathy has infrequently been associated with cirrhosis of the liver. Acute myelitis can follow inhalation or intravenous use of heroin.

Hereditary spastic paraparesis presents with a slowly progressive myelopathy and is most commonly inherited in an autosomal dominant pattern. Less likely to be confused with a pure myelopathy are the many different inherited spinocerebellar ataxias. There are multiple subtypes of both conditions and genetic testing is available for many. Hereditary leukodystrophies, especially adrenomyeloneuropathy, can present with myelopathy.

Vascular myelopathy

Spinal cord infarction can result from primary atherosclerotic occlusive disease or from embolism to the vessels that supply the cord. Emboli can arise from cardiac valves, the aorta, and fibrocartilaginous material from an acute disk rupture. Decompression sickness (caisson disease) causes myelopathy by the formation of nitrogen gas bubbles in blood vessels which impede spinal cord perfusion. Systemic hypotension or local hypoperfusion (e.g., due to clamping the aorta during surgery or arterial catheter procedures) can cause cord infarction. Infections such as syphilis, vasculitis, and tumor invasion can interrupt blood flow to the spinal cord. The prognosis of spinal cord infarction largely depends on the severity of the initial neurologic deficits.

Less commonly there can be bleeding into and around the spinal cord. Primary spinal subarachnoid hemorrhage is responsible for much less than 1% of all subarachnoid bleeds. The cause is often obscure: spinal vascular malformations are to blame in a minority of cases. Bleeding can occur within the spinal cord. Hematomyelia can be caused by trauma, spinal cord vascular malformations, a bleeding disorder, anticoagulant therapy, and hemorrhage into an intramedullary tumor.

Tumors

While tumors in and around the spine are much less common than other causes of spine and limb pain and neurologic symptoms, the possibility of a benign or malignant neoplasm must be considered and recognized in order to prevent eventual deterioration. Tumors can be primary to the spine or metastatic. Within the spine, they can arise from the bones, muscles, other soft tissues, meninges, spinal cord, and spinal nerves and nerve roots. Epidural tumors are more likely to be metastatic than primary, whereas those within the dura are more likely to be primary. As opposed to the more common causes of spine and limb pain, which tend to be acute and improve with or without treatment, tumors follow a gradually progressive course. The various tumor types are listed in Table 1.4. In general, MRI is the imaging procedure of choice for spine tumors. If the tumor is primary and accessible, surgical removal is usually performed which will also establish the pathologic diagnosis. For tumors which do not appear to be primary and/ or cannot be easily removed, an attempt to determine the pathology is usually made by CT-guided needle biopsy, open biopsy, or sometimes by spinal fluid cytology.

Pathophysiology – intrinsic, primary conditions of the spine

The above conditions account for only a small fraction of spine disorders. The vast majority of spine-related signs and symptoms are due to primary

19

Table 1.4. Tumor types

Benign non-neurogenic tumor of spine

    Osteoid osteoma

    Osteoblastoma

    Osteochondroma

    Chondroma

    Aneurysmal bone cyst

    Hemangioma

    Giant-cell tumor

    Eosinophilic granuloma

Malignant non-neurogenic tumors of spine

    Chordoma

    Chondrosarcoma

    Osteosarcoma

    Ewing sarcoma

    Multiple myeloma

    Lymphoma

    Metastatic tumors

        Extradural

            Often in bones of spine

        Meningeal

            Carcinomatosis and lymphomatosis

        Intradural/intramedullary

            Metastases within the spinal cord

Neurogenic tumors

    Intradural/extramedullary

        Nerve sheath tumors (schwannoma, neurofibroma) – can be extradural

        Meningioma

        Lipoma of filum terminale

        Paraganglioma – can be extradural and extraspinal

    Intradural/intramedullary

        Astrocytoma

        Ependymoma

        Hemangioblastoma

Extradural tumor-like conditions

    Extramedullary hematopoiesis

    Epidural lipomatosis

    Sarcoidosis

    Paget disease of bone

    Vertebral hemangioma

    Synovial cyst

Intradural tumor-like conditions

    Dural and spinal cord vascular malformations

    Syringomyelia not associated with intramedullary tumor

    Sarcoidosis

    Arachnoid cyst – can be extradural

congenital and acquired conditions which affect the spinal column and its component parts: the vertebrae, intervertebral disks, ligaments, joints (between C1 and the occiput, C1 and C2, the paired facet joints of the cervical, thoracic, and lumbar spine, the two sacroiliac joints, and the costovertebral joints that connect the ribs to the thoracic vertebrae), and paraspinal and other supporting muscles. These spinal structures work together as a functional unit. Trouble at one level of the spine can have a direct or indirect effect on other levels. Pathology of one component of the spine can have a direct or indirect effect on other elements at the same level or at higher or lower levels. Spine conditions can cause compression of or be associated with inflammation of the spinal cord and exiting nerve roots. Irritation of the neural structures can produce pain at a distance from the spine (referred limb and/or torso pain), making it difficult to be certain about the true origin of pain that occurs from the neck down. Many of the conditions which affect the spine are considered "wear and tear" or "degenerative." The term "spondylosis" is often applied nonspecifically to any lesion of the spine of a degenerative nature. Understanding the degenerative diseases of the spine which affect the bones, disks, and joints is critical to diagnosing and treating spine and referred limb pain.

Intervertebral disks

The intervertebral disks support the vertebrae and the entire weight of the upper body while providing limited rotational movement and bending in any direction. About 20%–25% of the entire height of the vertebral column comes from the aggregated disk heights. Compounded over the twenty-three intervertebral disks, there is a fairly significant total range of movement. The more superficial layers of the annulus fibrosus contain strong collagen fibers which attach to the surrounding vertical edges of the adjacent lower and upper vertebral bodies and to the apposing horizontal surfaces of the same vertebral bodies peripherally. The nucleus pulposus occupies roughly the middle half of the disk space and is nearly 90% water in the young adult. It is located closer to the back than the front of the disk. The intervertebral disk is compressible and helps to transmit vertical, horizontal, and torsional forces. The intervertebral disk has a blood supply in childhood which is lost with maturation of the spine, after which the tissue is dependent on diffusion for its supply of nutrients. Probably only the very superficial layers of the normal annulus fibrosus are innervated.

Over time and possibly influenced by more "wear and tear," degenerative changes take place in the annulus fibrosus and nucleus pulposus. The annulus develops tears or fissures, clefts, and bulges. The nucleus pulposus loses water, shrinks, and is less able to absorb and transmit posture-related changes in pressure. There is some evidence that damage to the annulus fibrosus allows the ingrowth of blood vessels and nerve fibers from the surface of the disk, which might then explain discogenic pain (pain of disk origin) and "internal disk disruption" as a cause of axial back pain.

Shrinkage due to degeneration of the intervertebral disk can narrow the intervertebral foramina at the same level. The annulus fibrosus can sustain tears, also termed fissures, that extend radially, transversely, or concentrically. Such fissures by definition are not associated with displacement of disk material beyond the intervertebral disk space. Fissures and tears typically occur without known trauma and their presence does not imply that significant trauma has occurred. More significantly, the intervertebral disk can herniate (also called rupture or prolapse) and if this occurs posteriorly or posterolaterally, there can be compression of the spinal cord, cauda equina, or, most commonly, a single spinal nerve or nerve root. The following definitions apply for the most part to the lumbar spine. A disk herniation is defined as a localized displacement of disk material beyond the limits of the intervertebral disk space. Disk herniations are divided into focal herniations (less than 25% of the disk circumference is involved) and broad-based herniations (25%–50% of the disk circumference is involved). Diffuse "disk bulging" of 50%–100% of the circumference is not considered a true disk herniation. Herniated disks are subdivided into protrusions or extrusions based on the size and shape of the displaced disk material. Measurements are made at the base of the disk and at the greatest width of the disk material beyond the disk space. The base is defined as the cross-sectional area of disk material at the periphery of the disk space of origin. The term disk protrusion is applied if the greatest width of the displaced disk material is less than that of the base of the herniated disk when measured in the same plane. A disk extrusion is defined as when the distance between the edges of the disk material beyond the disk space in any one plane is greater than the distance between the edges at the base or if there is loss of continuity between the disk material within and beyond the disk space. The term sequestration is applied to a disk extrusion that has completely lost continuity with its parent disk (see Figure 1.11). Displacement of disk material away from the parent disk is termed migration whether it is sequestered or not. Disk extrusions and sequestrations can migrate upward or downward so that they lie behind the same numbered or next lower vertebral body. Disk herniation can be further defined as contained if the disk protrusion is covered by annulus fibrosus and uncontained if not covered. Disks which herniate in a vertical, upward or downward direction into the adjacent

(a) Protrusion	(b) Extrusion	(c) Sequestration	(d) Migration
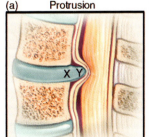	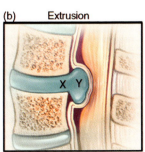	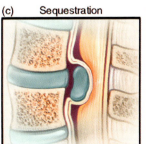	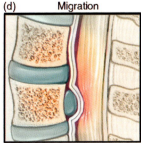

Figure 1.11. Disk herniations are divided into: (a) protrusion if the greatest distance between edges of the protruding disk material is less than the distance between the edges at the base of the protrusion (maximal diameter at Y is less than at X), and (b) extrusion, when the measurement in at least one plane beyond the disk space is greater than it is at its base (Y is wider or taller than X). (c) Disk extrusions can be further described as sequestrated if the displaced disk material has completely lost continuity with the parent disk. (d) The term migration is applied to disk material which has moved away from the parent disk, usually up or down, whether or not it is sequestered.

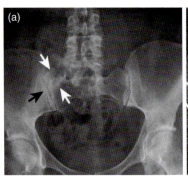
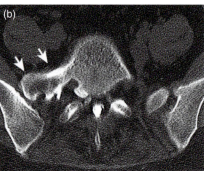

Figure 1.12. Partial sacralization of L5. (a) Anteroposterior plain X-ray and (b) axial CT scan at the L5 level which show partial sacralization of L5 on the right. The right "transverse process" of the fifth lumbar vertebra is enlarged and partially fused with the ilium and sacrum (arrows). The term Bertolotti syndrome is sometimes applied when a patient with partial sacralization of L5 develops low back symptoms. This 49-year-old woman did have a long history of low back pain and right lumbar radiculopathy.

the development of symptomatic disease later in life. Congenital anomalies are more common in the lumbar spine than in the cervical or thoracic spine. Sometimes one spine anomaly is associated with other anomalies. Congenital abnormalities are thought to cause front-to-back or side-to-side mechanical asymmetries and altered weight bearing that can result in musculoskeletal pain and premature and excessive degenerative changes. This is not always the case and many anomalies are not associated with any symptoms. In view of the commonness of spine symptoms, it can be difficult to attribute the adult onset of pain to a known or discovered congenital abnormality.

It is estimated that about 5% of normal people have a congenital abnormality in their lumbar spine. Probably the most common congenital abnormality in the lumbar spine is spina bifida occulta, which consists of failure of the posterior vertebral arch to fuse and form a spinous process. This occurs most commonly in the first sacral segment, but can occur at additional levels, usually in the lumbosacral spine. Spina bifida occulta is part of a spectrum of birth defects which are labeled as spina bifida and involve incomplete closure of the embryonic neural tube. In its most severe form, spina bifida is associated with myelomeningocele in which the spinal cord is exposed through an opening in the lower spine with associated partial or complete paralysis of the body below the abnormal spinal opening. Less commonly, there is a simple meningocele in which the meninges protrude through the spinal opening. Spina bifida occulta can be associated with other congenital anomalies such as a tethered spinal cord, an intraspinal lipoma, and Chiari malformation.

There is also congenital variation in the number of vertebra. This is especially likely to occur at the lumbar level where there can be six more often than four rather than five typical lumbar vertebrae. Much less commonly, there can be one too many or one too few thoracic vertebrae. "Counting" mistakes can occur when there is variation in the number of rib-bearing vertebrae or the number of lumbar vertebrae. When there are only four typical lumbar vertebrae, what would have been the fifth vertebra is said to be sacralized; conversely, when there are six lumbar-type vertebrae, what might be called the first sacral vertebra is said to be lumbarized. Whether there is one too many or one too few lumbar or thoracic vertebrae probably has no great effect on the development of spondylosis and symptoms but can give rise to problems with numbering and operating at the correct spinal level.

There may be more of a problem when sacralization of the fifth lumbar vertebra or lumbarization of the first sacral vertebra is incomplete and especially if it is unilateral or very asymmetric (see Figure 1.12). The anomalous enlargement of the transverse process of the caudal-most lumbar vertebra on one or both sides may then articulate with or fuse to the sacrum or ilium. In theory, pain could arise from this articulation, or altered mechanics associated with limitation and asymmetry of motion could cause increased stress and degenerative disk disease immediately above the level of the partially sacralized or lumbarized segment. About 5% of patients with low back pain have this type of anomaly which in combination is called Bertolotti syndrome.

In the cervical spine, one of the most common congenital abnormalities is congenital fusion of two or more vertebrae, termed Klippel–Feil syndrome. The congenital union of two adjacent vertebral bodies, also called a block vertebra, can also occur at the thoracic and lumbar levels. Typically, there is no intervertebral disk, and, as a result, the height of the two fused vertebrae is less than the height of two normal vertebrae. Patients with congenital cervical fusion affecting several levels often have associated congenital anomalies and characteristically have a short neck, very low hairline, and reduced neck range of motion. In theory, patients with congenital fusion may experience increased wear-and-tear changes in the adjacent normal segments above and below their fusion. Patients with a congenital fusion may be at increased risk of spinal cord injury due to hypermobility of spinal levels adjacent to the fusion.

Patients with congenital abnormalities of the upper cervical spine, such as fusion of the atlas to the occiput, and abnormalities of the odontoid process or the transverse ligament which holds the odontoid in place can develop canal stenosis with neurologic signs and symptoms or sustain spinal cord injury secondary to relatively minor trauma. Atlantoaxial instability occurs in 10%–20% of individuals with Down syndrome.

Abnormalities that can be congenital or acquired
Arachnoid and perineural cysts
Spinal arachnoid cysts can be congenital or acquired following trauma or possibly related to inflammation. They can occur at any level of the spine, but most occur in the thoracic region, more so posteriorly. They are typically intradural and extramedullary (between the dura and spinal cord), and the wall of the cyst may contain arachnoid and fibrous tissues. Many are asymptomatic, but they can cause local compression with back pain, radicular pain, and/or myelopathy. Presumably, the cysts grow via a ball-valve mechanism which traps CSF within the cyst. If symptomatic, they may require surgical removal. Possibly related to a silent intradural spinal arachnoid cyst, there are case reports of spinal cord herniation through an anterior defect in the dura in the mid to upper thoracic spine.

More commonly, cysts involve the meningeal covering of exiting spinal nerves. These CSF-filled cysts are frequent, can be bilateral, can occur at any level, most commonly occur at the lumbosacral level, and can occur within the sacrum. These perineural cysts are sometimes called nerve root sleeve diverticula or, if the cyst arises distal to the dorsal root ganglion, Tarlov cysts. Presumably, most of these are congenital in nature, although they may enlarge over time; some could follow trauma or inflammation. For the most part, these are incidental findings and should be ignored. There are two situations where nerve root sleeve diverticula may be

symptomatic. The first is that they may serve as a source of spinal fluid leakage and cause a low CSF pressure syndrome. In this situation, the discovery of a persistent spinal fluid leak related to a nerve root sleeve diverticulum may lend itself to surgical repair with restitution of normal CSF pressure. The other situation where they may cause symptoms is in the lumbosacral canal where, presumably through a ball-valve phenomenon in which spinal fluid can enter but not exit the cyst, a Tarlov cyst could cause a lumbosacral radiculopathy. Cyst aspiration and/or injection may help determine if the cyst is symptomatic. Intrasacral perineural cysts can cause localized areas of bone expansion which are usually asymptomatic. Nerve root sleeve diverticula are common and so is back and lower limb pain. While there may be a tendency to draw a causal connection between a prominent Tarlov cyst and a patient's spine and limb pain, in general these perineural cysts should be ignored.

Spinal stenosis
Probably the most significant congenital "abnormality" is variation in the size of one's spinal canal. Some people are born with a capacious spinal canal and others with one that barely accommodates the neural structures. There is often, but not always, an association between narrowing in the cervical and lumbar levels. There is a hereditary influence on the size of one's vertebral canal. In addition, patients with achondroplasia frequently have multi-level spinal stenosis. Typically, congenital narrowing is only discovered when the patient becomes symptomatic and imaging is obtained. No doubt, the narrowing was present long before this and is sometimes noted when the patient has imaging for another reason, perhaps because of trauma.

Superimposed degenerative spondylotic changes further compromise the size of the canal and can compress the spinal cord (in the cervical much more often than in the thoracic spine) or cauda equina (at the lumbar level). Facet joint hypertrophy, bulging and degenerated disks often with accompanying vertebral body spurring, thickening and bulging of the ligamenta flava, synovial cysts, enlargement of the posterior longitudinal ligament, and spondylolisthesis can all contribute to spinal canal narrowing. The intervertebral foramina can also be affected. Even a normal size spinal canal can be compromised by enlargement of the structures which surround and form the vertebral foramina or by the shift of

25

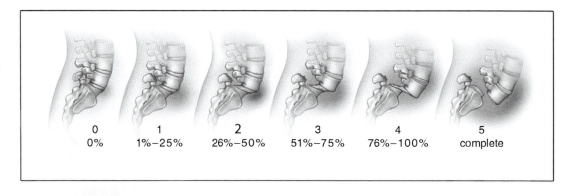

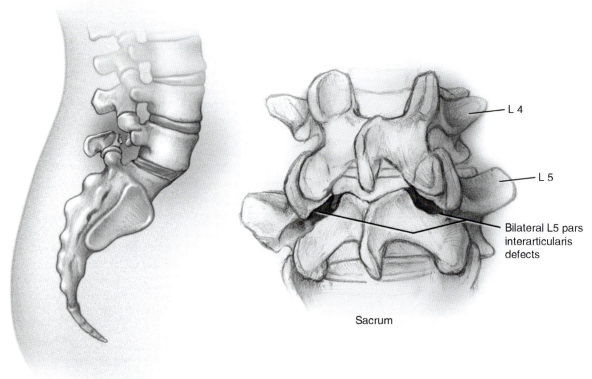

Figure 1.13. The six diagrams in the box at the top show the grades of spondylolisthesis ranging from normal (0 or no slippage) to greater than 100% slippage (grade 5, also termed spondyloptosis). The two figures at the bottom show lateral and posterior views of bilateral L5 spondylolysis (defects in the pars interarticularis).

one vertebral segment forward or backward in relation to the segment above or below (congenital or acquired spondylolisthesis).

Spondylolysis and spondylolisthesis

Spondylolysis is a bony defect in the pars interarticularis which lies between and connects the superior articular process and facet to the lamina of the same vertebral body (see Figure 1.13). The defect can be unilateral or bilateral and is seen most often at the L5 vertebral level. It is not clear whether spondylolysis is present at birth, but the propensity to develop a defect in the pars interarticularis does seem to be present from birth and may develop in childhood, presumably as a result of trauma which may or may not be associated with acute pain. The overall

Table 1.6. Classification of spondylolisthesis

Congenital or dysplastic

    Congenital defect which allows usually L5 to slip forward on S1

    Often associated with other congenital abnormalities

Isthmic spondylolisthesis

    Related to defect in pars interarticularis which is congenitally weak and may sustain a fatigue or acute fracture but can be due to an elongated, intact pars interarticularis

Degenerative spondylolisthesis

    Related to disk degeneration and degeneration and subluxation of the facet joints

Traumatic spondylolisthesis

    Due to severe trauma with fracture dislocation usually not involving the pars interarticularis

Pathologic spondylolisthesis

    Related to generalized or local bone disease

Iatrogenic spondylolisthesis

    Usually due to excessive removal of facet joints

prevalence is about 3%–6% of the adult population. Heredity is thought to play a role. Oblique X-rays and, better yet, CT scanning can demonstrate spondylolysis. Spondylolisthesis occurs when one vertebra slips forward (also called anterolisthesis) or, much less commonly, backward (also called retrolisthesis) on the vertebra below. The slippage can result from several different mechanisms (see Table 1.6). Spondylolisthesis is graded from 0 (normal – no slippage) to 5. Grade 1 is 1%–25% slippage of one vertebra on the next; 2 is 26%–50%; 3 is 51%–75%; 4 is 76%–100%; and 5 is greater than 100% or complete slippage. Complete slippage is sometimes termed spondyloptosis. Spondylolisthesis is a recognized cause of back pain and, if the degree of slippage is significant and impinges on the central canal or intervertebral foramina, it can cause radicular pain and neurologic deficits. Spondylolysis and spondylolisthesis need not be painful.

Scoliosis
Scoliosis is lateral, side-to-side curvature in the coronal plane of the spine and can be congenital or acquired. The term is typically applied to curves in excess of 10°. Curvatures of less than 30° usually will not progress after an individual's skeleton has matured. About 70% of all cases of scoliosis fall into the idiopathic category which are classified by age of onset: infantile (before age 3 years), juvenile

(age 3–10 years), and adolescent (age greater than 10 years) idiopathic scoliosis. Idiopathic scoliosis infrequently presents with pain. Aside from patients with trauma, inflammation, and tumors, patients with scoliosis develop discomfort and pain in their spine related to mechanical factors including muscle fatigue and myalgia and secondary disk and/or facet or sacroiliac joint degeneration. Radicular pain can occur secondary to root compression typically on the shortened side away from the side of convexity. In severe cases, the patient's ribs can rub against their iliac crest on the shortened side of their curve. Respiratory compromise can occur. Management consists of observation, orthotics (assistive devices such as a brace), and operative intervention. Congenital scoliosis is most likely to be recognized during or prior to adolescence. Causes of scoliosis are shown in Table 1.7. The prevalence of scoliosis tends to increase with age. About 3.9%–7.5% of adults have thoracolumbar scoliosis measuring 10° or more. Smaller curves are equally divided between men and women, but there is a female preponderance in patients with curves of 20° or more.

Kyphosis
Kyphosis is an abnormal curvature in the sagittal plane and can be congenital or acquired. Most commonly, this affects the thoracic spine with an excessive dorsal curvature of the spine (convex posterior), but can affect the cervical or lumbar spine. Potential causes of kyphosis are shown in Table 1.8. Except for patients with fractures, both traumatic and osteoporotic (or a combination), the pain associated with kyphosis usually develops gradually and is presumed to be secondary to the stress that the kyphosis places on the supporting musculoskeletal structures, possibly with superimposed degenerative changes in the disks and facet joints provoked by the spinal deformity.

Vertebral hemangioma
It is unclear whether vertebral hemangiomas are congenital abnormalities or benign vascular neoplasms. They can affect any level of the spine. They have been increasingly recognized with the advent of MRI because they show up very well with this imaging technique. They are occasionally symptomatic and can cause localized pain and tenderness. They can, rarely, cause nerve root and spinal cord compression. Larger hemangiomas, thoracic location, and evidence of expansion are associated with greater likelihood

Table 1.7. Classification of scoliosis

Nonstructural scoliosis

    Postural

    Compensatory

        Leg length discrepancy

Transient structural scoliosis

    "Sciatic scoliosis" – nerve root impingement causes list, usually to opposite side to reduce pain

    Related to temporary local inflammatory process

    Hysterical scoliosis

Structural scoliosis

    Idiopathic scoliosis

        Infantile – before age 3

        Juvenile – age 3–10

        Adolescent – age 10 to skeletal maturity

    Congenital scoliosis due to malformations of the spine

        Failure of vertebrae to fully form (hemi-vertebra – lateral aspect of vertebra is absent or incomplete)

        Failure of vertebrae to completely separate (unsegmented or block vertebrae – two or more vertebrae are connected laterally on one side)

        Combined failure of formation and failure of segmentation

    Neurologic

        Lower motor neuron disease (e.g., poliomyelitis, other viral illnesses, motor neuron disease)

        Upper motor neuron disease (e.g., cerebral palsy)

        Spinocerebellar degeneration

        Syringomyelia

        Spinal cord tumor

        Dystonia

    Myopathic disorders

        Muscular dystrophy

        Acquired myopathy

    Infectious (e.g., tuberculous, pyogenic)

    Inflammatory noninfectious (e.g., rheumatoid arthritis, ankylosing spondylitis)

    Post-traumatic

    Post-surgical

    Metabolic bone disease

        Osteoporosis

        Osteogenesis imperfecta

    Developmental

        Marfan syndrome

        Morquio syndrome

        Others

Table 1.8. Causes of kyphosis

Congenital disorders

    Defect of vertebral formation

    Defect of vertebral segmentation

    Myelomeningocele

Developmental

    Achondroplasia

Scheuermann disease

Paralytic disorder

    Lower motor neuron

        Poliomyelitis

        Motor neuron disease

    Myopathies affecting paraspinal muscles

    Upper motor neuron

        Cerebral palsy

Spondylosis

Post-traumatic

    Acute

    Chronic

Post-surgical

    Post-laminectomy

    Post-vertebrectomy

    Post-fusion

Tumor

    Benign

    Malignant

Post-irradiation

Infectious

    Tuberculous

    Pyogenic

Inflammatory noninfectious

    Ankylosing spondylitis

    Rheumatoid arthritis

Metabolic bone disease

    Osteoporosis

    Osteomalacia

    Osteogenesis imperfecta

Excess muscle contraction

    Muscle spasm

    Dystonia

Purely postural disorder

Other postural disorders with multiple causes, some of which are listed above

    Camptocormia (bent spine syndrome) – lumbar kyphosis

    Dropped head syndrome – cervical kyphosis

of cord compression. They are covered in greater detail in Chapter 3.

Syringomyelia

Syringomyelia can be congenital, related to a congenital condition, or acquired. Syringomyelia is the presence of a fluid-filled cystic cavity (syrinx) within the spinal cord. The term hydromyelia is used if the cyst is lined with ependymal cells. Although it may not develop or become symptomatic for many years, syringomyelia is frequently associated with Chiari malformation or hydrocephalus or both. Chiari malformation is a congenital abnormality of the hindbrain in which the brain stem and cerebellum are pushed downward into the foramen magnum and upper cervical spinal canal. Chiari I malformation is often an asymptomatic finding but can be associated with hydrocephalus and congenital malformations of the cervical spine and can cause lower cranial nerve dysfunction and Valsalva- and exercise-induced headache. Chiari I is defined as herniation of the cerebellar tonsils no more than 3 mm below the lower edge of the foramen magnum. Chiari II is a more severe hindbrain deformity which is associated with myelomeningocele in >90% and hydrocephalus in about 80% of patients. When associated with Chiari malformation or communicating hydrocephalus, syringomyelia is thought to develop because of altered CSF dynamics and increased pressure within the central canal of the spinal cord. Patients may develop secondary scoliosis. Syringomyelia can also occur following substantial trauma to the spinal cord, within a spinal cord tumor, following infection, following an inflammatory process, or for no apparent reason (idiopathic). Syringomyelia is more frequent in men than in women and often presents in the third or fourth decade of life. Signs and symptoms depend on the level of spinal cord involvement. Lower motor neuron weakness can occur at the level of the syrinx, while upper motor neuron weakness occurs below the syrinx. Because of the central location of the syrinx, crossing spinothalamic tract fibers are interrupted, while dorsal column sensory function is unimpaired. This results in "dissociated" sensory loss (loss of pain and temperature sensation in the dermatomes of the spinal levels affected by the syrinx with intact touch, joint position, and vibration sense). As a result of loss of pain perception, patients can develop painless skin ulcers and neurogenic arthropathy. So-called Charcot joints are characterized by joint effusion, destruction, and subluxation and commonly affect the shoulders if the syrinx involves the cervical spinal cord, which is common. Neurologic findings may be quite asymmetric. Syringomyelia most frequently affects the cervical level and can extend over many spinal cord levels. The cervical location often results in pain and temperature sensation loss in the upper extremities which extends up over the shoulders in a "shawl" distribution. Pain often, but not always, accompanies syringomyelia and can affect the spine or limbs or both. The pain can be deep and aching or have a dysesthetic quality. Syringomyelia tends to be slowly progressive over long periods of time. The diagnosis is established with MRI (see Figure 1.14). Surgical treatments

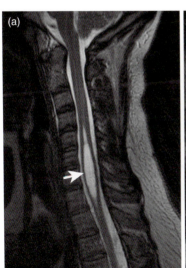
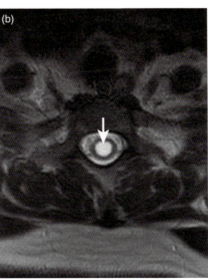

Figure 1.14. Syringomyelia. (a) Sagittal and (b) axial T$_2$-weighted MR images of a large cervical syrinx occupying the center of the spinal cord (arrows). The fluid in the syrinx has MRI signal characteristics very similar to those of the cerebrospinal fluid which surrounds the spinal cord. There is no accompanying Chiari malformation, which is often seen. This 28-year-old woman had multifocal pain but a normal neurologic examination. Her pain was not helped by shunting the fluid from the syrinx into her subarachnoid space.

include suboccipital craniectomy and upper cervical laminectomy to treat Chiari malformation if present, ventriculoperitoneal shunting if there is associated hydrocephalus, shunting of the syrinx fluid usually into the subarachnoid space, or directly approaching an associated spinal cord tumor or local scarring.

Muscles and other soft tissues

The muscles and ligaments of the spine are commonly blamed for axial pain. Indeed, acute injury to the muscles, more frequently than ligaments, is likely to be the mechanism for many patients with acute, self-limited axial spine pain. This is especially true if the patient has sustained either an acute traumatic injury or performed a single acute action such as lifting a very heavy object. Similar pain of muscle origin can follow repeated physical movement (e.g., shoveling), especially in the individual who is deconditioned. Subacute or acute pain sometimes accompanied by muscle spasm which follows these activities is blamed on mechanical failure, local ischemia, and disturbances of energy metabolism within the muscle. Muscle spasm can also occur as a reaction to pain originating from an adjacent nonmuscle structure. Acute pain following muscle and/or ligament injury usually rapidly subsides within days or a few weeks. Muscles have also been blamed for more chronic axial spine pain and for more widespread and chronic myofascial pain under the terms fibrositis and fibromyalgia. The underlying pathophysiology of chronic muscle, fascia, and ligament pain is elusive. This more chronic pain, presumed to be of muscle origin, is often associated with focal areas of tenderness which may be accompanied by small subcutaneous nodules or knots which come and go. Such chronic pain lacks electromyographic (EMG) abnormalities and any demonstrated muscle pathology. Nonetheless, chronic pain of muscle origin affecting the spine and limbs is a very genuine and relatively common condition.

So why does it hurt?

Pain of spine origin, whether felt in the spine or outside the spine, is related to stimulation of pain-sensitive tissues within the spine (see Table 1.9). Nerve structures that can transmit pain of spinal origin include the sinuvertebral nerves, the dorsal nerve roots, dorsal root ganglia, the mixed motor and sensory spinal nerves, and the dorsal and ventral rami which arise from the spinal nerves (see Figure 1.9).

Given the structures they innervate, the sinuvertebral nerves (which normally supply the posterior

Table 1.9. Potential sources of spine pain

Vertebra – chiefly the periosteum

Facet, sacroiliac, skull–C1, C1–C2, and costovertebral joints, especially the fibrous capsules

Various spinal ligaments

Superficial layers of the annulus fibrosus of the intervertebral disk

Paravertebral muscles

Dura mater, less so posteriorly

Skin and subcutaneous adipose tissue

Blood vessels

Sensory nerve structures

longitudinal ligament, superficial posterolateral annulus fibrosus, anterolateral dura, blood vessels, and some periosteum) and dorsal rami (which supply the paraspinal muscles, the interspinous ligament, the zygapophyseal joints, and cutaneous sensation of the posterior torso) would seem to be responsible for transmitting axial spine pain, whereas the ventral rami and spinal nerves supply sensation from the rest of the body below the neck.

Degeneration of the intervertebral disk, a common finding, should cause axial spine pain which, in turn, could be transmitted by the sinuvertebral nerves. Since the sinuvertebral nerves only innervate the superficial layers of the normal annulus fibrosus, it is postulated that degeneration and fragmentation of the annulus fibrosus allow nociceptive nerve fibers to grow inward and innervate deeper layers of the annulus and possibly the nucleus pulposus. The abnormal, deeper pain-sensitive nerves could then signal the presence of disk degeneration that is not normally felt. This mechanism of pain perception is not proven.

If degeneration and arthritis of the facet joints are responsible for some patients' pain and the medial branches of the dorsal rami innervate these joints, then treatments directed at the medial branches should help to reduce or eliminate pain. Facet joint changes are common on imaging studies, but there is a poor correlation between imaging findings and symptoms. A recognizable facet joint syndrome is elusive at best.

As noted above, it is postulated that axial spine pain can be of paraspinal muscle origin. This is likely to be the case, at least in part, for acute pain with muscle spasm, but there is no objective evidence supporting a muscular cause of chronic pain. Especially for axial spine pain, it is exceedingly difficult to determine which structure is causing an individual patient's pain and by what mechanism.

Pain due to pathology affecting the dorsal nerve roots, spinal ganglia, spinal nerves or their ventral rami is often perceived in the distribution of sensory supply of the affected nerve. Characteristically, this arises from compression of one of these nerves by a herniated intervertebral disk or osteophytic spur. Experimental evidence strongly suggests that compression alone will not cause radicular pain and that an additional inflammatory component is necessary in most instances. This may explain why some disk herniations with root compression are painless. The characteristic pain distribution for involvement at different levels of the spine is described in Chapters 2–4 and typically follows the dermatomal distribution of the injured nerve root. Involvement of these nerves is often associated with neurologic deficits and nerve root tension signs which have great localizing value. Radicular pain is often sharp and stabbing but can be aching or burning in character.

The cutaneous distribution of dermatomes is not absolute. There is some overlap from one dermatome to another, and there can be variation between individuals as well. In addition, patients with spine-related problems that do not affect the nerves can also have referred pain at some distance from their pathology. For example, injection of hypertonic saline into lumbar facet joints can cause pain in the flank, groin, buttock, or posterior thigh. Such nonradicular referred pain is variable and inconstant, and therefore not very helpful diagnostically. Such nonradicular referred pain can co-exist with radicular referred pain creating further confusion.

The concept of sclerotomes and myotomes is also used to help explain some referred pain. A sclerotome is the segmental, nerve root innervation of bones, and a myotome is the segmental, nerve root innervation of muscles. Both stem from embryonic development and innervation of these structures. The sclerotomal and myotomal distribution of pain related to nerve root disease is also somewhat variable and there is considerable overlap between different spinal levels. As a result, this type of referred pain does not have great localizing value except to signal its possible referred nature and spinal origin.

Pain arising from disease of internal organs can simulate referred pain of spinal origin. The classic example is chest and left upper limb pain secondary to myocardial ischemia. Visceral afferent sensory nerves from the thoracic, abdominal, and pelvic

internal organs travel through rami communicantes and pass through the spinal nerve and dorsal nerve root to enter the posterior horn of the spinal cord at their embryonic segment of origin. When they enter the spinal cord, they intermingle with and stimulate some of the same neurons as do the somatic sensory nerves that enter at the same spinal level. As a result, sensory stimulation of visceral origin may affect first- and second-order somatic sensory nerves and cause pain that is felt mostly or only in the somatic segmental distribution, which is usually dermatomal. For example, sensory fibers from the heart conduct impulses through the left C8 through T5 spinal levels, and myocardial ischemia can thus cause left upper limb pain as well as chest pain.

Myofascial pain can be multifocal and cause pain localized to the axial spine and/or one or more limbs. Rarely, disease of the central nervous system above the level of the pain can cause so-called central pain. This can be caused by irritation of or damage to the spinal cord (dorsal horns, posterior columns, or spinothalamic tracts), brain stem, thalamus, subcortical structures, or cerebral cortex. Such central pain is often burning, sometimes with superimposed sharp, jabbing pains and can be aggravated by cutaneous stimulation, movement, emotions, and temperature change, especially cold. Such central pain is characteristically accompanied by other neurologic symptoms and neurologic signs. Some pain can also be "central," but on a psychogenic basis. Purely psychogenic pain is uncommon.

Pain can be divided into nociceptive and neuropathic pain. Nociceptive pain is caused by the activation of peripheral primary sensory nerve endings. Myelinated A-δ nerve fibers (fast conduction) and unmyelinated C fibers (slow conduction) both have their cell bodies in the dorsal root ganglia of the spinal nerve roots and transmit sensory information into the spinal cord. Neuropathic pain is due to damage or dysfunction of peripheral sensory nerves, the spinal ganglia, or their central connections. Neuropathic pain characteristically has a burning, prickling, lancinating, or electric quality. Allodynia, pain caused by a nonpainful stimulus such as a light touch, and hyperalgesia, increased sensitivity to a normally painful stimulus, are common with neuropathic pain. Nociceptive pain typically indicates non-nervous system tissue damage. It is often aching and sometimes throbbing. Acute nerve root compression is characterized by nociceptive-type pain, whereas the residual of an old nerve root injury is more likely to exhibit neuropathic pain. Nociceptive pain is said to be more responsive to opioid analgesics, but recent evidence casts some doubt on this differentiating point. Some pain combines both nociceptive and neuropathic components. Central transmission of painful sensory input is affected by multiple layers of nerve cells in the dorsal horns of the spinal cord which serve to filter, amplify, or attenuate the information being sent to the brain. This processing and modulation greatly affects the perception of sensation in general and pain in particular.

These comments can help guide the clinician in understanding and diagnosing a given patient's pain. The next three chapters address the specific pain syndromes affecting the cervical, thoracic, and lumbar spine.

Further reading

1. Benarroch EE, Daube JR, Flemming KD, Westmoreland BF. *Mayo Clinic Medical Neurosciences: Organized by Neurologic Systems and Levels*, Fifth Edition. Rochester, Minnesota: Mayo Clinic Scientific Press. 2008.

2. Boden SD, Bohlman HH, eds. *The Failed Spine*. Philadelphia, PA: Lippincott Williams & Wilkins. 2003.

3. Byrne TN, Benzel EC, Waxman SG. *Diseases of the Spine and Spinal Cord*. New York: Oxford University Press, Inc. 2000.

4. Deyo RA, Mirza SK, Martin BI. Back pain prevalence and visit rates. *Spine* 2006; **31**(23):2724–2727.

5. Fardon DF, Milette PC. Nomenclature and classification of lumbar disc pathology: recommendations of the Combined Task Forces of the North American Spine Society, American Society of Spine Radiology, and American Society of Neuroradiology. *Spine* 2001; **26**(5):E93–E113.

6. Frymoyer JW, Wiesel SW, eds. *The Adult and Pediatric Spine, Third Edition*. Philadelphia, Pennsylvania: Lippincott Williams & Wilkins. 2004.

7. Kumar N, ed. Spinal cord, root, and plexus disorders. *Continuum Lifelong Learning Neurol* 2008; **14**(3):1–271.

8. Martin BI, Deyo RA, Mirza SK, et al. Expenditures and health status among adults with back and neck problems. *JAMA* 2008; **299**(6):656–664.

9. Masson C, Pruvo JP, Meder JF, et al. Spinal cord infarction: clinical and magnetic resonance findings and short term outcome. *J Neurol Neurosurg Psychiatry* 2004; **75**(10):1431–1435.

10. Slipman CW, Derby R, Simeone FA, Mayer TG, eds. *Interventional Spine: An Algorithmic Approach*. Philadelphia, PA: Saunders, 2008.

11. Standring S, ed. *Gray's Anatomy: The Anatomical Basis of Clinical Practice*, Thirty-ninth Edition. London: Elsevier Ltd., 2005.

Chapter

2 The cervical level

Introduction

An individual's spine-related complaints can usually be attributed to the cervical, thoracic, or lumbar level. Some patients will have multifocal symptoms, especially pain, and some patients will present with myelopathy, where there is a need to consider both the thoracic and cervical levels, or have a presentation localized to the conus medullaris and/or cauda equina wherein the lower thoracic and lumbar levels must both be considered. Because most patients present with signs and symptoms referable to one level, the clinical approaches to the patient with cervical, thoracic, and lumbar level disease will be presented separately. Within each level, there are three subtypes: radiculopathy, which is usually single but can be multiple; bilateral central injury, which affects the spinal cord at the cervical and thoracic levels and the cauda equina at the lumbar level; and axial spine pain. Radiculopathy, spinal cord or cauda equina injury, and axial spine pain can be combined. This chapter will begin with sections on the history and physical, neurologic, and special examinations that are pertinent to the cervical level, followed by sections dedicated to cervical radiculopathy, cervical myelopathy, and neck pain.

The history

The patient's chief complaint and history of their present illness are critical pieces of information for localizing the patient's problem and reaching a tentative diagnosis. Having said this, the patient's current medications, past medical history, social history, review of systems, and family history can be very helpful and should be reviewed.

At the outset of the interview, the patient should be given free rein to tell the physician about their chief symptoms and how they evolved. Inciting causes, especially trauma including minor, major, and that related to manipulation of the spine, should be sought. Antecedent procedures, injections, physical therapies, and medications should be reviewed. Recent interventions also raise the possibility of spinal infection. In particular, a history of neurologic symptoms (weakness, numbness, tingling, and incoordination) affecting the upper limbs and lower extremities should be obtained. Brain and cranial nerve symptoms indicate problems at a higher level of the nervous system that could be seen in patients, for example, with multiple sclerosis, who might present with spinal cord symptoms. Constitutional symptoms such as fever, chills, and weight loss could indicate an underlying systemic disease. A past history of cancer, acquired immunodeficiency syndrome (AIDS), or immunosuppressive therapy should be sought. All of the patient's ongoing medical problems should be documented. It is important to know if the patient is on a blood thinner. Pain that increases when the patient is supine or that wakes the patient from sleep suggests intraspinal nerve root or spinal cord impingement. A history of joint pain and/or swelling elsewhere in the body suggests a generalized arthritis or spondyloarthropathy.

Some patients are unable to hold their head up, which is usually due to severe weakness of the muscles that extend the neck. So-called dropped head syndrome may or may not be accompanied by neck pain and can be due to a focal or more generalized myopathic process including myositis or a congenital myopathy, motor neuron disease, myasthenia gravis, Parkinson disease and parkinsonian syndromes, and dystonia.

It is worthwhile inquiring whether certain neck positions make the patient's pain better or worse. Tingling down the spine and/or extremities with neck flexion, which is called Lhermitte sign, can be seen in many conditions that inflame or compress the cervical spinal cord including multiple sclerosis, pernicious anemia, and conditions that narrow the cervical spinal canal including spondylosis and tumors. Lhermitte sign with neck extension has the same significance. An increase in neurologic symptoms with an

Rate your pain:

0 = no pain
10 = worst pain you can imagine

Level of pain right now: 0 1 2 3 4 5 6 7 8 9 10
Level of pain at its best: 0 1 2 3 4 5 6 7 8 9 10
Level of pain at its worst: 0 1 2 3 4 5 6 7 8 9 10

Place appropriate symbols at the locations where you experience pain.

Burning = x
Deep ache = z
Sharp or stabbing = /
Pins and needles = o

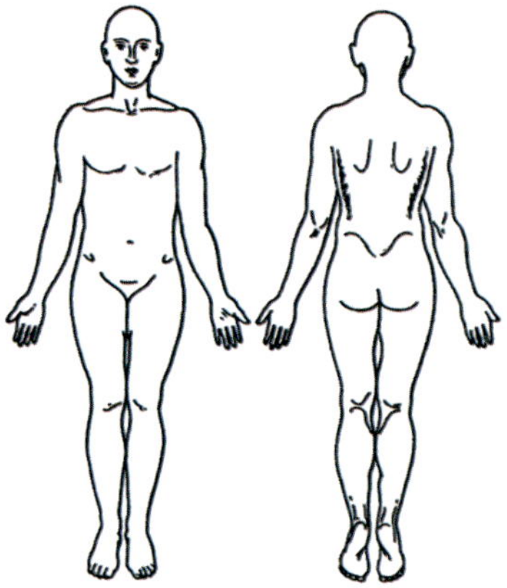

Figure 2.1. Example of a pain diagram which allows patients to graphically localize and describe their pain.

increase in body temperature (with exertion, fever, or a hot environment) is termed Uhthoff phenomenon and is often seen in patients with multiple sclerosis.

Localization of the patient's pain is important. Is it confined to the neck alone? Is it symmetric or asymmetric? Does it spread into the scapular region, trapezius muscle, shoulder, or anterior neck? Does the pain affect the upper limb and, if so, where? It can be helpful to have the patient fill out a pain diagram showing where on their body they have pain of different kinds (burning, aching, and sharp or stabbing) and where they experience paresthesias (see Figure 2.1). The rapidity of onset of the symptoms should be noted – the nervous system has a better tolerance for disks, osteophytic spurs, tumors, and other mass lesions that expand slowly. Some patients with cervical nerve root impingement report that their pain is reduced if they place their affected upper extremity in certain postures, which include abduction of the arm with flexion of the elbow and the hand held on top of or behind the patient's head or with the arm at their side and flexed at the elbow with the elbow held in the cupped hand of the

unaffected limb. Cervical nerve root impingement often causes referred pain in the scapula, shoulder, and/or upper extremity. Patients with mid and lower cervical root compression are more likely to experience pain in their arm or forearm or both. Recall that the arm is the part of the upper limb between the shoulder and elbow, and the forearm is between the elbow and wrist. Sensory symptoms (numbness and/or tingling) are usually in the distribution of the dermatome supplied by the nerve root (see Figure 2.2). The shoulder girdle pain that is a common accompaniment of cervical nerve root compression is thought to be related to the nerve root supply of sensation to cervicobrachial paraspinal and limb muscles (and thus on a myotomal basis) or possibly related to sensory supply of bone (sclerotomal). Typical pain distribution for various cervical radiculopathies is described in Table 2.1. The pain of cervical radiculopathy typically spares the hand. The distribution of upper limb sensory symptoms can be very useful in determining the level of nerve root involvement.

A key question is whether the patient is getting better, getting worse, or is about the same with or without treatment. Response or lack of response to previous treatments can be helpful. Were anti-inflammatory medications helpful? Were oral or injected corticosteroids beneficial? Was traction helpful? A history of cigarette smoking increases the risk of degenerative disk disease and reduces the likelihood of a solid fusion if the patient has previously undergone an attempt at cervical fusion. A shift from neck pain to upper limb pain may signal increased or new nerve root compression, especially by an extruded disk fragment. Sometimes there is improvement in pain with worsening of neurologic deficit as a consequence of increased nerve root compression. Patients are not always aware of their muscle weakness. Increased radicular pain with neck motion – rotation or bending or flexion or extension – suggests nerve root compression. Brief exacerbation of the patient's pain, especially radicular pain, brought on by coughing, sneezing, straining at stool, or by lifting an object also suggests cervical nerve root compression, often by a disk or osteophyte.

The examination
The general examination
The general examination can be helpful. Does the patient appear to be in significant pain? Do they have a fever? Do they have any skin lesions that might

Table 2.1. Symptoms and signs associated with cervical radiculopathy

Root	Disk level	Typical pain distribution	Dermatomal sensory distribution	Weakness	Affected reflex
C4	C3–C4	Neck	Suprascapular, supraclavicular, and top of shoulder	Usually none	None
C5	C4–C5	Neck, scapula, shoulder, anterior arm	Lateral aspect of arm and forearm	Shoulder abduction Elbow flexion	Biceps Brachioradialis
C6	C5–C6	Neck, scapula, shoulder, lateral arm and forearm	Anterolateral aspect of arm, forearm, hand, thumb and forefinger	Shoulder abduction Elbow flexion Forearm pronation	Biceps Brachioradialis
C7	C6–C7	Neck, shoulder, lateral arm, medial scapula, extensor surface of forearm	Dorsolateral forearm and hand, forefinger and long finger	Elbow extension Wrist extension Finger extension	Triceps
C8	C7–T1	Neck, medial scapula, medial aspect of arm and forearm	Medial forearm and hand, ring and little fingers	Finger abduction Finger adduction Finger flexion	None or finger flexor
T1	T1–T2	Anterior chest, medial arm and forearm	Medial arm and forearm	Finger abduction Finger adduction Finger flexion	None or finger flexor

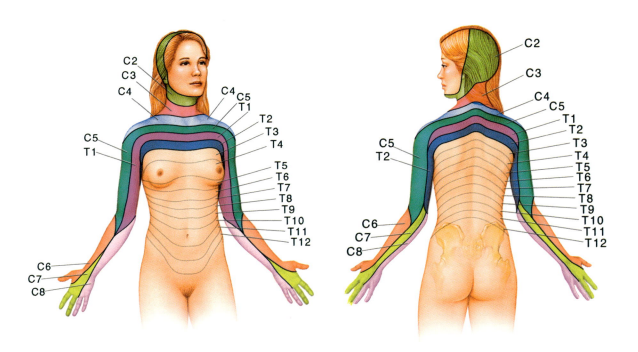

Figure 2.2. Depiction of cervical dermatomes. There is some overlap between dermatomes and variability from one individual to another. Not all authors agree about dermatomal territories and this illustration is offered as a consensus. Some authors show C4 meeting T2 instead of C5 meeting T1 across the upper anterior and posterior chest.

suggest an infectious illness (shingles or Lyme disease) or an underlying inflammatory arthritis (psoriasis)? Do they have iritis, which might suggest ankylosing spondylitis? Do they have a Horner syndrome that might suggest a Pancoast tumor? Do they have lymphadenopathy that might suggest a malignancy such as lymphoma? The musculoskeletal examination can show evidence of osteoarthritis, rheumatoid arthritis, or spondyloarthropathy. Patients with cervical spondylosis often have concomitant lumbar spondylosis and thoracic spondylosis, and the converse is true as well.

Evaluation of the cervical spine should start during the interview with simple observation before conducting a formal examination. The patient may hold their head tilted to one side or forward with nerve root impingement, bone and joint disease, or paraspinal muscle spasm which can be due to pain or dystonia (torticollis). Does the patient hold their head and neck stiffly? Some patients are unable to hold their head up due to severe weakness of the muscles which extend the neck. This so-called dropped head syndrome may or may not be accompanied by neck pain and can be due to the conditions listed earlier in this chapter. Is there any scoliosis of the entire spine? Is the normal cervical lordosis present or is it absent or exaggerated? Is torticollis present? Are the shoulders and scapulae even and symmetric? Does palpation of the paraspinal muscles reveal tenderness or spasm? Are there any masses or displaced bony structures? Are the spinous processes in alignment posteriorly?

Neurologic examination

The neurologic examination is critical in the assessment of patients with spine disease in general, and especially for the cervical spine. Except for spinal instability and severe deformity, the indications for surgical intervention on the cervical spine (and elsewhere in the spine) rest largely on evidence of spinal cord or significant spinal nerve root impingement. A complete description of the neurologic examination is beyond the purpose of this book. The signs and symptoms associated with specific cervical nerve root impingement syndromes and cervical myelopathy are listed in Tables 2.1 and 2.2. A few pertinent comments will be made regarding the findings on examination. On testing muscle strength, it is helpful to put the muscle being tested in a position of mechanical disadvantage, so that the examiner can actually overcome the muscle and compare its strength to the same muscle on the other side. For example, test the triceps muscle with the elbow flexed and not extended. Test the wrist extensors with the fingers extended, not fisted, and the wrist in a neutral or slightly flexed position. True weakness has a smooth quality when the muscle is overcome by manual strength testing. Give-way weakness can be seen in the presence of pain, lack of understanding, conversion disorder, malingering, suboptimal effort, or other reasons. Rather than guessing whether or not the muscle is truly weak or truly normal, it is best to consider the strength of the muscle that gives way as

Table 2.2. Symptoms and findings associated with cervical myelopathy

Symptoms

Neck pain

Unilateral or bilateral upper limb pain

Upper limb weakness, numbness, or loss of dexterity

Lower limb stiffness, weakness, or sensory loss

Urgency of bladder more often than bowel; urgency incontinence; frequency of urination

Lhermitte sign (shock-like sensations extending down the spine and out into the limbs with neck flexion or extension)

Findings

Increased lower and/or upper limb deep tendon reflexes

Loss of superficial reflexes below neck

Positive Hoffmann signs (thumb adduction and thumb and finger flexion after forced flexion and sudden release of the tip of the long finger)

Positive finger flexor reflex (brisk flexion of the patient's fingers when the examiner taps on the back of their own fingers while holding the patient's flexed fingertips)

Babinski and/or Chaddock signs

Upper limb weakness beyond the bounds of a single nerve root on one or both sides

Weakness in the lower limbs in an upper motor neuron distribution

Sensory loss in lower and/or upper limbs and/or torso

Spasticity in the limbs, especially the lower extremities

Gait disturbance, especially if suggestive of spasticity

being equal to or greater than the strength that was exerted just before the muscle gave way. The muscle could be normal or as weak as it was just before it gave way – we can't be sure. Using this approach, the examiner will not call a strong muscle weak, nor will they judge a truly weak muscle normal.

The biceps and brachioradialis reflexes are both innervated by the C5 and C6 nerve roots but by different peripheral nerves (the musculocutaneous and radial nerves respectively). A new or old C5 and/or C6 radiculopathy can cause reduced biceps and brachioradialis reflexes on one side. Sometimes this can cause the perception that all of the deep tendon reflexes are increased in the contralateral upper limb. Spondylotic myelopathy can be associated with increased triceps, but normal or even reduced biceps and brachioradialis reflexes. Alternatively, all of the upper limb and lower limb reflexes can be increased with spondylotic myelopathy. Especially with hyperreflexia in the upper limb, there can be pathological spread of reflexes such that muscles whose tendons were not stretched also contract. For example, the biceps reflex is tested and the brachioradialis and finger flexors contract at the same time as does the biceps muscle. Due to difficulty activating the muscles, upper motor neuron weakness tends to be more variable than lower motor neuron weakness. Upper motor neuron weakness is associated with increased muscle tone, lack of muscle atrophy, and greater impairment of fine movements and co-ordination than is lower motor neuron type weakness. The atrophy seen in lower motor neuron type weakness is often delayed for several weeks after the nerve root or peripheral nerve is injured. Hoffmann signs are more significant than Trömner signs. A positive finger flexor reflex (the examiner holds the patient's down-turned fingertips in their own up-turned fingertips and taps on the dorsal aspect of their own distal interphalangeal joints – brief brisk flexion of the patient's fingers is a positive response) is a sign of upper motor neuron dysfunction or generalized hyperreflexia. The finger flexor reflex is the equivalent of the Hoffmann sign. Babinski, Chaddock, and other so-called toe signs indicate a disturbance of the upper motor neurons which control the lower limbs. The upper motor neuron problem could be in the brain, brain stem, or spinal cord. Chaddock signs can be present in the absence of Babinski signs. Upper motor neuron type weakness of spinal origin typically does not cause true drift of the outstretched hands with the patient's eyes closed which occurs with supraspinal level lesions. Examination of higher functions and the cranial nerves is helpful when evaluating myelopathy and radiculopathy because intracranial processes can cause unilateral or bilateral corticospinal tract dysfunction, and inflammatory and neoplastic etiologies of spinal radiculopathy can also affect the cranial nerves.

The sensory examination is problematic because all sensory loss – partial or complete – is subjective. That is to say, we must rely on the patient's report of the diminished perception of a stimulus. Only they can tell us if the applied touch, pin, touch, vibration, or change in joint position is normal or reduced. The same is true for diminished hearing and vision. In contrast, the presence of sensation can be objectively documented. If the patient can always tell us with their eyes closed whether we are touching them with the sharp or dull end of a pin, if the stimulus is hot or cold, if the tuning fork is really vibrating (or actually placed against their bone), and which way the joint

has been moved, we can be sure that each sensory modality is qualitatively if not quantitatively intact. This subjectivity of the sensory examination is unlike other aspects of the neurologic examination, such as motor strength, co-ordination, deep tendon reflexes, and eye movements, where the examiner can make their own judgment. In fact, the patient's report of sensory symptoms, such as numbness or tingling in the characteristic distribution of, for example, the C7 nerve root, can be far more helpful in localization than trying to find sensory loss in the same distribution on examination. A map of the upper body dermatomes is shown in Figure 2.2. There is significant overlap in the sensory dermatomes and some variation in the dermatomal boundaries from one individual to another.

Tinel sign consists of applying pressure or percussion (with a reflex hammer or the tap of a fingertip) over a peripheral nerve. Tingling or electric-like paresthesias emanating proximally or distally from the site of pressure or percussion indicate nerve irritability. The damage could be occurring at the site of the tapping, or a positive sign could also indicate that nerves have regenerated to that point following a more proximal injury. It is most commonly used to test the median nerve in the anterior wrist, and a positive sign gives support for a diagnosis of carpal tunnel syndrome, which is frequently in the differential diagnosis of usually intermittent upper limb pain, sensory symptoms, and sometimes weakness. Phalen sign can also help look for carpal tunnel syndrome. In this test, the patient's wrist is held in forced flexion for 60 seconds. The test is often performed on both sides at the same time by having the patient press the backs of their hands together, forcing both wrists into extreme flexion. Provocation of hand numbness, tingling, or pain suggests median nerve entrapment at the wrist.

Special examinations
Cervical spine range of motion should be tested for forward flexion, extension, side bending to the right and left, and rotation to the right and left. Limitations in range of motion can be symmetric or asymmetric and relate to acute injury including possible fracture, muscle spasm, spondylosis, inflammatory arthritis, spondyloarthropathy, Parkinson disease, nuchal rigidity from infectious and neoplastic meningitis, torticollis (dystonia), congenital anomalies, and pain alone. Relief of symptoms, especially radicular pain, with manual upward traction on the cervical spine

can be helpful in determining if there is nerve root impingement and whether or not neck traction might have a beneficial effect on the patient's pain. The examiner puts one hand beneath the patient's chin and the other beneath the patient's occiput and gently lifts upward for 30–60 seconds while the patient monitors their pain level and other symptoms (e.g., numbness, tingling). Conversely, various compression tests can be performed to help determine the mechanism of an individual patient's pain. With their neck in a neutral position, downward pressure is applied to the top of the patient's head and they are asked if this increases their neck or upper limb pain or brings out pain or sensory symptoms not present beforehand. In the Spurling maneuver, or foraminal compression test, the patient's neck is extended and flexed (bent) laterally toward their symptomatic side (see Figure 2.3). Downward pressure is applied to the vertex; an increase in the patient's upper limb pain or paresthesias suggests nerve root impingement in the neck. Patients can also develop symptoms from assuming this position without applying pressure to the vertex. The Spurling test is not very sensitive, but it is fairly specific for cervical radiculopathy. In a modification of the Spurling maneuver, called the maximal compression test, rotation of the neck toward the symptomatic side is added to extension and lateral flexion.

The shoulder depression test can indicate ipsilateral nerve root irritation. The neck is laterally flexed to the asymptomatic side while downward pressure is placed on the shoulder on the symptomatic side. Increased radicular pain or paresthesias suggest abnormality of the spinal nerve roots, usually compression. In the shoulder abduction test (also known as the shoulder abduction relief sign), abduction of the arm at the shoulder (usually with placement of the patient's hand on top of the head) on the symptomatic side can reduce tension on the cervical nerve roots; improvement in the patient's symptoms with this test suggests cervical root impingement.

Bilateral jugular vein compression for up to two minutes (Naffziger test) can aggravate radicular pain at any level and suggests nerve root impingement from any cause. The patient can also be asked to perform a prolonged Valsalva maneuver to see if they experience an increase in their symptoms.

Lhermitte phenomenon, described above, can also be tested during the examination by having the patient flex the neck downward and extend it directly backward while the patient observes for tingling

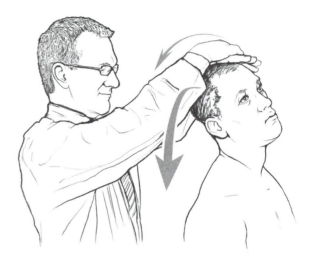

Figure 2.3. The Spurling maneuver is used to test for cervical nerve root irritability. The patient's head is bent backward and flexed (bent) laterally to their symptomatic side. Provocation of radicular pain or paresthesias with assumption of this position with or without downward pressure on the top of the patient's head suggests cervical nerve root compression. The test is better at confirming than screening for cervical radiculopathy. A modification of this test adds rotation of the patient's neck toward the side of pain.

or electric-like sensations down the spine and/or upper and/or lower extremities. While Lhermitte sign is classically described as symptoms provoked by neck flexion, some patients note the phenomenon with neck extension, which has the same clinical significance. Lhermitte sign can be positive in any condition that irritates the cervical spinal cord, including spondylotic narrowing of the cervical spinal canal, inflammatory demyelinating disease of the central nervous system (characteristically multiple sclerosis), tumors, Chiari malformation, syringomyelia, and pernicious anemia with subacute combined degeneration.

Adson and other so-called thoracic outlet maneuvers can help determine if the patient's upper limb symptoms are related to thoracic outlet syndrome. Adson maneuver is performed with the patient sitting and the hands resting on the thighs. The examiner palpates both radial arteries simultaneously while the patient takes a deep breath, hyperextends the neck, performs a Valsalva maneuver, and turns the head as far as possible to one side and then the other. A markedly reduced pulse on the side to which the head is turning is considered a positive result. In patients with thoracic outlet syndrome, the same maneuver may cause a bruit in the supraclavicular space which can be auscultated. Alternatively, one arm can be abducted and externally rotated; then the patient takes a deep breath and turns the head forcibly to the opposite side while the radial pulse in the abducted limb is palpated and the supraclavicular space auscultated. There are several other thoracic outlet maneuvers. Unfortunately, false positives abound.

Cervical radiculopathy

Radiculopathy is defined as disease of a spinal nerve or the ventral or dorsal nerve roots which form the spinal nerve. Radiculopathy usually presents with pain in the spine and limb (or torso with thoracic radiculopathy), and often with sensory disturbance, motor weakness, and/or reduced reflex(es) in an appropriate distribution. Cervical spondylosis (degenerative changes in the disks, vertebrae, and joints) is the most common cause of cervical radiculopathy. Cervical radiculopathy is less common than lumbar radiculopathy. Men are 50% more likely to experience cervical radiculopathy than women. A history of antecedent trauma is obtained in a minority of patients. The onset is acute to subacute over days to a few weeks.

The natural history of cervical radiculopathy is, like its lumbar cousin, one of improvement spontaneously and with medical or surgical treatment. While one-third of patients may experience recurrence over the course of years, most patients recover fully, and

there is less likelihood that a patient with cervical radiculopathy will develop chronic symptoms than is the case for patients with lumbar radiculopathy.

The most common mechanism of cervical radiculopathy is compression of the spinal nerve or nerve root in or near the intervertebral (neural) foramen. The usual causes are degenerative hypertrophic changes in the uncovertebral joints, similar changes in the zygapophyseal joints, and herniation of the intervertebral disk, which can occur alone or in combination (see Figure 2.4). Tumors, acute trauma, and infectious and noninfectious inflammatory conditions can also cause cervical radiculopathy.

Table 2.1 shows the characteristic symptoms and neurologic findings associated with the commonly affected cervical nerve root levels.

There are eight numbered cervical spinal nerves and only seven cervical vertebrae. The first cervical spinal nerve, which has little or no cutaneous sensory supply, emerges between the occiput and C1, and the eighth cervical nerve emerges between C7 and T1. The intervertebral foramina and disks in the cervical level are numbered according to the vertebra above, similar to the scheme used in the thoracic and lumbar spine. As a result of the "extra" cervical spinal nerve, the cervical nerve that emerges at a spinal level is one number higher than the number of the foramen and associated disk. In cervical spondylosis, C7 nerve

Figure 2.4. This axial view of a cervical level shows compression of an exiting cervical spinal nerve or nerve root by (A) uncovertebral joint hypertrophy, (B) herniation of a nucleus pulposus, and (C) hypertrophy of a facet (zygapophyseal) joint.

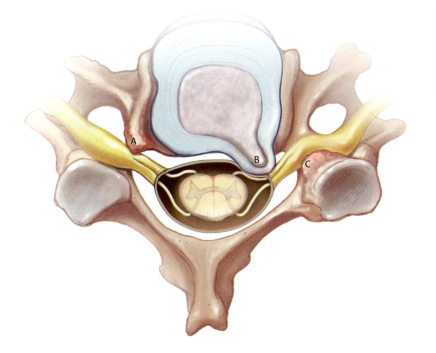

compression (by a C6–C7 disk or osteophyte and occurring at the C6–C7 intervertebral foramen) is most common. About 50% of all cervical radiculopathies affect the C7 spinal nerve. Next most common is the C6 nerve (which emerges through the C5–C6 intervertebral foramen) and accounts for about 20% of all cervical radiculopathies; C8 radiculopathy (which emerges between C7 and T1) is the next most common, accounting for about 10% of cervical radiculopathies, followed by C5 radiculopathy (which emerges between C4 and C5), accounting for another 10% of all cervical radiculopathies.

Differential diagnosis

The differential diagnosis of spondylotic cervical radiculopathy includes shoulder more likely than peripheral joint conditions, peripheral nerve entrapment, brachial plexus neuritis, thoracic outlet syndrome, herpes zoster, Pancoast syndrome, complex regional pain syndrome, and referred somatic pain from the neck structures. The differentiating points and tests which help to diagnose these cervical radiculopathy mimics are listed in Table 2.3.

Investigation

The diagnosis of cervical radiculopathy can usually be made, or least strongly suspected, after obtaining the patient's history and performing physical and neurologic examinations. In this setting, there may be no need for additional testing. However, as is the case with low back pain and lower extremity radiculopathy, there are red flag warning symptoms and signs which increase the likelihood of a serious underlying condition. These are shown in Table 2.4. The presence of one or more red flags should lead to earlier and more thorough investigation.

Magnetic resonance imaging (MRI) of the cervical spine is the diagnostic test of choice to confirm cervical nerve root impingement by spondylotic changes and to help exclude more worrisome causes. Without red flag warning signs, one can safely treat the patient who has cervical radiculopathy with conservative measures for a month or more. In patients unable to undergo MRI or who are intolerant of this methodology, computed tomography (CT) alone can be considered, but contrast myelography with CT is better for diagnosing compressive radiculopathy and planning surgery. CT myelography is sometimes useful as a complement to MRI. While plain X-rays of the cervical spine are often obtained, they are usually not very helpful in reaching a diagnosis.

Electromyography (EMG) with nerve conduction studies (NCS) can be helpful in confirming radiculopathy, but characteristic EMG changes may not be evident for up to 3–4 weeks after nerve injury onset. If the diagnosis of radiculopathy is clear, EMG is unnecessary. When there is doubt, EMG is very useful in confirming the presence of cervical radiculopathy and thus documenting a neurogenic process and, with NCS, differentiating between cervical radiculopathy, brachial plexopathy from any cause, and more peripheral nerve lesions. EMG can also be useful in determining if the radiculopathy is old or new, whether it is active or recovering, and the level of involvement if the clinical and imaging findings leave room for doubt. A normal EMG does not exclude cervical nerve root impingement.

Occasionally, additional tests are needed to help exclude cervical radiculopathy mimics. Some of these are listed in Table 2.3 and include imaging of the brachial plexus, upper chest, and neck; radionuclide bone scans; blood tests; and noninvasive studies of the upper limb vasculature.

Treatment

For most patients with cervical radiculopathy, nonsurgical management should be offered first. Because they are less common than low back disorders, evidence-based recommendations for cervical radiculopathy and neck pain are relatively lacking. Analgesics such as nonsteroidal anti-inflammatory drugs (NSAIDs), acetaminophen, and opioid-containing analgesics for severe pain can be used. Muscle relaxants can be used especially for acute pain apparently associated with muscle spasm. Translaminar and, increasingly in recent years, transforaminal epidural injections of a corticosteroid, usually with a local anesthetic, have been used to treat patients with subacute but persisting neck and radicular upper limb pain. Perhaps because cervical radiculopathy is less common than lumbar radiculopathy, there are fewer data upon which to judge the benefit of epidural steroid injections. Some 50% or more of patients report 50% or more improvement in their radicular more often than their axial neck pain, but the benefit is usually not sustained. Such injections require prior imaging of the cervical spine, typically with MRI. Complications of epidural corticosteroid injections include increased pain, post-dural puncture headache, infection, systemic corticosteroid side-effects, and rare cases of neurologic deficits due to nerve root injury, spinal cord damage from epidural hematoma, and spinal cord and posterior circulation cerebral infarction

Table 2.3. Differential diagnosis of signs and symptoms of cervical radiculopathy

Condition	Differentiating points	Helpful diagnostic studies
Rotator cuff disease and shoulder joint disease, more likely than more peripheral joints	Pain characteristically in the shoulder and not in the neck. Pain is aggravated by use of the shoulder including abduction and external rotation. Neck movements do not aggravate the pain. Neurologic examination should be normal except for weakness of external rotation and abduction of the shoulder.	Imaging of the shoulder joint and rotator cuff with plain X-rays and MRI. EMG/NCS should be normal and are helpful if there is any concern about a neurogenic cause.
Peripheral nerve entrapment (usually median nerve at wrist or ulnar nerve at elbow)	Characteristically causes intermittent symptoms, especially initially, with numbness and tingling and sometimes weakness and pain, usually in the distribution of the peripheral nerve. Can have fixed neurologic findings in the distribution of the affected peripheral nerve. Tinel's sign is often positive at the site of peripheral nerve compression. Phalen maneuver may be positive for carpal tunnel syndrome. Reflexes are usually normal.	EMG/NCS are usually conclusive, but 5% of patients with carpal tunnel syndrome may have normal EMG/NCS.
Acute brachial plexus neuritis (Parsonage–Turner syndrome)	Severe pain in neck, shoulder, and arm can simulate cervical radiculopathy. Weakness, usually affecting proximal muscles, is delayed by days to a few weeks, often starting as pain improves.	Imaging of the brachial plexus with MRI can be helpful (although not diagnostic), and MRI of the cervical spine should show incidental findings only. EMG is the most helpful diagnostic test, but abnormalities may take 3–4 weeks to fully emerge.
Thoracic outlet syndrome	Intermittent paresthesias, weakness, and sometimes shoulder and arm pain are typically caused by use of one or both upper extremities with the arms extended or abducted. Neurologic examination is usually normal but can show lower brachial plexus deficits. Positional testing of the upper extremities looking for reduction in radial pulse with provocative posture can be helpful, but false positives and negatives abound.	Noninvasive testing of upper limb arteries in a vascular laboratory can be helpful, but can be falsely positive or negative. EMG/NCS are usually normal, but if abnormal, point to a problem in the brachial plexus.
Shingles (herpes zoster)	Severe pain is present in a dermatomal distribution, but neck pain is typically absent. The typical vesicular rash soon follows the onset of pain.	EMG/NCS are not helpful acutely. Culture of the vesicles or acute and convalescent serologies can be useful but are usually unnecessary.
Fibromyalgia	The pain is typically bilateral and often affects the lower extremities as well. Characteristic tender points are usually present.	EMG/NCS should be normal. Imaging of the cervical spine should show incidental spondylosis only.
Pancoast syndrome (pulmonary apex syndrome)	Typically the lower brachial plexus and sympathetic chain are affected with medial hand and forearm sensory loss, intrinsic hand muscle weakness and ipsilateral Horner syndrome (miosis, ptosis, and forehead hypohidrosis).	Imaging of the upper chest and brachial plexus with CT or MRI should be abnormal. EMG/NCS can help to confirm lower brachial plexus involvement.
Complex regional pain syndrome (CRPS)	Distal upper limb, usually burning pain associated with swelling, superficial temperature and skin color changes, and hypersensitivity with allodynia.	Response to sympathetic blocks may be helpful diagnostically. EMG/NCS can be abnormal if the provoking cause was nerve injury (CRPS type 2), which is usually peripheral and not at the level of the brachial plexus or spinal nerve.
Pain from musculoskeletal neck structures	Radicular pain and neurologic findings are usually absent. Tenderness and limited range of motion are common.	Imaging can show musculoskeletal abnormalities but no significant neural impingement. EMG/NCS should be normal.

Notes:
CT, computed tomography; EMG, electromyography; MRI, magnetic resonance imaging; NCS, nerve conduction studies.

related to needle injury of the vertebral artery causing dissection, clot, or vasospasm. Serious complications are very rare. Alternatively, patients with acute pain are sometimes treated with a short course of an oral corticosteroid. A typical dose might be 60–70 mg of prednisone per day tapered to zero over 1 week. There are anecdotal reports of benefit. Transient systemic corticosteroid effects can occur.

Table 2.4. Red flag warning signs for potentially serious conditions in patients with neck and/or upper limb pain

Significant trauma or minor trauma in a patient with or at risk for osteoporosis

Age over 50 or under 20

History of cancer, fever or chills, unexplained weight loss, recent bacterial infection, intravenous drug use, immunosuppression from any cause, or pain that worsens when the patient is supine

A significant or progressive radicular neurologic deficit

Profound pain

Progressively worsening pain

Evidence of myelopathy from history and/or examination

Physical measures can be recommended. These include short-term use of a cervical collar, use of a cervical pillow at night, heat and/or ice, and intermittent cervical traction. Neck exercises should be reserved for the recovery period in an effort to help strengthen neck muscles and prevent future recurrence.

The indications for surgical treatment of compressive cervical radiculopathy include persistent pain in the upper extremity with strong physiologic evidence of dysfunction of a specific cervical nerve root coupled with confirmation of nerve root compression at the appropriate level and side on an imaging study, usually an MRI. Symptoms should usually have persisted for 4–6 weeks, but factors that can influence earlier surgical consultation and surgical intervention include a severe or progressive radicular deficit (usually motor), any signs or symptoms of spinal cord impingement, a larger-sized disk on the imaging study, profound pain, or weakness that is critical to the patient's work or favorite leisure activity.

Surgery for cervical radiculopathy can be from a posterior or anterior approach. Posterior surgery includes laminectomy and removal of disk and/or bony spur usually without fusion. Anterior surgery involves complete discectomy, interbody fusion using bone from the patient or a cadaver, and usually placement of a plate and screws. Both approaches are associated with good outcomes in 75% or more of patients. Perhaps because of lack of dual innervation from adjacent nerve roots, recovery from C5 radiculopathy is not as good as for other cervical levels.

In July, 2007, the U.S. Food and Drug Administration approved the Prestige ST artificial cervical disk made by Medtronic Sofamor Danek and in December 2007 they approved the ProDisc-C made by Synthes, Inc. Additional artificial cervical disks are in the pipeline for approval. The approval is based on evidence showing that placement of the artificial disk was as safe and as effective as a cervical fusion. Placement requires removal of the damaged and/or protruding cervical disk from an anterior approach and replacement with the artificial disk. The Prestige ST and ProDisc-C artificial cervical disks are said to be indicated for single-level disk replacement from C3 through C7 in skeletally mature patients for intractable radiculopathy and/or myelopathy (see Chapter 13). The artificial cervical disk is attractive in that it preserves motion at the segment where it is placed and thus does not put undue stress on adjacent cervical spine levels. Surgical treatment of cervical radiculopathy is further described in Chapter 9.

Cervical myelopathy

Cervical spondylosis is the most common cause of myelopathy in general, especially in individuals who are middle-aged and older. The peak age of onset of cervical spondylotic myelopathy is 40–60 years, and men are more often affected than women in a ratio of about 3 to 2. Spondylotic myelopathy is due to stenosis caused by degenerative disk and joint disease with hypertrophic changes with the addition of a dynamic component related to movement of the cervical spine, chiefly flexion and extension. Degeneration of the cervical disks, especially at C5–C6, C6–C7, and C4–C5, coupled with hypertrophic bony changes adjacent to the posterior aspects of the protruding and degenerating cervical disks produces spondylotic bars that compress the spinal cord, often at more than one level. The spondylotic changes are often superimposed upon a congenitally narrowed cervical spinal canal. There may be a superimposed acute disk protrusion or extrusion.

The presentation of cervical myelopathy depends on the cause and localization of the pathologic process. Patients with spondylotic myelopathy typically present with combinations of a spastic ataxic gait, upper limb numbness often affecting the hands, loss of hand strength and dexterity, hyperreflexia in the lower extremities and often of the triceps if not other upper extremity reflexes, and Babinski and/or Chaddock signs. Patients may or may not have neck and/or upper limb pain. It is important to stress that spondylotic myelopathy can be painless. Frequency and urgency of urination are common while urinary incontinence and rectal sphincter symptoms are infrequent. Depending upon the level(s) of compression, there can be upper and/or lower motor neuron signs in the upper limbs. Upper limb reflexes can thus be decreased or increased (especially the triceps reflexes). Hoffmann and/or Trömner signs may be present. Weakness and wasting of hand and forearm muscles are often seen. Patients may report Lhermitte sign. Sensory findings can be complex. Vibration and joint position sense are often decreased in the lower limbs due to posterior column compression; pain and temperature sensation reduction can be seen in the upper and lower limbs. If present, upper limb pain can be aching, sharp, or even burning and can affect one or both upper extremities. Neck range of motion may be reduced. Severe neck pain is uncommon. The onset and course are usually gradual, but sudden worsening can occur after even mild neck injury usually with abrupt flexion and/or extension. Signs and symptoms can be asymmetric, and a Brown–Séquard syndrome can be seen. Common symptoms and signs associated with myelopathy are shown in Table 2.2.

Differential diagnosis

While cervical spondylosis is the most common cause of cervical myelopathy, there are many other potential causes which are listed in Table 2.5. Many of these were described in Chapter 1. In the younger patient, multiple sclerosis, neuromyelitis optica, and acute transverse myelitis must be considered. In the older patient, motor neuron disease and subacute

Table 2.5. Differential diagnosis of myelopathy

Extrinsic to spinal cord
  Cervical spondylosis with stenosis
  Cervical disk herniation
  Congenital spinal stenosis
  Synovial cyst
  Extramedullary and extradural tumors
  Epidural abscess
  Osteomyelitis
  Diffuse idiopathic skeletal hyperostosis
  Rheumatoid arthritis or ankylosing spondylitis with upper cervical subluxation
  Trauma
    Fracture
    Central cord syndrome
  Ossification of posterior longitudinal ligament
  Extramedullary hematopoiesis
  Paget disease
  Arachnoid cyst
  Fluorosis
Intrinsic to spinal cord
  Intramedullary spinal cord tumor
  Infection
    Viral including HIV, HTLV, herpes zoster, West Nile
    Syphilis
    Rarely, intramedullary abscess
  Inflammatory demyelinating
    Multiple sclerosis
    Neuromyelitis optica
    Acute transverse myelitis
    Acute disseminated encephalomyelitis
  Noninfectious inflammatory
    Systemic lupus erythematosus
    Sjögren syndrome
    Behçet disease
    Sarcoidosis
    Paraneoplastic
  Toxic, metabolic, hereditary
    B_{12} deficiency
    Folic acid deficiency
    Nitrous oxide toxicity
    Copper deficiency
    Vitamin E deficiency
    Superficial siderosis
    Radiation myelopathy
    Hereditary spastic paraparesis
    Adrenomyeloneuropathy
  Vascular
    Spinal cord infarction
    Arteriovenous malformation
    Hematomyelia
    Decompression sickness (caisson disease)
  Other
    Syringomyelia
    Conversion disorder
    Motor neuron disease
  Mimics
    Parasagittal cerebral lesion such as a tumor
    Multiple strokes, brain stem stroke
    Guillain–Barré syndrome

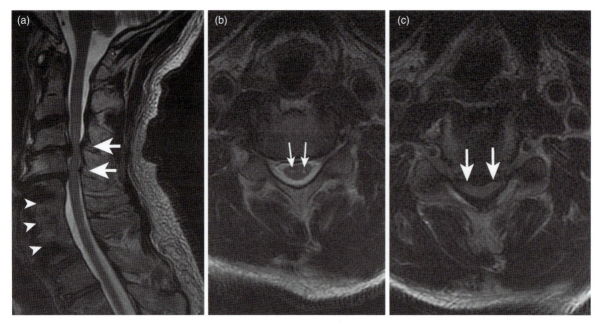

Figure 2.5. Cervical spondylotic myelopathy. (a) Sagittal T_2-weighted MRI shows severe cervical stenosis at C3–C4 and moderate stenosis at C4–C5 (large arrows) which are just above a previous C5–C7 anterior cervical discectomies with interbody fusion and instrumentation (arrowheads). There is subtle increased T_2 signal within the spinal cord just above the level of maximal stenosis. (b) Axial T_2-weighted image just above and (c) a similar image at the level of severe stenosis. (b) shows small areas of increased T_2 signal within the spinal cord representing edema or myelomalacia (arrows). (c) Significant deformity of the spinal cord (arrows). This 56-year-old former football player presented with subtle evidence of a painless cervical myelopathy.

combined degeneration are potential confounders, especially in the patient with coincidental, asymptomatic cervical spondylosis. Syringomyelia and tumor are possible.

Investigation

A more rapid onset will point to an acute infectious, inflammatory, demyelinating, traumatic, or vascular cause; a gradual onset is more typical of spondylosis, tumor, syrinx, and toxic–metabolic etiologies. Imaging will determine whether or not there is spinal cord compression and often provides a diagnosis or greatly limits the diagnostic possibilities. MRI is the initial diagnostic test of choice in a patient presenting with myelopathy at any level or of uncertain level (see Figure 2.5). MRI will confirm cervical spondylosis with stenosis, spinal cord tumor, many cases of multiple sclerosis, syringomyelia, and arteriovenous malformation. Myelography with CT scanning is recommended if MRI is not possible. Abnormal T_2 signal within the cervical spinal cord at the levels of spondylotic narrowing is thought to indicate that the spinal cord impingement is significant and suggests

edema or myelomalacia. Plain CT and plain X-rays of the cervical spine are not usually helpful, but can show fracture, stenosis due to osteophytic spurring, and cervical spinal instability. Blood tests help to confirm or rule out vitamin B_{12} deficiency, HTLV-1 and HIV infection, neurosyphilis, copper deficiency, paraneoplastic syndromes, and neuromyelitis optica which affects the spinal cord and optic nerves, and was previously thought to be a form of multiple sclerosis but is now recognized as a distinct condition. EMG can help to exclude motor neuron disease, brachial plexopathy, and peripheral nerve disease. EMG would be expected to show abnormalities related to compression of cervical nerve roots and/ or anterior horn cells within the cervical spinal cord. To the extent that EMG shows evidence of multiple cervical radiculopathies, it can lend support to the diagnosis of compressive spondylotic myeloradiculopathy. Because cervical spondylosis is ubiquitous, especially in the older patient, imaging studies will frequently show cervical spondylosis and sometimes cervical spinal stenosis with apparent, albeit usually mild, spinal cord compression. These findings may be asymptomatic, and clinical correlation between the patient's signs and symptoms and imaging studies is critical. Somatosensory evoked potentials (SSEPs) are occasionally helpful in the evaluation of the patient with cervical spondylotic myelopathy. Abnormalities include loss of amplitude, degradation of waveforms, or slight interpeak delays which help to confirm the presence of cervical spinal cord disease but not its etiology. There is not a good correlation between the severity of SSEP abnormalities and clinical evidence of myelopathy. In general, SSEPs do not improve, despite spinal cord decompression. Motor evoked potentials are even less frequently used to assess spinal cord function.

Treatment

For some of the conditions causing myelopathy and listed in Table 2.5, specific treatment is available, whereas for others it is not. With regard to treatment for the most common cause of cervical myelopathy, cervical spondylosis, most experts recommend consideration of surgical decompression with or without simultaneous fusion. However, the natural history of spondylotic myelopathy shows that many patients follow an indolent course. On the other hand, few patients improve with time, and many worsen. Those who worsen usually do so gradually, sometimes punctuated by a sudden decline, which in turn can be related to a fall. Most would surely advocate decompression for patients with moderate to severe neurologic deficits and historical and/or examination-documented progression. Surgical results are influenced by the duration of pre-operative signs and symptoms: those with a shorter duration tend to do better. While many patients, especially those with a short duration of symptoms, do experience improvement in their pre-operative neurologic signs and symptoms, for some patients all that is achieved by surgery is stabilization of their deficits. Because surgical decompression helps prevent progression but may not restore lost spinal cord function, many advocate for earlier surgery rather than taking a wait-and-see approach to observe for worsening. However, there are only two studies that have prospectively compared surgical versus nonsurgical treatment for cervical spondylotic myelopathy, and neither showed significant benefit from surgery. Nonetheless, most spine specialists offer decompressive surgery for clear-cut spondylotic cervical myelopathy in patients who are otherwise in good health.

As is the case for spondylotic cervical radiculopathy, surgery for spondylotic cervical myelopathy can be performed from a posterior or anterior approach. Posterior surgery entails decompressive laminectomies or laminoplasty, which may need to be done at several levels. Anterior surgery involves discectomy and fusion, typically with instrumentation (plates and screws) at one or two levels. With either approach, about 70% of patients experience initial improvement. Whether or not they improve or stabilize, some patients will later worsen in the absence of recurrent spinal cord compression.

As was mentioned in the section on cervical radiculopathy, placement of an artificial cervical disk is also an option for patients with single-level myelopathy secondary to cervical spondylosis. Surgical treatment of cervical myelopathy is described further in Chapter 9.

Nonoperative, conservative treatment consists of use of a cervical collar with the neck in a neutral or slightly flexed position and physical therapy directed at the patient's neurologic signs and symptoms. The patient should be cautioned to reduce the risk of falling or otherwise injuring the neck. NSAIDs can be used for pain control but are not thought to be disease-modifying. Injections directed at the cervical spine for myelopathy are best avoided.

Neck pain

This section deals with pain that affects the anterior, lateral, and posterior neck from the external occipital protuberance and superior nuchal line posteriorly and the lower jaw line anteriorly down to the spine of the scapula, superior border of the clavicle, and suprasternal notch. As is the case with acute low back pain, many patients with acute neck pain, even with accompanying muscle spasm, defy precise diagnosis.

Neck pain without significant upper limb pain or neurologic deficit is more common than cervical radiculopathy or cervical spondylotic myelopathy. While acute neck pain is not as common as acute low back pain, 12-month prevalence estimates in adults range from 30% to 50% and are only slightly less prevalent in children and adolescents (21%–42%). Neck pain which limits activities is less common, with 12-month estimates ranging from 2% to 11%. Somewhat surprisingly, there is little evidence to support the assumption that degenerative disk changes are a risk factor for neck pain without radiculopathy. As is the case with low back pain, some patients experience chronic neck pain which can begin after one or a series of discrete episodes of acute neck pain or follow a chronic course from first onset. Patients with neck pain following a whiplash-type of injury are especially likely to experience a protracted episode of pain.

Many patients for no apparent reason will awaken in the morning with a "wry" neck or a "crick" in the neck. They may have trouble moving the neck and often have acute muscle spasm. Their pain and limited range of motion subside typically in a matter of a few days without or perhaps more quickly with treatment.

The same red flag warning signs and symptoms that were listed for cervical radiculopathy should be sought in the patient who presents with primarily neck pain (see Table 2.4). In addition, for patients with significant axial spine pain, additional red flags include possible signs and symptoms of ankylosing spondylitis, another spondyloarthropathy, or rheumatoid arthritis such as spine or peripheral joint deformity or obvious signs of joint inflammation and limited joint range of motion.

Differential diagnosis

There are, obviously, many possible causes for neck pain. The patient's history (e.g., trauma) or accompanying symptoms (e.g., fibromyalgia) will be most helpful in determining the cause of an individual patient's neck pain. The possible causes of neck pain are shown in Table 2.6.

Investigation

For most patients with acute neck pain, in the absence of red flag warning signs or symptoms, no diagnostic studies are needed for the first 4–6 weeks after onset of pain. During this time, symptomatic treatment should be offered. If the patient's pain persists or they develop any red flag signs or symptoms, their

Table 2.6. Causes of acute and chronic neck pain

Spondylotic (degenerative from the spine)
  Bones
  Muscles, including myofascial pain
  Ligaments
  Facet joints
    Degenerative joint disease
    Synovial cyst
  Intervertebral disks
Rheumatologic conditions
  Fibromyalgia
  Polymyalgia rheumatica
  Rheumatoid arthritis
  Ankylosing spondylitis
    Other spondyloarthropathies
  Crystal deposition diseases
  Diffuse idiopathic skeletal hyperostosis
Trauma
  Fractures and dislocations
  Sprains
  Soft tissue injuries
Neurogenic
  Meninges
  Nerve roots
  Spinal cord
  Cerebral palsy with increased muscle activity
  Torticollis
Tumor
  Spine
    Vertebra
      Primary
      Metastatic
    Meninges, nerve roots, spinal cord
      Primary
      Metastatic
  Neck
  Pulmonary apex (Pancoast syndrome)
Infection
  Osteomyelitis
  Disk space infection
  Epidural
  Meninges
  Dorsal root ganglion
  Nerve roots
  Spinal cord
Viscerogenic
  Thyroid disease
  Carotid or vertebral artery dissection
  Upper esophagus
  Throat and larynx
Psychogenic
  With an additional source of pain
  Rarely, without an additional source of pain
Malingering

pain worsens, or their pain becomes severe, additional diagnostic testing is warranted. Many references advocate obtaining plain X-rays (three views – lateral, anteroposterior, and open mouth) as the initial diagnostic test of choice. Flexion and extension views of the cervical spine can be added to help exclude instability. While plain X-rays will usually show evidence of cervical spondylosis and this will be the presumed underlying cause of most patients' neck pain, plain X-rays do not show many of the worrisome causes of neck pain, expose the patient to a small dose of radiation, and may provide false reassurance that the patient's pain is due to the demonstrated spondylosis seen in most adults and not due to some underlying, undiscovered, sinister cause. MRI will reveal more and exclude most of the worrisome causes of neck pain. On the other hand, MRI will not show evidence of fracture as well as plain X-rays or CT and will not show evidence of subluxation as readily either. One might consider both MRI and plain X-rays. CT is useful in patients with a suspected fracture. Additional tests, including blood tests such as blood count with sedimentation rate, rheumatoid factor, and a radionuclide bone scan, should be considered in selected cases.

Treatment

Comfort control treatment that are safe can be offered to most patients with acute neck pain. Over-the-counter analgesics, heat, ice, and prescription analgesics and muscle relaxants (cyclobenzaprine, benzodiazepines, tizanidine, and carisoprodol) can be offered. Muscle relaxants should be considered, especially for those with muscle spasm. Uncommonly, opioid analgesics may be needed. Ample doses of reassurance should be provided as well. Physical activity may need to be temporarily restricted or modified. For patients with a self-limited attack of acute neck pain, no ongoing physical therapy is required.

More problematic is the patient who has chronic or recurrent neck pain, often associated with trapezius muscle, upper scapula, and suboccipital head pain. Many of these patients have myofascial pain which may or may not be related to an underlying demonstrated cervical spondylosis. Imaging will probably be required in these patients, but is unlikely to show anything beyond age-related cervical spondylosis. These patients should be considered for an ongoing program of physical therapy including modalities which they find helpful. Rather than relying on treatment provided at the therapist's office, the therapist,

patient, and their family should strive for an ongoing home program of therapy which the patient can do twice a day, 7 days a week. Use of a cervical pillow at night helps some patients. There is no good evidence that cervical collars are beneficial for acute, chronic, or recurrent neck pain alone in the absence of instability or recent surgery.

Pharmacologic therapy for patients with chronic neck pain includes NSAIDs, neuromodulating medications such as gabapentin or pregabalin, and tricyclic agents such as amitriptyline or nortriptyline. Opioid analgesics are best avoided if at all possible. Muscle relaxants are much less likely to be helpful for patients with chronic neck pain.

Injection therapy for chronic cervical pain is typically unhelpful. Epidural corticosteroid injections will provide little or no benefit as most patients' pain is myofascial and not directly related to their disk and facet joint disease. Injections directed at the facet joints can be used both to provide short-term symptomatic relief and to search for a "pain generator." If injections of local anesthetics with or without a corticosteroid directed at target facet joints or the medial branch nerves which supply them provide temporary relief of the patient's neck pain, radiofrequency lesioning of the same medial branches is performed in an effort to produce more lasting pain relief. Several medial branches on one or both sides of the neck may need to be treated. Such lesioning is reported to help some patients with chronic neck pain, especially those who experience pain after a whiplash-type of injury. However, the nerves that are lesioned are very short and, in theory, should be able to grow back in a matter of a month or two. Destroying the sensory innervation of joints is not practiced anywhere else in the body except the spinal facet joints. In addition, the injections and lesioning are associated with a low rate of complications which include increased pain, allergic reactions, bleeding, infection, and rare cases of neurologic injury. These injections and radiofrequency lesioning should be performed only in experienced pain centers.

Surgery, chiefly anterior cervical discectomy and interbody fusion usually with instrumentation, should probably not be considered for patients with significant chronic, chiefly posterior axial neck pain alone. In this situation, the provocative procedure of discography is sometimes used to help determine which level (or levels) of disk degeneration is responsible for the patient's pain. Depending upon the results from discography, anterior cervical discectomy and fusion (and much less commonly posterior fusion) at one or two levels may be recommended. Discography is fraught with false positives and requires injection of likely symptomatic and likely asymptomatic disk levels to help ensure accurate results. The results from fusion for axial neck pain alone are imperfect at best. Cervical fusion is associated with some significant operative and post-operative risks. If the cervical fusion is successful, it will theoretically and practically subject the adjacent unfused disk levels to increased motion and accelerated degenerative changes in the disks and facet joints. Cervical fusion for neck pain alone is best avoided if at all possible. Cervical fusion is discussed further in Chapter 9.

Further reading

1. The Bone and Joint Decade 2000–2010 Task Force on Neck Pain and its Associated Disorders. *Spine* 2008; **33**(4S):S1–S220.

2. Borenstein DG, Wiesel SW, Boden SD. *Low Back and Neck Pain: Comprehensive Diagnosis and Management*, Third Edition. Philadelphia, Pennsylvania: Elsevier Inc., 2004.

3. Carette S, Fehlings MG. Cervical radiculopathy. *New Engl J Med* 2005; **353**(4):392–399.

4. Ebersold MJ, Pare MC, Quast LM. Surgical treatment for cervical spondylitic myelopathy. *J Neurosurg* 1995; **82**:745–751.

5. Fouyas IP, Sandercock PAG, Statham PF, Lynch C. Surgery for cervical radiculomyelopathy. *Cochrane Database Syst Rev* 2008; **4**.

6. Levin KH, ed. *Neurologic Clinics: Neck and Back Pain*, Vol. 25, No. 2. Philadelphia, Pennsylvania: W. B. Saunders Company. 2007, pp. 331–575.

7. Lunsford LD, Bissonette DJ, Zorub DS. Anterior surgery for cervical disc disease. Part 2: Treatment of cervical spondylotic myelopathy in 32 cases. *J Neurosurg* 1980; **53**:12–29.

8. Nachemson AL, Jonsson E, eds. *Neck and Back Pain: The Scientific Evidence of Causes, Diagnosis, and Treatment*. Philadelphia, Pennsylvania: Lippincott Williams & Wilkins, 2000.

9. Radhakrishnan K, Litchy WJ, O'Fallon WM, Kurland LT. Epidemiology of cervical radiculopathy: a population-based study from Rochester, Minnesota, 1976 through 1990. *Brain* 1994; **117**:325–335.

10. Slipman CW, Derby R, Simeone FA, Mayer TG. *Interventional Spine: An Algorithmic Approach*. Philadelphia, Pennsylvania: Saunders, 2008.

11. Yoss RE, Corbin KB, MacCarty CS, Love JG. Significance of symptoms and signs in localization of involved root in cervical disk protrusion. *Neurology* 1957; **7**(10):673–683.

Chapter 3

The thoracic level

Thoracic level spine problems are much less common than cervical, which in turn are less frequent than lumbar level problems. For every patient with a thoracic level problem, there are probably ten with a cervical level problem and thirty with a lumbar level process. All of the terrible conditions that befall the spine can occur at the thoracic level, and there is a significant potential for confusion with diseases that affect the adjacent chest and abdomen.

The thoracic level will be divided, like the cervical, into sections on the history, physical, neurologic, and special examinations that are pertinent to the thoracic spine, followed by thoracic radiculopathy, thoracic myelopathy, and thoracic spine pain. Of course, these three entities do not always present in pure form, and there is often an admixture of two or all three problems, especially thoracic radiculopathy and midline thoracic spine pain.

The history

The general suggestions given regarding obtaining the history in the preceding chapter on the cervical level hold true for patients with thoracic level complaints. Therefore, in this section historical points specifically related to thoracic level problems will be stressed.

The red flag warning signs and symptoms listed in Table 2.4 also apply to the patient with thoracic (and lumbar) level problems. In particular, the patient's age should be noted. Scheuermann disease characteristically affects teenagers, and compression fractures typically present after the age of 50, more so in women, and especially in patients with risk factors for osteoporosis. Pain which worsens when the patient is supine or is increased by cough, sneeze, strain, and other Valsalva maneuvers suggests an intraspinal compressive process. The T1 nerve roots along with the C8 roots innervate the intrinsic hand muscles and supply sensation along the medial arms and forearms. Thus, it is worthwhile asking about upper limb function. In addition, some conditions that affect predominantly the thoracic spinal cord, such as dural arteriovenous fistulas and syringomyelia, can simultaneously affect the cervical spinal cord. The spinal cord characteristically ends at about the level of the L1 vertebral body. Virtually all of the thoracic and much of the lumbar spinal cord lies within the bony thoracic spine. Lower thoracic and lumbar spinal cord compression or intrinsic spinal cord disease can affect lower motor neurons as well as upper motor neurons and give rise to lower limb and sphincter disturbances that can be difficult to differentiate from a cauda equina syndrome (see below). Topics to cover in the patient with potential thoracic spine disease include: motor and sensory function of the chest, abdomen, and lower extremities; gait; bowel and bladder control; and sexual function. One should ask about chest and abdominal pain, especially that which suggests a dermatomal pattern around the chest, into the flank, and/or into the abdomen on one or both sides (see Figure 3.1). Upper thoracic radiculopathy can present with pain in the axilla.

The patient and their family should be questioned about any long-standing abnormality of or recent change in their posture. Is there a history of scoliosis, kyphosis, a list, or change in height? Is there any history of trauma? Injuries involving a torsional movement can increase the risk of thoracic disk herniation.

Respiratory symptoms should be sought, as thoracic spinal deformities, intercostal muscular weakness, and weakness of abdominal muscles innervated by the lower thoracic nerve roots can all affect respiratory function. Increased difficulty breathing when supine suggests unilateral or bilateral phrenic nerve damage with paralysis of the diaphragm.

Increase in neurologic symptoms with the Valsalva maneuver can suggest an intraspinal neurologic process such as a large disk, tumor, or dural arteriovenous fistula. Patients with spinal cord arteriovenous malformations or spinal stenosis of any cause may report that standing and walking aggravate their neurologic symptoms. An increase in neurologic symptoms associated with an increase in body temperature caused by

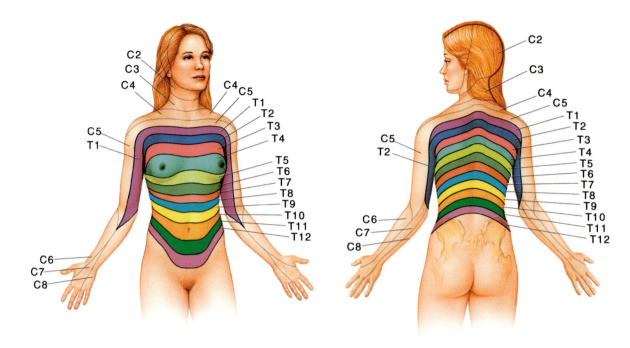

Figure 3.1. Diagram showing thoracic dermatomes. Damage to a single thoracic nerve root rarely causes demonstrable sensory loss. There is overlap of individual nerve root territories and variation between individuals. There is greater agreement about the distribution of thoracic than cervical or lumbosacral dermatomes.

exertion, fever, or environmental heat is characteristic of multiple sclerosis (Uhthoff phenomenon).

The examination
The general examination
Throughout the interview and formal examination, the patient's spinal posture should be observed. Is there any scoliosis, list, or kyphosis? The causes of scoliosis and kyphosis are listed in Tables 1.7 and 1.8 respectively. Is the chest asymmetric? The patient and their family should be able to help in determining the duration of any spinal deformities noted. Lying and standing blood pressure may be useful because patients with upper thoracic cord lesions can have impaired blood pressure control. Are there any skin lesions – shingles in the case of acute radicular torso pain or café-au-lait spots that may suggest neurofibromatosis and an underlying spinal tumor?

Neurologic examination
As noted above, the first thoracic nerve root innervates intrinsic hand muscles and sensation in the medial arm and forearm. T1 level lesions (as well as C8) can cause an ipsilateral Horner syndrome.

Intercostal muscle paralysis is difficult to observe clinically. In some thin patients, retraction of the intercostal space with inspiration and outward bulging with coughing or Valsalva maneuver may indicate weakness of the appropriate intercostal nerve which is supplied by the same level thoracic nerve root. The degree of chest wall movement on deep breathing helps to assess intercostal muscle function generally, which in turn reflects function of the upper thoracic roots. The abdominal muscles are supplied by the lower thoracic spinal nerves. The umbilicus is supplied by the T10 nerve root. In general, the abdominal muscles above the umbilicus are supplied by the T5–T10 thoracic nerve roots, while the lower abdomen is supplied by T11, T12, and L1. The abdominal muscles may be tested by having the supine patient attempt to sit up against resistance with their hands held behind their head or with their arms held against their chest. If there is weakness on one side, the umbilicus will shift to the normal side on attempts to sit up and on inspiration, while the weak side will bulge with coughing and straining. If there is paralysis of the upper half of the abdominal muscles (T10 and above on both sides), there will be downward movement of the umbilicus with attempts to sit up; with paralysis of the lower half (T10 and below on both sides), there will be upward movement of the umbilicus with attempts to sit up. Beevor sign is the upward movement of the umbilicus with contraction of the abdominal muscles on attempts to sit up and indicates a cord lesion at the T10 level. If the abdominal muscles are paralyzed diffusely on both sides, attempts at sitting up and coughing will cause the umbilicus to bulge outward. Palpation of the abdominal muscles is valuable in determining which muscles are innervated and can be contracted, and which are paralyzed and cannot. Spinal cord lesions above T6 typically cause weakness of the abdominal muscles diffusely. Diffuse abdominal wall muscle weakness makes it difficult to strain and empty the bladder and rectum.

The abdominal reflexes are elicited by stroking or scratching the abdominal wall diagonally in each of the four quadrants or lateral to the umbilicus in a vertical or horizontal direction while watching for movement of the umbilicus toward the stimulus. They are elicited with the patient supine and the abdominal wall thoroughly relaxed. A blunt point such as a split tongue blade or fingernail or dragging a pin lightly across the skin elicits the reflex. Abdominal reflexes are so-called superficial reflexes and are reduced in both upper motor neuron and lower motor neuron processes. The upper abdominal reflex is innervated by the intercostal nerves from the T7 through T9 thoracic segments; the middle abdominal reflex (lateral to the umbilicus) is innervated by the T9 through T11 thoracic segments; and the lower abdominal reflex is innervated by T11, T12, and L1. Spinal cord lesions above T6 can cause a loss of all abdominal reflexes, while lesions at T10 preserve only the upper and middle abdominal reflexes.

Some general comments regarding the subjective nature of the sensory examination and reduced and absent sensation were made in the preceding chapter. Detecting sensory loss in the distribution of a single thoracic nerve root is unusual. The dermatome supplied by a single thoracic nerve root is rather narrow, and there is some overlap in sensory innervation from adjacent roots, which makes it difficult to demonstrate reduced sensation in the distribution of a single thoracic nerve root. The distribution of sensory symptoms can be very helpful in diagnosis (see Figure 3.1). The innervation of certain anatomic landmarks is useful when interpreting findings and symptoms. The nipple is supplied by the fourth thoracic nerve root; the xiphoid process is supplied by the seventh

thoracic nerve root; the umbilicus by the tenth thoracic nerve root; and the inguinal region by the twelfth thoracic and first lumbar nerve roots. Nerve fibers which carry joint position and vibration sense remain ipsilateral in the spinal cord, while those serving pain and temperature ascend for one or two segments on the same side of the spinal cord before crossing over and ascending to the brain stem on the contralateral side. In spinal cord disease, unless the cord lesion is complete, touch perception may be preserved.

Special examinations
Evidence of scoliosis, smooth or angled kyphosis, impaired thoracic range of motion, and reduced chest expansion should all be assessed. Range of motion includes flexion, extension, lateral bending, and rotation. Observe the gait for evidence of spasticity or a truncal list; patients will often lean away from the side of a herniated thoracic disk. Impaired chest expansion can be seen in ankylosing spondylitis, other chronic inflammatory arthritides, severe thoracic spondylosis, and neuromuscular weakness. Chest expansion can be assessed using a tape measure around the chest and comparing the girth at rest to that with maximal inspiration. A difference of less than 3 cm is abnormal and suggests ankylosing spondylitis or another condition. Spinal, paraspinal, chest, and abdominal tenderness and evidence of muscle spasm should be sought. Occasionally, one can auscultate a bruit over the spinal cord in patients with arteriovenous malformations. If nothing else, listening to the spinal cord sometimes impresses patients.

Thoracic radiculopathy
Thoracic radiculopathy is much less common than cervical or lumbar radiculopathy. Spondylotic thoracic radiculopathy is usually due to a lateral disk herniation, but many thoracic disk herniations are asymptomatic and found incidentally on imaging studies. Unlike cervical and lumbar radiculopathy, where the vast majority of radiculopathies are due to spinal spondylosis, in the thoracic spine, shingles and diabetic radiculopathy are nearly as common as those due to degenerative joint and disk disease. Shingles can almost always be recognized by its characteristic rash (which is rarely absent), and diabetic radiculopathy usually involves multiple spinal nerves. Patients with diabetic polyradiculopathy can have mild diabetes that is only discovered after they present with this complication.

51

Most thoracic radiculopathies, especially those due to spondylosis, will be accompanied by spine pain. More so than is the case with upper or lower limb pain due to radiculopathy, in the thoracic spine radicular pain can often be confused with viscerogenic pain. As is the case elsewhere in the spine, thoracic radiculopathy can also be mistaken for pain arising in musculoskeletal structures.

As noted above, it is rare to find motor or sensory deficits in the distribution of a single thoracic nerve root on examination. Thus, the patient with radiculopathy usually presents with unilateral chest or abdominal pain with or without thoracic spine pain. They may or may not have sensory symptoms but characteristically have no sensory findings on examination. They usually do not report weakness. As is the case with cervical radiculopathy, symptoms and signs of myelopathy should be sought.

Patients with thoracic radiculopathy are usually in middle age, in their fourth to sixth decades of life. Men and women are affected roughly equally. Most isolated radiculopathies secondary to herniated thoracic disks affect the lower thoracic nerve roots with three-fourths occurring below the T8 level. The T11–T12 level is most frequently affected. A history of trauma may or may not be obtained.

The natural history of thoracic radiculopathy secondary to spondylotic disease is typically one of improvement.

Differential diagnosis

The differential diagnosis of torso and thoracic spine pain is lengthy and shown in Table 3.1. True radiculopathy can be due to thoracic spondylosis (usually a lateral disk protrusion), shingles, diabetes, Lyme disease, other inflammatory processes, primary and metastatic tumors, and acute trauma. Axillary pain has been reported as the initial manifestation of malignancy affecting the upper thoracic nerve roots. Simulated radicular pain can arise from almost any internal organ. In the chest, this includes the heart (myocardial infarction, pericarditis, myocarditis), thoracic aortic aneurysm, aneurysmal dissection, lung tumors, pleurisy, pleural effusion, pulmonary embolus, pulmonary infarction, bacterial pneumonia, tuberculosis, sarcoidosis, esophageal tumors, esophagitis including gastroesophageal reflux disease, mediastinal tumors, and mediastinitis. Abdominal problems include hepatitis, cholecystitis, peptic ulcer disease, hiatal hernia, pancreatitis, splenomegaly, intra-abdominal lymphadenopathy, pyelonephritis,

Table 3.1. Differential diagnosis of thoracic radiculopathy and mid back pain

I. In or near thoracic spine

  A. Spondylosis

    1. Disk herniation

    2. Stenosis

    3. Facet joint arthritis and other diseases

    4. Local ligaments and muscles

    5. Synovial cyst

    6. Costovertebral joints

  B. Trauma

    1. Acute fracture with or without dislocation

    2. Osteoporotic compression fracture

    3. Soft tissue injury

  C. Tumors (benign and malignant)

    1. Spine

      a. Bone

      b. Epidural

      c. Vertebral hemangioma

    2. Nervous system

      a. Spinal cord

      b. Nerve root

      c. Meninges

  D. Infectious

    1. Osteomyelitis

    2. Disk space infection

    3. Epidural abscess

    4. Herpes zoster (shingles)

    5. Lyme disease

  E. Vascular

    1. Various arteriovenous malformations

    2. Spinal cord ischemia, infarction

  F. Associated with spine deformities

    1. Kyphosis

    2. Scoliosis

    3. Scheuermann disease

  G. Rheumatologic

    1. Ankylosing spondylitis and other spondyloarthropathies

    2. Rheumatoid arthritis

    3. Fibromyalgia

    4. Diffuse idiopathic skeletal hyperostosis

  H. Miscellaneous

    1. Diabetic radiculoplexus neuropathy

    2. Syringomyelia

3. Arachnoid cyst

4. Sarcoidosis

5. Notalgia paresthetica

II. External to spine

A. Cardiovascular

1. Myocardial ischemia (angina pectoris and myocardial infarction)

2. Myocarditis

3. Pericarditis

4. Thoracic aortic aneurysm and dissection

5. Abdominal aortic aneurysm

B. Pulmonary

1. Pulmonary embolus

2. Pneumonia

3. Tuberculosis

4. Pleurisy and other pleuritic chest pains

5. Pneumothorax

6. Pulmonary infarction

7. Tumor

C. Hepatobiliary

1. Hepatitis

2. Cholecystitis

3. Cholangitis

4. Tumor

D. Gastrointestinal

1. Gastroesophageal reflux disease

2. Esophagitis

3. Esophageal spasm

4. Peptic ulcer disease

5. Pancreatitis

6. Diverticulitis

7. Appendicitis

8. Colitis and enteritis

9. Tumor

E. Retroperitoneal

1. Pyelonephritis

2. Nephrolithiasis

3. Hydronephrosis

4. Ovarian cyst

5. Ectopic pregnancy

6. Tumor

III. Other musculoskeletal

A. Rib fracture

B. Costochondritis

C. Rib tip or slipping rib syndrome

D. Post-incisional pain

E. Referred from cervical spine structures, especially the C5–C7 level facet joints, disks, and nerve roots

nephrolithiasis, abdominal aortic aneurysm, and sundry abdominal tumors. Musculoskeletal problems include rib fractures, rib tumors, costochondritis, muscle pulls and other pains of muscle origin, and pain following thoracotomy or abdominal incisions. A lower rib pain syndrome has also been described. This condition is usually attributed to lower ribs that are unattached, can "slip," and are tender, and presents with pain along the course of the "loose" rib or ribs. Notalgia paresthetica consists of itching, pain, and paresthesias sometimes accompanied by hyperpigmentation in the thoracic paraspinal region usually on one side. It is thought to be due to a sensory neuropathy involving thoracic spinal nerves or their dorsal rami, can sometimes be associated with spondylotic changes in the adjacent spine, and should be treated conservatively.

Investigation

In some situations, no testing may be needed. For example, if the patient presents with an apparent spondylotic thoracic radiculopathy which is stable and has no red flag warning signs, one could treat them with comfort control measures and reassurance, and only investigate in the event of progression or the development of new and worrisome signs or symptoms. In order to confirm the presence of a suspected thoracic disk and to rule out more sinister causes such as tumor, magnetic resonance imaging (MRI) is the imaging procedure of choice (see Figure 3.2). Plain X-rays will not add much, computed tomography (CT) will not show all of the potential soft tissue causes, and both expose the patient to radiation. If the patient is unable to undergo MRI for whatever reason, plain CT can be utilized. CT myelography will better demonstrate thoracic disk disease and intraspinal tumors and will be needed in patients who are surgical candidates who cannot undergo MRI. MRIs will show thoracic disk herniations in 10%–20% of asymptomatic individuals. As a result, correlation of the patient's imaging with their symptoms and findings is critical.

Electromyography (EMG) can be helpful in documenting the presence of radiculopathy by showing

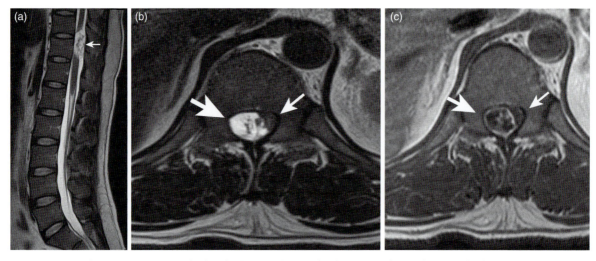

Figure 3.2. Spinal tumor presenting as radiculopathy. (a) Sagittal T_2-weighted MR image shows a large intradural extramedullary tumor at T10–T11 (arrow). Note the very normal bones and intervertebral disks. (b) Axial T_2-weighted image shows the large right-sided tumor (large arrow) compressing and displacing the spinal cord (small arrow) to the patient's left. (c) Axial T_1-weighted post-gadolinium image shows that the tumor (large arrow), which proved to be a schwannoma, enhances peripherally while the spinal cord (small arrow) does not. This 33-year-old man had an 18-month history of right lower quadrant abdominal pain followed by right thoracolumbar junction back and flank pain and a 5-month history of progressive bilateral lower extremity numbness and weakness. He had undergone extensive evaluation of his abdomen and pelvis before he developed paraparesis.

abnormality in intercostal or abdominal and paraspinal muscles at the same spinal level. EMG findings may take 3–4 weeks to appear after nerve injury, and thus the EMG may not be very helpful in the acute setting. For lower thoracic radiculopathies, where most occur, EMG findings may be seen in abdominal wall muscles, but localization is not as good as it is for the mid and upper thoracic levels, where individual intercostal muscles can be sampled, albeit with difficulty.

If there is concern about an intrathoracic, intra-abdominal, or retroperitoneal process mimicking radiculopathy, imaging studies of the various visceral structures mentioned in Table 3.1 will be needed.

Treatment

For most patients with spondylotic thoracic radiculopathy, conservative treatment measures including analgesics, some restriction of physical activities, and possibly physical therapy will provide the patient with time for their symptoms to improve. Shingles should be treated with an oral anti-viral medication. Diabetic radiculopathy usually affects multiple thoracic and lumbar nerve roots and can also affect the lumbar plexus. There may or may not be an accompanying, often mild, diabetic peripheral neuropathy. Recently, the term diabetic radiculoplexus neuropathy has been used. This condition runs a benign but protracted

course and can leave behind residual deficits. There is recent evidence that immunotherapy may speed up the rate of recovery in patients with diabetic radiculoplexus neuropathy.

Physical therapies can be helpful. The patient can be instructed in posture and body mechanics to reduce their symptoms. Heat and/or cold, ultrasound, massage, and transcutaneous electrical stimulation can be used. Active muscle strengthening exercises should probably be delayed until the patient's pain has subsided.

Surgery on the thoracic spine for spondylotic disease is difficult and described in Chapter 10. If there is no myelopathy present, conservative treatment should be continued unless the patient's pain is very severe and protracted. Evidence of spinal cord compression on an imaging study might influence the decision to operate on a significant radiculopathy in the absence of signs of a myelopathy. For longer-duration pain, neuromodulating agents such as gabapentin or pregabalin, a tricyclic agent such as amitriptyline or nortriptyline, or duloxetine can be tried.

Epidural corticosteroid injections, often given transforaminally, are used in the treatment of spondylotic thoracic radiculopathy. Because thoracic disk disease is much less common than cervical or lumbar disk disease, much less is written about epidural injections for thoracic radiculopathy. Injection of a local

Table 3.2. Conus medullaris versus cauda equina syndrome

	Conus medullaris	Cauda equina
Vertebral level of injury	Depends on level of termination of spinal cord, usually vertebral level T12–L1; injury is usually to sacral spinal cord (S1–S5)	Between L1 or L2 and the sacrum with injury to multiple lumbosacral nerve roots
Causes	Fracture, primary and secondary tumors, vascular injury, infection, spondylosis (usually disk)	Fractures, primary and secondary tumors, infection, spondylosis (disk or spondylolisthesis), ankylosing spondylitis (rarely)
Pain	Less common and less severe; usually bilateral and affecting perineum and/or thighs	Often and more severe, can be symmetric or asymmetric and typically radicular (sciatica)
Motor findings	Less severe, more symmetric, fasciculations more likely, usually restricted to sacral roots	Less symmetric, can be more severe, fasciculations less common
Reflex loss	Ankle reflex only	Ankle and knee reflexes may be absent
Sensory findings	Bilateral perineal, more likely symmetric, loss of pain and temperature with possible retention of touch	Less symmetric, perineal and lower limb may be affected, all types of sensation can be affected
Bowel and bladder function	Usually early and prominent for both urinary and rectal sphincters	Occurs later and is less severe for both bowel and bladder
Sexual function	Erection and ejaculation more likely to be affected	Less likely to be affected
Onset (depends on cause)	More likely to be acute	More likely to be gradual
EMG findings	Restricted to sacral myotomes, usually bilateral	Multiple lumbosacral levels, usually bilateral root involvement
Prognosis (depends on etiology)	Relatively worse	Relatively better

anesthetic alone is sometimes used to help determine if the patient's pain is mediated by the same level thoracic spinal nerve. Transforaminal thoracic injections are associated with a small risk of nerve root and even spinal cord injury. Pre-injection imaging of the thoracic spine with MRI, CT myelography, or plain CT is required. To date, objective evidence of benefit from thoracic level transforaminal epidural injections is lacking.

Thoracic myelopathy

Thoracic myelopathy may or may not be accompanied by unilateral or bilateral radicular symptoms and findings. Thoracic myelopathy is less common than cervical myelopathy and somewhat less likely to be secondary to spondylosis. Thoracic spondylosis can cause myelopathy by a central or paracentral thoracic disk protrusion, spondylotic changes with spurring and thoracic spinal stenosis, or a combination of the two. Thoracic myelopathy may or may not be associated with thoracic spine pain. Thoracic myelopathy can be completely painless.

Except for intrinsic hand muscle weakness and numbness along the medial upper extremity with T1 involvement, the upper limbs should be spared in patients with thoracic myelopathy. The conus medullaris contains the lower motor neurons supplying the lower limbs and bowel and bladder sphincters. Compression of the conus medullaris can be confused with a cauda equina syndrome. As mentioned earlier, the spinal cord usually ends at the level of the L1 vertebral body. A very lower thoracic spine process affecting the bottom of the spinal cord can produce a conus medullaris syndrome. Differentiation between conus medullaris syndrome and cauda equina syndrome can be difficult. The differences are described in Table 3.2.

Differential diagnosis

The differential diagnosis of thoracic myelopathy is essentially the same as that presented for cervical myelopathy in the preceding chapter (see Table 2.5). In addition to tumors which are listed in Table 1.4, some of the more common causes of thoracic myelopathy are discussed below.

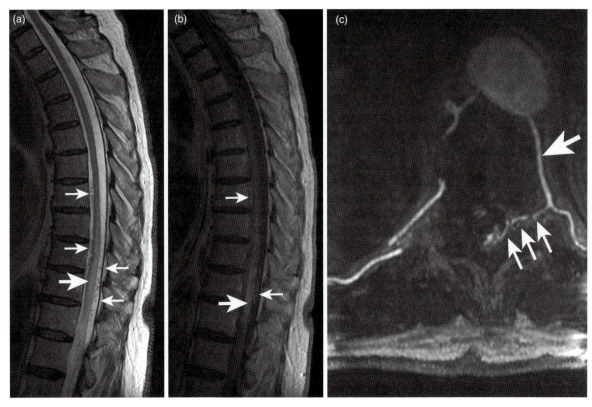

Figure 3.3. Dural arteriovenous fistula of the thoracic spinal cord. (a) Sagittal T_2-weighted MRI shows increased T_2 signal in the lower spinal cord (large arrow) and serpiginous flow voids representing arterialized veins in front of and dorsal to the spinal cord (small arrows). (b) Sagittal T_1-weighted MRI with gadolinium reveals enhancement of lower spinal cord (large arrow) and superficial blood vessels (small arrows). (c) Axial view of gadolinium bolus MR angiogram demonstrates a posterior intercostal artery (large arrow) which supplies a large left-sided spinal branch and radicular artery (small arrows), which in turn supply the fistula. This 72-year-old man presented with a 5-year history of progressive standing- and walking-induced lower limb numbness and weakness. On examination, he had evidence of a thoracic myelopathy.

Dural arteriovenous fistulas (DAVF) are the most common spinal cord vascular malformation and most often affect the thoracic spinal cord, although any level can be affected. Sometimes, more than one spinal level (e.g., thoracic and cervical) is involved. Patients with DAVF present with symmetric or asymmetric sensory loss, lower limb weakness, and sometimes pain in their lower back and lower limbs that can worsen with standing, walking, and Valsalva maneuver. DAVF affect middle-aged and older men more often than women. It is thought that high-pressure arterial flow from a radicular artery causes venous hypertension, engorgement, and secondary spinal cord ischemia. Burning dysesthetic pain in the lower limbs and/or perineum can occur. The evidence of myelopathy may be subtle. Bowel and bladder dysfunction usually occur late. DAVF can affect long segments of the spinal cord, and patients sometimes report upper limb as well as lower

extremity symptoms. Patients with DAVF may have intramedullary areas of increased T_2 signal in the spinal cord, enlarged pial vessels on the surface of the cord, and post-gadolinium spinal cord enhancement (see Figure 3.3). Occasionally in DAVF, only the MRI with contrast is abnormal.

Arachnoid cysts most commonly occur in the thoracic spine. They are intradural and more often posterior than anterior to the spinal cord. They can be congenital, follow trauma, or be secondary to inflammation from any cause. Many arachnoid cysts remain asymptomatic and are incidental findings. However, some can cause pressure on the spinal cord with secondary mid back pain, radicular pain, and/or thoracic myelopathy.

Spinal cord infarction causes spine pain, weakness, sensory loss, and sphincter disturbance beginning suddenly and reaching a peak in about 12 hours. Any level of the cord can be affected but the lower thoracic is most common. Transient cord ischemia is uncommon. Common causes of spinal cord infarction include regional hypotension (e.g., aortic surgery), systemic hypotension, atherosclerotic occlusive disease, thromboemboli from the heart or aorta, fibrocartilaginous emboli from a disk, infectious or inflammatory vasculitis, endovascular procedures, arterial dissection, and venous occlusive disease. The pattern of infarction within the cord is variable. Many involve the distribution of the anterior spinal artery and affect the anterolateral two-thirds of the cord with resulting paraparesis or paraplegia, neurogenic sphincter dysfunction, and loss of pain and temperature sensation with preservation of touch and posterior column function. MRI may be normal but usually shows cord enlargement and increased T_2 signal, the occurrence of which may be delayed by a few days. Adequate spinal cord perfusion should be maintained, but there is no specific treatment.

Extramedullary hematopoiesis (EMH) is a response to deficient production by blood forming cells within the bone marrow and can affect many tissues in the body. EMH frequently affects the thoracic spine and can accompany a wide variety of hematologic conditions including hemoglobinopathies (thalassemia, sickle cell anemia), hereditary spherocytosis, myelofibrosis, myelodysplastic syndrome, polycythemia vera, and Gaucher disease among others. EMH affecting the thoracic spine can cause mid back pain, radiculopathy, and most commonly myelopathy which is frequently painless.

Investigation

Again, MRI is the initial diagnostic test of choice in patients presenting with thoracic myelopathy. CT myelography is used in patients who are intolerant of closed spaces or who cannot undergo MRI. MRI with and without gadolinium is better than CT myelography in diagnosing tumors, inflammation, demyelination, spondylosis, infection, ischemia, syringomyelia, and other spine conditions. Because patients with cervical myelopathy may have a paucity of upper extremity signs and symptoms, the cervical spine is often imaged along with the thoracic spine. For patients in whom MRI or CT myelography shows evidence of an arteriovenous malformation and in patients with spinal cord ischemia, MR angiography or conventional transfemoral angiography is used to confirm the diagnosis, map out the blood supply, and potentially plan surgical intervention.

The same blood tests that were mentioned for cervical myelopathy are useful in excluding medical causes of thoracic myelopathy. Electromyography can help to exclude motor neuron disease and confirm the presence of a diabetic or other polyradiculopathy or lumbar plexopathy. Somatosensory evoked potentials are occasionally helpful, but are more often used for monitoring during cervical and thoracic spine surgery.

Treatment

Specific treatment is available for some of the causes of thoracic myelopathy. For spondylotic disease with disk protrusion and/or spinal stenosis, surgery may need to be considered. However, if the patient's history is that of acute or subacute onset, they have subsequently been stable, their deficits are mild, and the degree of cord compression is not severe, one could take a conservative, wait-and-see approach and defer surgery until, or unless, the patient worsened. Operating on the thoracic spine is more difficult than operating on the cervical or lumbar level and is associated with higher complication rates. If surgery is not pursued, the patient's activity should be modified and consideration given to bracing with a thoracolumbar orthosis. For patients with significant spinal cord compression and/or a progressive course, surgery will need to be strongly considered as described in Chapter 10. Pain control with analgesics and physical therapy directed at any neurologic deficits should be offered before and after surgical intervention. Proper bowel and bladder function should be ensured.

Thoracic spine pain

Pain in the mid back without significant radicular-type pain extending into the chest or abdomen is less common than neck pain alone and far less common than low back pain without lower limb pain. Because it is less common, mid back pain is less commonly investigated and less commonly treated. As a result, there is less evidence in terms of how thoracic spine pain should be evaluated and treated.

This section deals with pain that affects the mid back from the cervicothoracic junction to the top of the lumbar spine and extending out several inches in either direction from the midline. Patients may have accompanying, significant muscle spasm on one or both sides irrespective of the underlying etiology. As is the case with isolated cervical and lumbar spine pain, mid back pain alone can be difficult to accurately diagnose.

57

Differential diagnosis

Possible underlying causes of mid back pain are listed in Table 3.1. Musculoskeletal conditions are the most frequent cause of thoracic spine pain. Primary muscle pain, degenerative disk disease, facet joint arthritis, costovertebral arthritis, and compression fracture frequently affect the thoracic spine. Conditions in the cervical spine can cause pain that is felt in the upper mid back. This is especially true of cervical radiculopathy affecting the mid and lower cervical nerve roots. There are a number of worrisome internal causes such as cardiovascular, pulmonary, mediastinal, hepatobiliary, and gastrointestinal conditions that can present with pain that is felt chiefly or partially in the thoracic spine or suggest referred pain arising in the spine. Pain referred from the viscera to the thoracic spine is often accompanied by pain elsewhere in the chest or abdomen or by other symptoms specific to the symptomatic internal organ. Myocardial ischemia usually presents with anterior chest pain or heaviness or left upper limb pain and often nausea, but can present with pain radiating to the mid back or felt exclusively in the thoracic spine. A dissecting thoracic aortic aneurysm is typically felt in the chest but can radiate to or be felt only in the mid back. A gastric or duodenal ulcer on the posterior wall of the stomach or duodenum can also radiate to the back, but there is often a relationship to food ingestion which can make the pain worse or better. Gallbladder pain can be referred to the right infrascapular area and is often accompanied by nausea and vomiting. Pain of pancreas origin can also be felt in the back, typically at the thoracolumbar junction, and can be severe. Pain of renal origin is usually felt in the flank or costovertebral angle. Conversely, pain originating in the thoracic spine can be referred to the posterior and anterior chest wall, flank, abdomen, and even the upper or lower limb. Acute thoracic disk herniation without neurologic features is a relatively uncommon cause of mid back pain.

Scheuermann disease, also known as vertebral osteochondritis, is worthwhile mentioning here. Adolescent boys more often than girls present with kyphosis of the thoracic or thoracolumbar spine often, but not always, associated with back pain. The etiology is unclear, although there may be a hereditary component. A few or many vertebrae may be involved, and there may be more than one pathogenic mechanism. The kyphosis is occasionally associated with scoliosis. Neurologic examination is normal. Plain X-rays show wedging of vertebral bodies, intravertebral disk herniations (Schmorl nodes), irregular vertebral end plates, and kyphosis. Diagnostic criteria include anterior wedging of three contiguous thoracolumbar vertebrae, each of which measures 5° or more. Patients are treated with analgesics, orthotics, and exercises. Surgery may be needed for rare patients with spinal cord compression, impaired cardiopulmonary function, or for cosmesis. The prognosis is favorable, but residual spinal deformity can lead to altered spinal biomechanics with an increased risk of symptomatic spondylosis later in life.

Vertebral hemangiomas are benign dysembryogenic or hamartomatous vascular lesions that are discovered in the spine in 10%–12% of people. They have a predilection for the thoracolumbar segments but can occur at any level, may be multiple, are more commonly symptomatic in women, and can present in middle age with mid back pain more likely than neurologic symptoms. Pregnancy may have an adverse effect. Only about 1% of these tumors are ever symptomatic. Most symptomatic hemangiomas affect the thoracic spine. Many patients have mid back pain without developing neurologic symptoms. The major complication is neural compression by fracture, expansion, or bleeding. The hemangiomas can be seen with plain X-rays, CT, or MRI. While surgery can be performed if compressive myelopathy develops, the bone bleeds easily, and other less invasive treatment options such as radiation therapy or injection of the vertebral body with polymethylmethacrylate or alcohol are usually beneficial.

Investigation

It is probable that the same red flag warning signs and symptoms that were listed for cervical spine pain apply to thoracic spine pain (see Table 2.4). In addition, signs or symptoms of a significant inflammatory arthritis (e.g., ankylosing spondylitis, rheumatoid arthritis), such as limited spine range of motion or evidence of joint inflammation affecting the axial or appendicular joints, are important in the patient presenting with midline mid back pain and should prompt additional testing.

Patients with acute or subacute thoracic spine pain in the absence of red flag warning symptoms can be treated symptomatically and investigated only if their symptoms progress. The advice to take a conservative approach is especially true if the pain occurs in the setting of a minor injury, be it direct trauma or some sort of overactivity with twisting and/or bending of the torso so long as there is a low likelihood that the patient has osteoporosis.

For patients with more significant pain, pain that persists, and certainly for patients with associated red flag warning signs or symptoms, investigation is prudent. If there is a history of trauma or concern about compression fracture, plain X-rays may be the first line of investigation. Having said this, patients with a history of trauma who are awake and alert and have no clinical evidence of injury, including absence of localized spine tenderness, are unlikely to show significant abnormalities on plain X-rays. Anterior and posterior views are usually all that is needed; oblique and flexion-extension views do not add very much in most instances. For any patients where there is concern about underlying tumor, infection, arteriovenous malformation, or nerve root or spinal cord impingement, MRI should be considered. Unless the only concern is a herniated disk, the MRI is usually performed with and without gadolinium if kidney function is normal. CT of the thoracic spine is a reasonable alternative to MRI and is better than MRI at looking for spinal fracture and proximal rib disease. If there is any concern about disease arising in the chest, abdomen, or pelvis, appropriate imaging of these areas often with CT should be obtained. When there is concern about bony tumors, in addition to plain X-rays and an MRI scan, a radionuclide bone scan should be considered.

Blood testing such as for tumor markers [e.g., prostate-specific antigen (PSA), carcinoembryonic antigen (CEA), and CA-125] should be obtained in appropriate patients. If there is concern about infection or significant inflammatory arthritis, then inflammatory markers such as blood count with sedimentation rate, rheumatoid factor, C-reactive protein, and HLA-B27 status can be obtained.

Electromyography is basically unhelpful in patients with pain confined to the mid back region. Even if the EMG were abnormal, suggesting thoracic nerve root disease, there would be no guarantee that the patient's mid back pain was due to radiculopathy or the same process causing the nerve root injury. While EMG can be abnormal in notalgia paresthetica (showing only paraspinal muscle denervation in the mid thoracic level on the side of discomfort), the diagnosis is based on clinical grounds and does not require electrophysiologic testing. Patients with notalgia paresthetica usually report pruritus with or without pain on one

side of the midline in the mid thoracic region and follow a benign course. Somatosensory evoked potentials are also unhelpful in the absence of signs or symptoms suggestive of myelopathy.

Treatment

For patients with acute, subacute, and chronic mid back pain, comfort control treatment should be employed. This can range from over-the-counter analgesics to prescription analgesics and muscle relaxants to heat, ice, and massage. Opioid analgesics are probably best limited to patients with acute and subacute severe pain and for a limited period of time.

Formal physical therapy is probably not needed for most patients with acute mid back pain, but can be offered to those with subacute and certainly to those with lingering and chronic thoracic spine pain.

Many patients with chronic mid back pain alone are difficult to accurately diagnose. Most probably have myofascial pain which may or may not be caused by thoracic spondylosis or another musculoskeletal condition seen on an imaging study. For patients with chronic mid back pain, nonsteroidal anti-inflammatory drugs and acetaminophen can be recommended. Neuromodulating medications, such as gabapentin or pregabalin, and tricyclic agents, such as amitriptyline or nortriptyline, can be used. Opioid analgesics should be avoided but tramadol could be considered. Muscle relaxants are not helpful unless there is significant associated muscle spasm.

Especially for mid back pain that is limited in area, injection therapy may be of temporary benefit and may provide some help diagnostically. Intra-articular injections of a few thoracic zygapophyseal joints or blocks of the medial branches of the dorsal rami which supply those zygapophyseal joints with sensory innervation may help to determine if the anesthetized or blocked facet joints are responsible for a given patient's localized unilateral or bilateral mid back pain. If the patient obtains consistent and very substantial, if not complete, relief of their pain by these injections, a pain specialist may consider radiofrequency lesioning of the medial branches supplying the apparent pain-generating facet joints on one or both sides in an effort to provide the patient with longer-lasting relief. However, there is no good evidence of benefit from radiofrequency lesioning of medial branches supplying facet joints in the thoracic spine.

A thoracolumbar orthosis is sometimes employed to help mid back pain alone when it is thought to be due to associated, significant spondylosis, but there is concern that wearing such a device will result in weakening of the paraspinal and abdominal muscles. In addition, such orthotics are cumbersome to don and doff and miserable to wear in hot weather.

For patients with acute and subacute compression fractures who do not respond to conservative measures, vertebroplasty and kyphoplasty can be of prompt and sustained benefit. The presence of a compression fracture can be suggested from the history, and confirmed with plain X-rays and MRI.

Magnetic resonance imaging can provide some information about whether the compression fracture is new or old. Apparent edema seen within a compressed vertebra on routine T_2-weighted and especially on fat-saturated T_2-weighted MRI suggests that the compression fracture is relatively new. However, such edema can linger for many months after the injury is sustained. If edema is still present within the vertebral body, vertebroplasty is more likely to help relieve the patient's pain than if there is no edema present.

Should surgery on the thoracic spine ever be performed for mid back pain alone in the absence of compression fracture, nerve root or spinal cord impingement, instability, or severe deformity? The answer is probably no. As a result, there is no indication to perform discography which is unproven in thoracic disk disease.

Further reading

1. Atkinson JL, Miller GM, Krauss WE, et al. Clinical and radiographic features of dural arteriovenous fistula: a treatable cause of myelopathy. *Mayo Clin Proc* 2001; **76**(11):1120–1130.

2. DeJong RN. *The Neurologic Examination: Incorporating the Fundamentals of Neuroanatomy and Neurophysiology*, 4th edn. Hagerstown, MD: Harper & Row, 1979.

3. Fox MW, Onofrio MB. The natural history and management of symptomatic and asymptomatic vertebral hemangiomas. *J Neurosurg* 1993; **78**:36–45.

4. Frymoyer JW, Wiesel SW, eds. *The Adult and Pediatric Spine*, Third Edition. Philadelphia, PA: Lippincott Williams & Wilkins, 2004.

5. Koch CA, Chin-Yang L, Mesa RA, Tefferi A. Nonhepatosplenic extramedullary hematopoiesis: associated diseases, pathology, clinical course, and treatment. *Mayo Clin Proc* 2003; **78**:1223–1233.

6. O'Connor RC, Andary MT, Russo RB, DeLano M. Thoracic radiculopathy. *Phys Med Rehabil Clin N Am* 2002; **13**:623–644.

7. Rubin DI, Shuster EA. Axillary pain as a heralding sign of neoplasm involving the upper thoracic root. *Neurology* 2006; **66**:1760–1762.

8. Slipman CW, Derby R, Simeone FA, Mayer TG. *Interventional Spine: An Algorithmic Approach.* Philadelphia, PA: Saunders, 2008.

9. Tracy JA, Dyck PJB. The spectrum of diabetic neuropathies. *Phys Med Rehabil Clin N Am* 2008; **19**(1):1–26.

10. Wang MY, Levi ADO, Green BA. Intradural spinal arachnoid cysts in adults. *Surg Neurol* 2003; **60**:49–56.

The lumbar level

Introduction

Low back problems are extraordinarily common. Virtually every person is affected at some point during their life. Low back problems are the second-most common reason for a symptom-related visit to a healthcare provider. Despite the commonness of low back pain, reaching a diagnosis can be difficult. Many causes are not revealed by the diagnostic tests we have available. In many cases, the diagnostic studies reveal abnormalities that are unrelated to the patient's presenting complaint. Moreover, the natural history of many patients' lower back problem is one of spontaneous recovery and frequently no diagnostic studies and no therapeutic intervention are needed. Even though they might not be needed, diagnostic studies are frequently performed on the patient with lower back pain. Evidence suggests that there is marked variation in the performance of diagnostic testing between countries and within the United States. U.S. healthcare providers are probably the most aggressive in the world in terms of subjecting their low back pain patients to testing.

There are also marked variations in treatment between countries and between regions within the United States. While prevalence rates of lumbar spine disorders are not dissimilar between countries or between regions within the United States, there is extreme variation in the use of expensive, invasive surgical procedures including laminectomy and fusion. Recent Medicare data document a nearly eight-fold variation in regional rates of lumbar discectomy and laminectomy in the United States; for lumbar fusion, the variation was nearly twenty-fold between the lowest and the highest rate regions. These regional variations were stable from the early 1990s through the early 2000s and were higher than for any other surgical procedure in the United States. There is absolutely no documented difference in the incidence and prevalence rates of spine disorders in different regions that could justify the huge variation in surgical treatment. No doubt, similar variations exist for

invasive tests such as discography and treatments with equivocal efficacy such as epidural steroid injections. All of this suggests that the care of patients with low back disorders is highly variable, and much of the care that is provided is unnecessary and subjects patients to needless risk. It is hoped that this chapter will help to reduce the waste and harm of unnecessary testing and intervention on the patient with low back pain.

The lumbar level will also be divided into sections on the history and examinations that are pertinent to the lumbar spine, followed by sections directed at the main clinical presentations: lumbosacral radiculopathy, cauda equina syndrome, lumbar spinal canal stenosis, and low back pain.

The history

As is true for all of medicine, the low back patient's history is critical to reaching an accurate diagnosis. The patient's age is helpful in that spondylotic spine disease reaches a peak between the ages of 30 and 55. The prevalence of low back pain is roughly the same between men and women. It is important to have the patient describe their symptoms, how they began, and if anything might have triggered their onset. Be sure to determine their chief complaint. Especially for complaints of pain, numbness, and tingling, it is important to have the patient demonstrate exactly where they feel each of these symptoms. Having the patient complete a pain diagram can provide useful information about the character and location of the patient's pain and sensory symptoms (see Figure 2.1). The pain drawing can also suggest exaggerated and/or nonanatomic complaints. The location of the patient's sensory symptoms can aid in localization of the patient's problem (e.g., to a specific peripheral nerve or lumbosacral nerve root). Ask if they have weakness in their lower limbs, and, if so, where. Weakness can be hard for the patient to localize. Favoring one lower limb or a limp is nonspecific and could be due to pain and/or weakness. Ask if symptoms are made worse by standing, walking, both standing and walking, sitting, or lying down. If symptoms are brought on by walking and standing, ask if they are delayed in onset by use of a cart, walker, or lawn mower, which suggests lumbar spinal stenosis. If they are made worse by walking, ask if they are also brought on by use of a stationary or regular bicycle which would favor vascular claudication over neurogenic claudication (pseudoclaudication) due to lumbar spinal stenosis. If walking brings on symptoms, do they subside when the patient stands still (favoring vascular claudication) or does the patient need to sit down or lean against an object (favoring pseudoclaudication)? If walking provokes symptoms, do they occur sooner if the patient walks uphill (favoring true claudication) or downhill (favoring pseudoclaudication)? Table 4.1 describes the characteristic differences in the demographics, typical symptoms, and physical examination findings between vascular and pseudoclaudication.

Determine if the pain is made worse by coughing, sneezing, or Valsalva maneuver which suggests nerve root impingement especially by a herniated lumbar disk. Ask if their symptoms are getting better, worse, or staying about the same. Ask if the patient has had similar symptoms in the past. Inquire about previous testing and treatment and the benefit or lack of benefit from prior and current therapies.

Ask if their pain wakes them from sleep or increases if they lie down. Back or limb pain which awakens the patient from sleep at night is characteristic of or at least highly suggestive of an intraspinal mass lesion such as a disk or tumor or a spinal infection often with nerve root compression or inflammation. The patient may report that they have taken to sleeping in a recliner instead of in bed. Why does the patient with an intraspinal lesion note an increase in their pain at night? Some have suggested that the spinal column shortens in the daytime when we are upright due to the effect of gravity and lengthens at night when we are supine and that this lengthening could result in traction on nerve roots that emerge from the spinal cord, travel some distance, and then leave the spine. In the thoracic and especially in the lumbar and sacral regions, the nerve roots course downward some distance and laterally before emerging from their respective intervertebral foramina. One can imagine how lengthening of the spinal column could put traction on an impinged lumbosacral nerve root. However, in the cervical region, the nerve roots travel horizontally for the most part to leave the spine, and patients with cervical

Table 4.1. Differentiating vascular from neurogenic claudication

	Vascular	Neurogenic
Age	Older	Older
Gender	Male > female	Male = female
Current or previous low back pain	Less common	Very common
Lower limb symptoms		
Pain	Buttock, thigh, and/or leg	Buttock, thigh, and/or leg
Character of pain	Ache, cramp, tight	Ache, sharp, electric, burn
Spread of symptoms	± Distal to proximal	± Proximal to distal
Numbness, tingling	No	Frequent
One or both sides	Yes	Yes
Provoking factors		
Walking	Yes	Yes
Up an incline	± More likely	± Less likely
Down an incline	± Less likely	± More likely
Distance to symptoms	More fixed	More variable
Standing	No	Yes
Bicycling	Yes	No
Relieving factors		
Stand still	Helps	No help
Lean	Helps	Helps
Time to relief	Slightly quicker	Slightly slower
Preventive factor		
Flexed posture (cart, mower)	± No difference	Helps
Examination findings		
Pulses	Reduced	Usually normal
Bruits	Often present	Usually absent
Trophic skin changes	May be present	Absent
Neurologic exam	Usually normal	Some findings
Straight leg raise test	Negative	Usually negative
Lumbar extension	May be limited	Usually limited
Standing posture	Erect	Often flexed at waist

nerve root impingement also report that pain wakes them from sleep at night. Alternatively, it is possible that the increase in pain at night is related to redistribution of body water. At the end of the day, our feet and ankles are a bit swollen, and overnight this water is redistributed throughout the body. As a result, in the morning, our feet and ankles are normal, but our eyes are puffy. The redistribution of fluid could cause slight swelling of the spinal column and adjacent structures and an increase in any existing mass effect and nerve root irritation.

A neurogenic mechanism for the patient's symptoms is suggested by a history of sciatica (pain in the distribution of the sciatic nerve), other persistent referred radicular pain, or pseudoclaudication which can be defined as buttock, thigh, or leg pain; numbness; tingling; or weakness with standing or walking that mimics ischemic vascular claudication. The presence of sciatica is highly suggestive of lumbosacral nerve root impingement and has a sensitivity of 0.95 and a specificity of 0.88 that the patient harbors a herniated lumbar disk. Deyo et al. (1992) estimated the likelihood of a surgically important lumbar disk in the patient without sciatica as being 1 in 1000.

Sciatica is defined as pain in the distribution of the sciatic nerve which supplies the buttock, posterior thigh, the posterior and lateral leg, and the foot. Recall that the thigh is the segment of the lower limb between the hip and knee, and the leg is the part between the knee and ankle. Many authors argue that the patient's pain must go below the knee and into the leg in order for it to be true sciatica. However, adherence to the definition that sciatica is pain in the distribution of the sciatic nerve does not mandate that the pain extend into the leg; pain in the buttock and/or thigh alone could be due to disturbance of the lumbosacral nerve roots that comprise the sciatic nerve (part of L4, L5, S1, S2, and S3), the lumbosacral plexus, or the sciatic nerve itself. Alternatively, the patient with sciatica could have pain in their leg alone. Of course, irritation of the nerve roots above L4 (L1, L2, and L3) commonly produces pain that does not go below the knee.

A history of pain, especially burning pain and/or numbness and/or tingling in one or both lateral thighs, suggests entrapment of the lateral femoral cutaneous nerve. The term meralgia paresthetica is applied to symptoms arising from entrapment of this nerve.

It is very important to ask about the possibility of cauda equina syndrome in patients with low back disorders. Multiple nerve roots in the cauda equina can be compressed by a large disk or tumor. It is imperative to ask if the patient has numbness and/or tingling in the perineum, perianal region, and buttocks (saddle distribution). Inquire about bladder and bowel function. Urinary retention with overflow incontinence is characteristic of cauda equina syndrome. Patients may report incontinence of bladder and/or bowel, inability to sense bladder or bowel fullness, reduced ability to sense passage of urine or stool, or a decreased sense of having emptied their bladder or bowel.

It is also important to inquire about the presence of certain systemic symptoms and specific significant medical problems in the patient's history. These inquiries help to determine whether or not the patient has an increased risk of harboring a current cancer or spine infection, or has osteoporosis and an increased risk of spinal fracture. The specific questions that need to be asked are whether the patient has had any recent fever or chills, whether or not they have had unexplained weight loss, if they have had a recent bacterial infection, if they have recently used intravenous drugs, if they have any relatively recent or ongoing immunosuppression, and if they have a past history of cancer or acquired immunodeficiency syndrome (AIDS). Diabetes mellitus is a risk factor for infection. Questions that get at the risk of osteoporosis include the patient's gender (women are more likely to develop osteoporosis), the patient's age (increasing age makes osteoporosis more likely), a history of corticosteroid therapy now or in the past, low calcium intake, or premature gonadal steroid hormone deficiency.

Some authors advise asking the patient about factors which would suggest that they have ankylosing spondylitis. This would include age (the younger patient is more likely), male gender, morning stiffness, improvement in pain with exercise, uveitis, and arthralgias.

More so than is the case for cervical and thoracic spine disease, evaluation of the patient with low back pain often includes assessment of psychologic and socioeconomic factors. This is especially true for patients with recurrent or chronic pain. Substance abuse, anxiety, depression, job dissatisfaction, family problems, financial issues, workers' compensation entanglement, involvement in litigation, and stress can contribute to more severe symptoms, prolonged symptoms, greater disability, and worse outcomes from interventions. Some authorities recommend the routine use of screening tests to assess for psychologic factors, but they are not mandatory (see Chapter 7).

The examination
The general examination

Does the patient appear to be in pain? Are they febrile? Do they have limited chest expansion suggesting ankylosing spondylitis? Do they have skin lesions (or a history of same) that are characteristic of shingles, Lyme disease, psoriasis, café-au-lait spots (suggesting neurofibromatosis), or a mass or tuft of hair in the lumbosacral region that could indicate deeper lesions including spina bifida with or without an associated tumor such as a dermoid that might include the spinal canal? How is the patient's posture while seated and while standing and walking? Are they flexed forward at the waist? Do they have scoliosis? Do they have a list (acute sideward angulation in the lumbar region which often suggests an acute or subacute disk protrusion or extrusion)? Are they markedly flexed forward at the waist (camptocormia)? The inability to stand erect in the absence of a fixed spine deformity was originally described in conversion hysteria, but can be seen in Parkinson disease and parkinsonian syndromes, dystonia, and severe weakness of the thoracolumbar paraspinal muscles which, in turn, can be seen in focal and generalized myopathies, motor neuron disease, and myasthenia gravis. Bent spine syndrome is a synonym for camptocormia. Camptocormia or bent spine syndrome is similar to the previously described dropped head syndrome (Chapter 2) but affects the thoracolumbar spine instead of the cervical spine. Are they modestly flexed forward at the waist when standing and walking which suggests lumbar spinal stenosis whether or not they are having symptoms? Is there percussion tenderness of the spine which can suggest infection more likely than compression fracture or tumor?

Neurologic examination

The neurologic examination complements the history and is essential in determining if there is major motor weakness in the distribution of one or multiple lumbosacral nerve roots or perineal sensory loss or sphincter weakness suggesting a cauda equina syndrome. Such deficits help determine whether or not red flags are present and whether investigation and ultimately surgery should be considered (see below). If the patient's symptoms are confined to their low back and lower extremities, one could consider performing only a neurologic examination from the waist down. If higher levels of the nervous system are suggested from the history, a complete neurologic examination is advisable. Neurologic screening tests for patients with low back and lower limb pain are listed in Table 4.2.

Table 4.2. Neurologic screening tests for patients with low back and lower limb pain and suspected lumbar radiculopathy

Finding	Lumbosacral Nerve Root
Weakness or atrophy of anterior thigh	L2, L3, and/or L4
Weakness or atrophy of posterior thigh	L4, L5, S1, and/or S2
Weakness or atrophy of anterior leg	Mostly L5
Weakness or atrophy of posterior leg	Mostly S1
Reduced/absent knee reflex	L2, L3, and/or L4
Reduced/absent hamstring reflex	L4, L5, S1, and/or S2
Reduced/absent ankle reflex	S1
Sensory loss of proximal anteromedial thigh	L2
Sensory loss of anteromedial thigh	L3
Sensory loss of anterior knee, medial leg	L4
Sensory loss of anterolateral leg/ dorsum foot	L5
Sensory loss posterior leg/ lateral foot	S1
Perineal/perianal sensory loss	Cauda equina syndrome
Rectal sphincter weakness	Cauda equina syndrome
Reduced/absent perianal wink	Cauda equina syndrome
Positive reverse straight leg raise	L2, L3, and/or L4
Positive straight leg raise	L4 (±), L5, S1, S2, and/or S3

The signs and symptoms associated with specific lumbar nerve root syndromes are listed in Table 4.3. The signs and symptoms of cauda equina syndrome are listed in Table 3.2. Fixed neurologic deficits are seen in a minority of patients with lumbar spinal stenosis and are described under that section later in this chapter.

The comments in Chapter 2 (The cervical level) regarding muscle strength testing and the sensory examination apply equally to the lumbosacral level, and the reader is referred back to those sections on pages 36–37. A diagram of the lumbosacral dermatomes is shown in Figure 4.1. A few comments regarding the neurologic examination of the low back and lower limbs follow.

Can the patient arise from a seated position without the use of their upper limbs? Difficulty performing this maneuver suggests bilateral proximal lower limb weakness or a tendency to retropulsion as is seen

Table 4.3. Symptoms and signs associated with lumbosacral radiculopathy

Root	Typical pain distribution	Dermatomal sensory distribution	Weakness	Affected reflex
L1	Inguinal region	Inguinal region	None	Cremasteric
L2	Inguinal region and anterior thigh	Proximal anterior and medial thigh	Hip flexion Hip adduction Some knee extension	Cremasteric Thigh adductor
L3	Anterior thigh and knee	Anterior and medial thigh	Knee extension Hip flexion Hip adduction	Knee Thigh adductor
L4	Anterior thigh, anteromedial leg	Anterior knee and medial leg	Knee extension Hip flexion Hip adduction	Knee
L5	Posterolateral thigh Lateral leg Medial foot	Anterolateral leg, top of foot, great toe	Foot dorsiflexion, inversion and eversion Knee flexion Hip abduction Toe extension and flexion	Possibly internal hamstring
S1	Posterior thigh and leg, heel, and lateral foot	Posterolateral leg, lateral foot, heel	Foot plantar flexion Toe flexion Knee flexion Hip extension	Ankle Possibly external hamstring
S2	Buttock	Posterior leg and thigh, buttock	Possibly foot plantar flexion Possibly hip extension	Anal reflex Possibly ankle

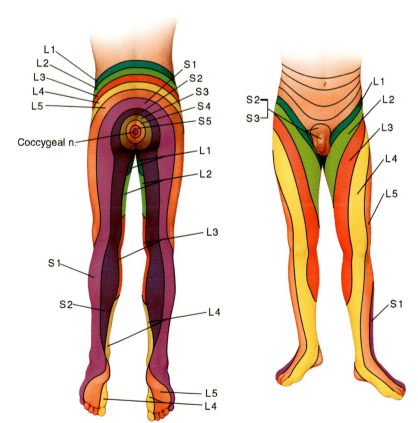

Figure 4.1. Diagram of lumbosacral dermatomes. There is lack of agreement about dermatomal boundaries and this depiction is meant to be a compromise. There is overlap of dermatomal territories and variation from person to person.

in basal ganglia disorders and hydrocephalus. The casual gait can suggest hip abductor weakness (Trendelenburg sign), a foot drop or difficulty with toe push-off. Trendelenburg sign can be seen when the patient is casually walking or if they are asked to stand or balance on one leg. A positive Trendelenburg sign occurs when the patient is standing on one leg or walking and their pelvis on the opposite, nonweight-bearing side droops downward. A positive Trendelenburg sign is an indication of weakness or instability of the hip abductor muscles, primarily the gluteus medius, on the patient's weight-bearing side. Heel walking and toe walking assess for L5 and S1 distribution weakness respectively. Difficulty with toe walking out of proportion to difficulty with heel walking suggests bilateral radiculopathies (especially S1) rather than peripheral neuropathy, even if the patient has numb feet. The gastrocnemius muscle is very strong, and weakness may only be noted by having the patient stand on one foot and do repeated toe lifts while holding on to the wall or table for help with balance. An asymmetry between the two sides in the number and ease of toe lifts performed may be significant. Testing muscle strength when the muscle is placed in a position of mechanical disadvantage may reveal weakness which is inapparent when the muscle is held in a position of mechanical advantage to the patient when it cannot be overcome. Atrophy of the leg muscles can be determined by measuring the maximum girth of both legs. A difference of 2 cm or more between the two sides is thought to be significant and usually indicates S1 nerve root damage because the gastrocnemius and soleus muscles are larger than the anterior tibialis and posterior tibialis muscles in size. It is more difficult to measure thigh circumference, but the same 2 cm rule difference is suggested. Thigh atrophy is typically due to quadriceps atrophy and suggests L2, L3, or L4 radiculopathy.

The knee reflex can be reduced in L2, L3, or L4 root disease, and the ankle reflex is typically reduced in S1 nerve root disease. The internal hamstrings are innervated more by the L5 than the L4, S1, and S2 roots, and the lateral hamstring reflex is more innervated by the S1 than the L4, L5, and S2 roots. However, because multiple roots contribute to both the internal and external hamstring reflexes, asymmetries may not occur in the presence of isolated nerve root compression, or differences may be present that do not fit with the typical root distribution patterns described. In general, abnormalities of the internal and external hamstring reflexes are not helpful and they need not

be tested. Sensory loss in the lateral thigh suggests entrapment of the lateral femoral cutaneous nerve. Perianal sensation should be checked. Rectal examination is recommended, especially if there is any possible question of cauda equina syndrome and in older men when the possibility of prostate cancer is present. One checks the tone and strength of the rectal sphincter muscle by palpation and by asking the patient to squeeze down firmly on the examiner's glove-covered finger. The superficial anal reflex checks the S2, S3, and S4 nerve roots. With a finger in the rectum, the perianal region is pricked with a pin or scratched, and the reflex contraction of the sphincter is palpated via the inserted finger. The contraction can also be observed without finger palpation. As a superficial reflex, the anal reflex is diminished in lower motor neuron conditions and with upper motor neuron, corticospinal tract lesions. Rectal examination also allows for palpation of the very lower rectum, a small portion of the posterior pelvis in women, as well as the prostate gland in men.

The cremasteric reflex is elicited by stroking or pricking the skin on the upper inner thigh, which causes contraction of the ipsilateral cremasteric muscle and elevation of the ipsilateral testicle. This superficial reflex is innervated by L1 and L2, but as a superficial reflex can also be lost in corticospinal tract lesions. The bulbocavernosus reflex consists of contraction of the bulbocavernosus muscle when the foreskin or glans of the penis is flicked or pinched or pricked. The contraction can be felt by placing a finger on the perineum behind the scrotum. This reflex is supplied by the third and fourth sacral nerves.

Finally, if there is severe weakness of toe flexion as might be seen in a severe S1 radiculopathy, Babinski testing may be falsely positive – the great toe may extend because there is no counterbalancing toe flexion function.

Special examinations

The patient's spine should be directly examined. A gown that opens at the back should suffice, or the patient can be examined in their undergarments. When just standing, the patient may show a "list" in which there is an acute sideward bend in the lumbar spine, which is often seen with disk herniation and nerve root impingement on the opposite side, away from the one they are leaning toward. Presumably, the list opens the intervertebral foramen on the contralateral, painful side. There may be loss of the normal lumbar lordosis with acute pain, especially if there is associated involuntary muscle spasm. Lumbar lordosis is often reduced in patients with lumbar spinal stenosis. Muscle spasm can be observed and palpated. The patient with active radiculopathy may prefer to keep their weight on the sound limb and may flex the hip and knee and plantar flex the ankle on the side of pain. Assuming this posture presumably reduces tension on their compressed nerve root. Look for scoliosis which may be accentuated or more noticeable when the patient bends forward at the waist.

Forward bending, backward bending, lateral bending to both sides, and rotation to both sides with the pelvis held stationary should all be checked. Impaired flexion of the lumbar spine can be seen with disk herniation with or without nerve root impingement. Patients with root impingement often show "corkscrewing" on attempts to flex at the waist; the lumbar spine makes a sharp lateral movement, then returns to a straight position as the patient bends forward, and the same typically occurs when they stand back upright. Rigidity of the entire spine is seen in ankylosing spondylitis. Limitation of extension suggests lumbar spinal stenosis or facet joint disease at one or more levels. Lateral flexion can be measured by seeing how far the patient can slide the ipsilateral hand down their lateral thigh. This will narrow neural foramina on the side to which the patient is bending; there may be limitation on the side of nerve root impingement, and the maneuver can bring out referred limb pain and/or paresthesias. Limited rotation can indicate facet joint disease or significant, more widespread arthritis including ankylosing spondylitis. In patients with spondylolisthesis, one may observe or palpate a "step-off" – a significant forward, more likely than backward, displacement of one spinous process on the one below. Depending upon the direction of the spondylolisthesis and its stability, this step-off can increase with attempts to flex or extend the lumbar spine. Significant percussion tenderness can indicate infection or fracture.

The sciatic nerve can be palpated in the buttock just lateral to the ischial tuberosity and its tibial nerve branch can be palpated in the popliteal fossa. The peroneal nerve lateral to the head of the fibula can also sometimes be palpated. Masses within or irritability of these peripheral nerves as manifest by tenderness or positive Tinel sign with palpation or percussion can aid in the diagnosis of neurologic findings and neurogenic pain.

There are a variety of tests that are meant to stretch the lumbosacral nerve roots and provoke pain

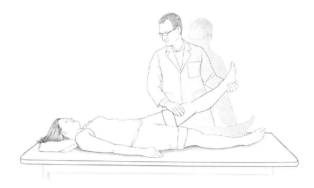

Figure 4.2. The Lasègue sign (straight leg raising test) is accomplished by passively flexing the hip with the knee extended. Provocation of the patient's radicular ipsilateral lower extremity pain is highly suggestive of nerve root impingement. Provocation of the patient's pain by testing the contralateral lower limb is even more suggestive of nerve root compression by a herniated or extruded lumbar disk.

if they are compressed. They are very useful in the patient with possible referred buttock and lower limb pain. Broadly, they can be divided into straight leg raising (SLR) and reverse straight leg raising tests. Straight leg raising stretches the sciatic nerve and will be positive if one or more of the nerve roots comprising the sciatic nerve (L4–S3) is irritated, usually by compression from a herniated lumbar disk. Classically, this is tested by the Lasègue sign. The patient lies supine, and the examiner gradually flexes the thigh at the hip, while the leg is held in extension at the knee by the examiner (see Figure 4.2). The test is positive if the maneuver elicits pain along the course of the sciatic nerve, especially leg pain, with elevations of 70° or less. Provocation of low back pain alone is not highly suggestive of nerve root impingement. Crossed SLR in which pain in the affected lower extremity is brought out by SLR of the contralateral asymptomatic limb is highly suggestive of nerve root compression by a herniated or possibly extruded lumbar disk. These tests are "more positive" if they bring out the patient's usual pain and if the pain is provoked with lower elevation of the lower limb.

A variation of this test is the Kernig sign in which the thigh is flexed to 90° at the hip with the knee in flexion. The examiner then tries to extend the leg at the knee. The test is positive if sciatica is provoked and there is resistance to full extension of the knee. Dorsiflexion of the foot or even the great toe while performing the Lasègue and Kernig tests increases tension on the sciatic nerve, which can accentuate pain and provide further evidence of lumbosacral root impingement (see Figure 4.3). SLR can also be

67

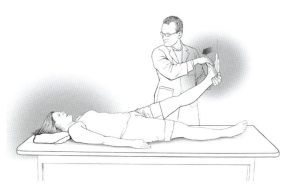

Figure 4.3. Dorsiflexion of the foot when performing a straight leg raising test (either Lasègue or Kernig sign) will increase tension on the nerve roots which form the sciatic nerve. Provocation of the patient's radicular pain with this maneuver increases the likelihood of lumbosacral nerve root irritation or impingement.

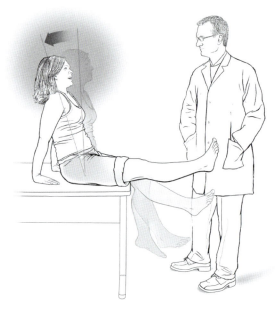

Figure 4.4. Asking the patient to extend one knee then the other while seated is a modified straight leg raising (SLR) test and is equivalent to about 65° of supine SLR. The patient may lean back and grimace when asked to perform this maneuver. If they do not show evidence of pain, you can ask them if their pain was provoked or worsened by assuming this position.

surreptitiously tested during the routine neurologic examination. With the patient seated, they can be asked to extend one, then the other lower limb fully at the knee, for example, to perform heel to knee to shin testing (see Figure 4.4). This position is the same as 90° of SLR when supine, but the degree of traction on the sciatic nerve and roots which supply the sciatic nerve is not as great as when the patient is supine. Some have suggested that a positive SLR when the patient is seated carries about the same significance as pain at 65° of elevation when the patient is supine. Sitting SLR is more convincing if the uncoached patient extends their lumbar spine or shows obvious pain when they are asked to extend the knee on the side of their sciatica. One can also ask the patient if they experience pain with this maneuver. Better yet, to "blind" the patient, you can ask them if extending their leg makes their pain better or worse.

Another test of organic root compression involves elevating both lower limbs at the same time. This causes less traction on the lumbosacral nerve roots comprising the sciatic nerve than single-leg raising, and one can reach a higher degree of elevation when raising both lower limbs at the same time than when testing one leg at a time. If the examiner lifts both lower limbs simultaneously to just below the point where it brings out the patient's referred pain and then lowers the asymptomatic extremity, this should provoke the patient's sciatica and a noticeable grimace is often observed.

The bowstring sign also gives evidence of lumbosacral nerve root impingement. In this test, SLR is carried out until pain is produced. Then, the knee is slightly flexed until the pain abates. The hip can then be flexed further, and the patient's heel is rested on the examiner's shoulder. Using both thumbs, the examiner applies pressure in the popliteal space over the tibial nerve. The test is positive if compression of the tibial nerve causes pain in the low back, ipsilateral buttock, or along the course of the sciatic nerve. Tenderness of the sciatic nerve in the sciatic notch is also suggestive of compression of the roots contributing to the sciatic nerve. Tenderness in the soft tissues of the lower extremity apart from the sciatic and tibial nerves can be seen in patients with radicular pain. The mechanism of this tenderness is unknown, but the presence of such tenderness does not eliminate the possibility of true radiculopathy due to nerve root compression.

Reverse SLR is performed with the patient prone. The knee on one side is passively flexed maximally. Provocation of the patient's same-sided limb pain is highly suggestive of impingement of the L2, L3, or L4 nerve roots (see Figure 4.5). These three roots contribute to the femoral nerve and are stretched by the reverse SLR maneuver. Hip and/or knee pathology can limit the utility of the reverse SLR test.

The Patrick or FABER (Flexion, ABduction, and External Rotation) test helps assess for hip and sacroiliac joint pathology. With the patient supine, the heel

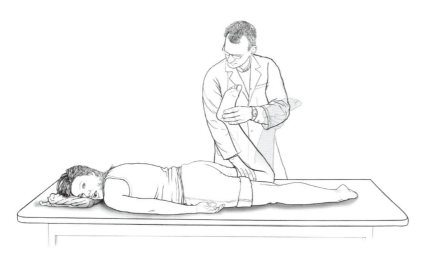

Figure 4.5. Reverse straight leg raising. With the patient prone, the knee ipsilateral to the patient's lower limb pain is passively, maximally flexed. Provocation of the patient's radicular pain suggests impingement of the L2, L3, or L4 nerve root.

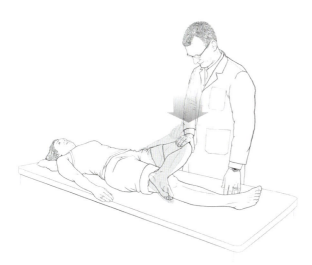

Figure 4.6. The Patrick or FABER test is performed with the patient supine and the ankle of the painful lower limb placed on the opposite knee. The knee on the side of pain is pushed downward; provoked pain is suggestive of hip or sacroiliac joint origin.

or lateral ankle of the painful lower limb is placed on the opposite knee, and the medial knee on the side of pain is pushed downward (see Figure 4.6). Thus, an attempt is made to provoke pain with simultaneous flexion, abduction, and external rotation of the involved hip. Pain in the groin (typically provoked by slow downward pressure) indicates probable hip joint disease, and pain in the sacroiliac area (typically provoked by quick downward pressure on the knee) indicates a possible problem with the sacroiliac joint. Pain of spine origin is usually not reproduced by this test.

Tenderness over the lateral hip region, especially if marked, suggests trochanteric bursitis.

For patients with possible lumbar spinal stenosis, there are two suggested office tests. The first is to check the effect of spine posture on their symptoms by having them stand during the interview or walk in the hall until they are symptomatic and then asking them to bend forward at their waist without putting their hands on, or in any other way bearing their upper body weight on, a stationary object. If the patient's provoked symptoms are relieved by forward flexion at the waist, this is very suggestive that they have lumbar spinal stenosis. The other technique is to re-examine the patient neurologically after they have developed symptoms and look for the emergence of new radicular lower limb neurologic deficits, the presence of which suggests lumbar spinal stenosis.

Finally, Waddell signs for nonorganic pathology and pain magnification are specifically meant for patients with low back pain. If three or more of the five tests listed in Table 4.4 are positive, there is a high probability of nonorganic disease.

Lumbar radiculopathy

This section will deal with lumbar radiculopathy without and, more commonly, with low back pain. Cauda equina syndrome, usually due to the compression of multiple lumbosacral nerve roots, will be covered in the following section. Subsequent sections deal with lumbar spinal stenosis and low back pain alone.

The large majority of patients with acute low back problems, 90% or more, recover within one month of onset of their symptoms with very conservative management. This is true whether they have low back pain alone or accompanying lower extremity pain. Because so many patients recover on their own with

69

Table 4.4. Waddell nonorganic physical signs in low back pain

If three or more of the following tests are positive, there is a high probability of nonorganic disease:

Tenderness: Tender to superficial pinch in the lumbar area or deep tenderness in a wide, nonanatomic distribution

Simulation of an organic test: Low back pain caused by axial loading (pressure on top of the standing patient's head) or rotation of the pelvis and shoulders in the same plane while the patient is standing

Distraction: A positive finding demonstrated in the routine manner (e.g., straight leg raising when supine) is not present when the patient is distracted or tested in a different way (e.g., straight leg raising when seated)

Regional disturbances: Weakness or sensory loss that follows a regional, nonanatomic distribution

Overreaction: Dramatic verbalization, facial expression, muscle tension, tremor, and collapse – "an academy award performance"

Table 4.5. Red flag warning signs for potentially serious conditions in patients with low back and/or lower limb pain

Possible fracture	Major trauma such as motor vehicle accident or fall from height Minor trauma or lifting a weight in an older or potentially osteoporotic patient
Possible tumor or infection	Age >50 or <20 Past history of cancer History of AIDS Recent fever or chills or unexplained weight loss Recent bacterial infection, intravenous drug use, or immunosuppression Pain that worsens when supine or wakes patient from sleep at night
Possible cauda equina syndrome	History or examination evidence of perianal/perineal sensory loss Recent onset of bladder or bowel dysfunction or unexpected weakness of anal sphincter on examination History of severe or progressive lower limb neurologic deficit

Major lower limb motor weakness on examination

conservative comfort control measures, studies have shown that there is little need to investigate most patients who present with acute low back and/or lower limb pain. In fact, diagnostic studies are expensive, sometimes invasive, and may give false evidence about the cause of the patient's symptoms which, in turn, can lead to unfounded concern, prompt unnecessary restriction of work and leisure activities, and lead to premature intervention which is associated with a risk of harm.

For these reasons, the role of the clinician is to make certain that there are no worrisome symptoms in the history or worrisome findings on examination (which are often suggested from the history) that should lead to additional investigation sooner rather than later. The so-called red flags for potentially serious conditions causing low back pain often but not always with lower limb pain are similar to those presented for cervical radiculopathy and are listed in Table 4.5. The red flags indicate an increased likelihood of possible fracture, possible tumor or spinal infection, or significant neurologic disease (e.g., severe or progressive weakness, evidence of cauda equina syndrome) where consideration should be given to early investigation and intervention in order to preserve neurologic function. Some would add to this list of red flags symptoms suggestive of ankylosing spondylitis.

As noted above, the presence of sciatica [pain in the distribution of the sciatic nerve (and the nerve roots which supply it)], while nonspecific, is highly suggestive of lumbosacral radiculopathy. Almost any pain in the lower extremity when accompanied by low back pain in an otherwise healthy individual suggests lumbosacral radiculopathy, especially if the onset is acute or subacute. The most common cause for acute lumbosacral radiculopathy is impingement of an exiting lumbosacral nerve root by a protruded intervertebral disk. Low back and lower limb pain secondary to lumbar disk herniation is likely to be acute or subacute in onset, more likely to be aching than sharp, is typically aggravated by sitting, and is often worsened temporarily by cough, sneeze, and Valsalva maneuver.

Lumbosacral radiculopathy and low back pain affect men and women equally. The peak incidence is from age 30 to 55. The natural history of acute lumbosacral radiculopathy due to lumbar spondylosis with nerve root compression is one of spontaneous improvement and recovery in the majority of patients. Patients with radiculopathy improve more slowly than those with low back pain alone as a rule. Even with sciatica, the majority of patients recover within one to two months of onset of their symptoms, and 90% within three months. However, recurrences are common, and perhaps 10% of patients go on to experience chronic symptoms.

As described in Chapter 1, lumbosacral ventral and dorsal nerve roots join to form a spinal nerve (taken together these structures are commonly termed a nerve root) which exits beneath the pedicle of the vertebral body with the same number as the nerve (the L4 root exits beneath the pedicle of the L4

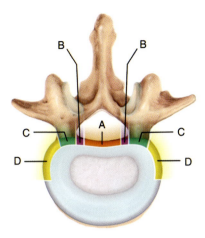

Figure 4.7. This axial view of a lumbar vertebra shows the anatomic zones where the disk can protrude and cause lumbosacral nerve root impingement. The central zone (A) lies between the medial edges of the two facet joints. The lateral recess lies between the medial edge of one facet and the medial edge of the pedicle on the same side (B). The foraminal zone is from the medial to the lateral edge of the pedicle (C). The extraforaminal or far lateral zone is lateral to the pedicle (D). Central canal compromise can be further described as mild (one-third of the cross-sectional area), moderate (two-thirds of the canal), and severe (complete or nearly complete narrowing).

vertebral body). The pedicle is well above the interspinal disk. A herniated lumbar disk characteristically occurs posterolaterally and impinges on the nerve root that is migrating laterally to exit beneath the pedicle of the next lower vertebral segment. For this reason, in the lumbar region, a lumbar disk rupture characteristically compresses the nerve root that is one higher in number (and one lower within the spinal canal). Therefore, an L4 disk typically impinges on the L5 nerve root. However, a very far lateral disk protrusion or extrusion can compress the nerve root at the same level as the protruded disk. Figure 4.7 shows an axial view of a lumbar level showing the different anatomic zones where disks can protrude posteriorly and potentially cause nerve root impingement.

More than 90% of disk herniations occur at L4–L5 (and usually cause L5 radiculopathy) and L5–S1 (and typically cause S1 nerve root impingement). Less commonly, disk protrusions can occur at L3–L4 (causing L4 radiculopathy), L2–L3 (causing L3 radiculopathy), and L1–L2 (usually causing L2 radiculopathy). The symptoms and signs associated with single lumbosacral radiculopathies are shown in Table 4.3.

Of course, large disk herniations can compress more than one nerve root on one side, especially if the nerve roots are conjoined and, if large enough,

a disk herniation can cause bilateral root compression and result in a cauda equina syndrome.

Differential diagnosis

The differential diagnosis of lower extremity pain or "sciatica" includes both neurogenic and non-neurogenic causes. Potential nerve root, plexus, peripheral nerve, and non-neurogenic causes of lower limb pain suggesting sciatica are shown in Table 4.6. Especially if there is little or no low back pain, it can be difficult to differentiate between nerve root, lumbosacral plexus, and unilateral peripheral nerve origin. The main non-neurogenic mimics are orthopedic conditions (especially arthritis of the hip or knee and soft tissue disease) and peripheral vascular disease. The elusive piriformis syndrome and resulting pain merit mention. The piriformis muscle arises largely from the front of the sacrum, passes out of the pelvis through the greater sciatic foramen, and attaches to the greater trochanter of the femur. The sciatic nerve is usually anterior to the piriformis muscles, but portions of the nerve can pierce the muscle. Excess contraction of the piriformis muscle can then compress the sciatic nerve against anterior structures or within the muscle. Alternatively, trauma could cause a local hematoma with subsequent scarring and sciatic nerve irritation. Patients may present with "pseudosciatica" with relatively little or no low back pain, typically negative straight leg raising signs, and possible evidence of denervation in muscles supplied by the sciatic nerve at and below the piriformis. Reproduction of the patient's pain may occur with internal rotation of the ipsilateral hip. Various nonoperative therapies are used, and surgery is very rarely performed. The differentiating points and tests which help to diagnose lumbar radiculopathy mimics are listed in Table 4.7.

Investigation

The diagnosis of lumbosacral radiculopathy is often straightforward, especially in the younger patient without accompanying medical conditions. Based on the history and physical and neurologic examinations, if it is clear that the patient has lumbosacral radiculopathy, in view of the benign natural history of the condition when it is due to lumbar disk protrusion, there is usually no need for additional testing. Clinical practice guidelines have been developed to direct the clinician in the evaluation and treatment of patients who present with low back pain with and without referred lower limb pain. In the absence of red flags

Table 4.6. Differential diagnosis of lower limb pain suggestive of sciatica

Neurogenic at level of conus medullaris, cauda equina or exiting nerve roots

Spondylotic

    Herniated nucleus pulposus

    Stenosis of central canal, lateral recess, or intervertebral foramen

    Synovial cyst

Arachnoid cyst

Perineural cyst

Sterile inflammatory arachnoiditis

Tumor

    Primary, e.g., neurofibroma, ependymoma

    Metastatic to bone or epidural space

    Meningeal involvement by cancer or lymphoma

Infection

    Disk space

    Epidural space

    Ganglionitis (herpes zoster)

    Lyme

Inflammatory radiculopathy

Various vascular malformations

Sarcoidosis

Neurogenic outside the spine

Lumbosacral plexus

    Tumor

    Idiopathic inflammatory

Sciatic neuropathy

    Compression

    Tumor

Diabetic radiculoplexus neuropathy

Peripheral neuropathy

Non-neurogenic

Musculoskeletal

    Arthritis

    Bursitis

    Myofascial

    Myogenic

    Post-traumatic

Bone disease

    Injury including fracture

    Tumor

    Osteoporosis

Peripheral vascular disease

    Arterial

    Venous

Genitourinary

for potentially serious conditions underlying low back pain with referred lower limb pain, the guidelines recommend conservative, symptom-control measures and no diagnostic testing for the first 4–6 weeks after onset of symptoms.

Some of the earlier practice guidelines focused on when to obtain plain X-rays of the lumbar spine, but plain X-rays are not very sensitive for some of the worrisome underlying conditions such as infection or cancer and do not typically show the most common causes for nerve root impingement, including herniated lumbar disks and foraminal and central spinal canal narrowing. Most authors agree that MRI is the diagnostic imaging study of choice for the patient with recent-onset low back and lower limb pain who has red flag warning signs or symptoms, and for the patient who has persistent symptoms of lumbar radiculopathy without red flags after 4–6 weeks of conservative management (see Figure 4.8). Plain X-rays should probably be limited initially to patients whose history and findings suggest systemic disease or fracture due to trauma or osteoporosis. Plain films can show congenital anomalies and help determine the "number" (spinal level) of the vertebrae and disks showing pathology on other imaging studies. Plain CT does not reveal as much as MRI. CT with myelography is nearly as good as MRI and, for some conditions, better, but is more invasive. MRI can also be utilized to image the lumbosacral plexus and large peripheral nerves such as the sciatic nerve. However, MRI often shows degenerated, bulging, and herniated disks in patients without spine and limb pain. These "false-positive" findings can mislead the clinician and alarm the patient, their family, and their employer.

Compared to CT, MRI does not use X-rays and shows soft tissues, including disk material, to much better advantage. The iodinated contrast used with CT has a greater risk of complications, including allergic reactions and renal damage. However, nephrogenic systemic fibrosis has recently been recognized in patients with renal impairment who are given gadolinium, the contrast agent used with MRI. Nephrogenic systemic fibrosis includes dermal fibrosis which can cause severe contractures and limited mobility and involvement of internal organs such as the liver, heart, lungs, and diaphragm, as well as skeletal muscle.

Electromyography (EMG) with nerve conduction velocity testing is helpful in confirming the presence of lumbosacral radiculopathy but is often unnecessary in the patient with a clear-cut root syndrome. EMG is

Table 4.7. Differential diagnosis of signs and symptoms of lumbar radiculopathy

Condition	Differentiating points	Helpful diagnostic studies
Diabetic radiculoplexus neuropathy	Pain and neurologic findings go beyond boundaries of a single nerve root or peripheral nerve. Natural history is one of eventual improvement.	EMG/NCS can be diagnostic. Imaging studies exclude compressive and infiltrative lesions of plexus and roots.
Lumbosacral plexopathy	Findings go beyond boundaries of single nerve root or peripheral nerve. Often little or no back pain.	EMG/NCS usually helpful. Imaging studies needed to exclude compressive and infiltrative lesions and exclude spine disease.
Sciatic neuropathy	Should not have back pain. Should have more than one root involved.	EMG/NCS can be helpful, but absence of abnormalities in paraspinal muscles is unreliable. Imaging of spine should be normal. Imaging of sciatic nerve may be abnormal.
Peroneal neuropathy	Findings are all below the knee. Usually painless. There should be no non peroneal innervated weakness (e.g., posterior tibialis). Absence of positive straight leg raising and absence of reflex loss are helpful. More common with recent weight loss and in leg-crossers.	EMG/NCS should confirm diagnosis. Imaging can exclude proximal causes.
Meralgia paresthetica	Only finding is possible sensory loss in distribution of lateral femoral cutaneous nerve.	Imaging and EMG/NCS are normal.
Degenerative joint disease of hip or knee	Pain is more localized to joint. May be limited range of motion, swelling, tenderness, pain with weight-bearing. Neurologic examination should be normal.	Imaging of joint is usually diagnostic. Response to joint injection may be helpful. EMG/NCS should be normal.
Trochanteric bursitis	Limited area of pain as a rule. Local tenderness, normal neurologic examination, imaging usually normal.	Imaging and EMG/NCS are normal.
Piriformis syndrome	Usually no back pain, negative straight leg raising, and no neurologic findings. Women may have dyspareunia. May have sciatic notch tenderness. Pain provoked by internal rotation of hip.	EMG of sciatic innervated muscles below piriformis may show denervation. Abnormal H reflex may be present with limb in symptomatic position. MRI may show enlargement of piriformis muscle.
Coccydynia	Pain usually confined to tailbone area with prominent tenderness and aversion to sitting. Usually no back pain. Neurologic examination is normal.	EMG/NCS and imaging studies if obtained are normal.
Iliotibial band syndrome	Pain, often stinging, above and lateral to knee. Often seen in runners and cyclists. May occur during or after exercise. Positive Ober test. Normal neurologic examination.	EMG/NCS normal. MRI may show thickened iliotibial band.
Deep vein thrombophlebitis	Local swelling, tenderness, and sometimes palpable abnormal vein. Positive Homans sign. Normal neurologic and musculoskeletal examinations.	Ultrasound of leg is usually diagnostic. EMG/NCS and other imaging studies are normal but usually unnecessary.

Notes:
EMG, electromyography; NCS, nerve conduction studies.

very helpful in differentiating nerve root from plexus and peripheral nerve disease. EMG changes may not be evident for 3–4 weeks after the onset of nerve injury, and therefore may be unrevealing in the face of significant root damage. EMG can also be helpful in the patient with longer-standing pain by determining if the radiculopathy is old or new and whether it is active or recovering. EMG can also shed light on the level of involvement in the spine when imaging studies leave room for doubt or show findings at more than one level.

Additional tests to consider are radionuclide bone scans which can help look for conditions such as osteoid osteoma and abscess, bone densitometry to evaluate for osteoporosis, imaging of lower limb joints with several different techniques (X-ray, MRI, arthroscopy), noninvasive and imaging studies of the arterial and venous circulation of the lower extremity, and blood tests such as sedimentation rate, C-reactive protein, serologies (Lyme, HIV), prostate-specific antigen, and rheumatoid factor.

Treatment

For some patients with lumbar radiculopathy, the cause or suspected cause will lead to early, specific therapy. This could be the case, for example, with shingles or significant trauma with fracture or known metastatic cancer. However, for most patients who have a suspected lumbar disk herniation, in the absence of cauda equina syndrome or a severe or

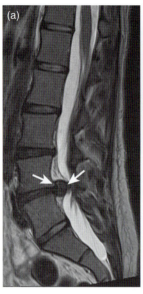 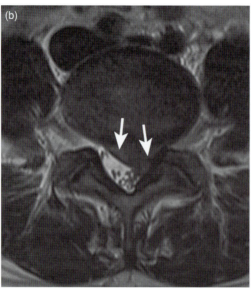

Figure 4.8. MRI in acute lumbar radiculopathy. (a) Sagittal and (b) axial T$_2$-weighted images show a very large left L4–L5 disk extrusion compressing the thecal sac (arrows). Note on the sagittal view that the protruding disk is taller than the disk at the edge of the disk space and is therefore an extrusion. There is also slight bulging of the L3–L4 disk. This 31-year-old woman experienced acute low back pain followed by left sciatica after pulling on a 100-pound weight. She had only left greater than right positive straight leg raising on examination. She recovered completely with simple analgesics. The MRI scan was obtained prematurely, just 10 days after onset of symptoms.

progressive neurologic deficit or other red flags, patients should be treated nonsurgically for at least 1 month. Treatment for acute and subacute lumbar radiculopathy is similar to that for acute and subacute low back pain (see below). Treatment can be divided into activity modification, medications given through various routes including by injection, physical therapies including manipulation, and surgery.

Patients with fresh radiculopathy should be advised to avoid activities which aggravate their pain, and they should probably be advised to avoid lifting significant weight, bending, twisting, and stooping. Bed rest is not recommended any longer for the treatment of acute lumbar radiculopathy or acute low back pain. Patients can be advised to remain as physically active as possible to help prevent inactivity-induced debilitation and reduce the risk of lower limb deep vein thrombophlebitis.

Nonsteroidal anti-inflammatory drugs (NSAIDs) are effective in the treatment of acute low back pain and probably the pain of lumbar radiculopathy as well. No specific NSAID is clearly superior. The benefits are modest. Acetaminophen has not been studied as much as NSAIDs, but it is reasonably safe and acceptable. For severe pain, time-limited use of opioid analgesics is reasonable. Muscle relaxants are of some help for acute low back pain and lumbar radiculopathy, especially in the patient with apparent muscle spasm, but the benefit is probably not additive to the use of analgesic medication. No one muscle relaxant is favored. Epidural corticosteroid injections are commonly administered to patients

with acute and subacute low back and lower limb pain. There is evidence that these injections do help to relieve referred, lumbosacral nerve root pain for a matter of weeks after the injection is given. The evidence is unclear, but the injections may "buy time" and enable some patients to defer and avoid surgical intervention. Transforaminal epidural steroid injections may be more effective than interlaminar injections of the same substances. The risk of epidural steroid injection is very low and includes increased back and lower limb pain, headache, infection, bleeding, and nerve injury. Some patients do experience transient systemic side-effects from the injected corticosteroid which can last for a few weeks. These injections should be performed with fluoroscopic guidance and only after an imaging study, almost always an MRI, has excluded a mass lesion and infection. The need to obtain an MRI before performing an epidural injection presents a dilemma in the patient who has had symptoms for a short period of time. A patient without red flags will be subjected to an expensive imaging study and an expensive treatment in an effort to hasten recovery which is likely to occur spontaneously.

Various physical therapies may provide temporary benefit to the patient with radiculopathy. These include ice, heat, massage, and ultrasound. Specific back exercises are not recommended in the acute phase for patients with lumbosacral radiculopathy. Exercise physical therapies initiated after the patient has recovered from their acute lumbar radiculopathy or bout of low back pain may be of help in preventing future recurrences. Spinal manipulation can be helpful for patients with acute low back pain, but its usefulness for the patient with acute lumbar radiculopathy is unclear.

Investigation, necessary in the patient with lumbar radiculopathy and evidence of cauda equina syndrome, progressive or severe neurologic deficit, other red flag warning signs, or persistence of signs and symptoms beyond 1 month, may lead to the discovery of conditions that require or lend themselves to surgery including infection, tumor, fracture, or most likely a herniated lumbar disk. Infection such as discitis or epidural abscess will require culture and possibly drainage. Primary and metastatic tumors may require biopsy and removal. Compression fractures or fracture dislocations may be discovered and can require surgical intervention or vertebroplasty or kyphoplasty. In the patient with smoldering radiculopathy and especially in the patient with a severe neurologic deficit, a progressive neurologic deficit, or the cauda equina syndrome, surgery must be considered (see Chapter 11). Lumbar laminectomy and removal of the protruding or extruded disk material without fusion is the most commonly performed operation for lumbar radiculopathy.

While it is clear that the patient with a severe or progressive deficit or profound pain or cauda equina syndrome should be strongly considered for surgery, what about the patient with lingering, stable, painful lumbosacral radiculopathy with only a mild to moderate deficit? Surgery in this setting has been long studied. A preponderance of evidence indicates that surgery for subacute and persistent pain will give the patient quicker relief of their pain but may not improve their neurologic outcome. The benefit from operative intervention probably persists for about 1 year or less before the natural recovery catches up with the improvement provided by an operation. There is evidence that patient preference results in better outcomes from surgery for lumbar radiculopathy. The risks of surgery are low (less than 5%) and include increased pain or neurologic deficit, dural tear, infection, and chronic low back pain (failed back surgery syndrome).

Cauda equina syndrome

Cauda equina syndrome is usually due to a large herniated lumbar disk, most frequently at either L4–L5 or L5–S1 (90%), and represents a true medical/surgical emergency. Patients usually present with low back pain with unilateral or bilateral sciatica, saddle sensory loss, sexual dysfunction, bladder more likely than bowel dysfunction (urinary retention, overflow incontinence, difficulty starting or stopping the urinary stream, reduced sensation, bowel incontinence), and variable lower limb motor and sensory loss. Symptoms and findings of cauda equina syndrome are also described in Table 3.2.

Differential diagnosis and investigation

The differential diagnosis of cauda equina syndrome is shown in Table 4.8. The time course of the patient's history will help give some indication about the cause. A very slowly expanding tumor, arachnoiditis, and the cauda equina syndrome secondary to long-standing ankylosing spondylitis usually present with a very leisurely onset of symptoms. Trauma, lumbar disk herniation, epidural abscess, epidural hematoma, and metastatic tumor have a much more rapid course. Even in patients with a chronic lumbar disk herniation, the evolution of symptoms may accelerate dramatically as the nerve roots within the confines of the thecal sac run out of room and experience increased compression and a decrease in blood flow.

If the symptoms have been at all progressive, cauda equina syndrome should be considered an urgent, if not emergent, situation calling for immediate imaging and possible surgical intervention. In this setting, imaging must be arranged as soon as possible and simultaneous with arrangements for evaluation by a spine surgeon. MRI without and often with gadolinium is the diagnostic imaging procedure of choice, but if this cannot be obtained on an emergent basis, then CT with or CT without myelography should be obtained. Plain X-rays have limited utility but may show evidence of fracture or tumor. In patients with a leisurely course, the timing of the imaging study is less critical. In the patient with a leisurely course, EMG may help to confirm the presence of a cauda equina syndrome and rule out a more peripheral disease affecting the lumbosacral plexus and peripheral nerves. Measurement of residual urine volume or, if needed, full urodynamic study can be helpful in evaluating bladder dysfunction.

Treatment

For patients with compressive cauda equina syndrome, especially those related to a large lumbar disk, there is evidence that surgical decompression within 24–48 hours of recognition of the cauda equina syndrome improves clinical outcomes. Therefore,

Table 4.8. Differential diagnosis of cauda equina syndrome

Spondylogenic

    Acute and subacute large lumbar disk herniation

    Synovial cyst

    Spondylolisthesis

    Lumbar spinal stenosis

    Arachnoid cyst

Trauma

    Fracture with displaced fragment

    Subluxation

    Penetrating trauma (e.g., gunshot wound)

Tumor

    Primary (e.g., schwannoma)

    Metastatic (prostate most frequent)

    Meningeal including infiltration of nerve roots (various cancers, lymphoma)

Infectious

    Epidural abscess with or without disk space infection

Epidural hematoma

    Spontaneous

    Following lumbar puncture, injection therapy, or surgery

    In patient on anticoagulant or antiplatelet therapy or with a bleeding diathesis

Miscellaneous

    Sarcoidosis

    Cauda equina syndrome secondary to long-standing ankylosing spondylitis

    Arachnoiditis (often following surgery, myelography, or misplaced injection therapy)

    Inferior vena cava thrombosis

    Aortic dissection

    Tethered cord syndrome

    Spinal manipulation with subluxation

    Paget disease of bone

    Extramedullary hematopoiesis

because of the urgent/emergent nature of this situation, a spine surgeon should be contacted when a progressive cauda equina syndrome is recognized. In this situation, the most expeditious management may be to send the patient to the emergency room of a hospital capable of performing emergency spine surgery where imaging and surgical consultation can be obtained rapidly.

There are two causes of cauda equina syndrome where surgery is clearly not indicated. One situation is the patient with chronic adhesive spinal arachnoiditis often due to previous spine intervention, and the other is the cauda equina syndrome seen in some patients with very long-standing ankylosing spondylitis. For patients with cauda equina syndrome secondary to chronic adhesive spinal arachnoiditis, the diagnosis can often be established with MRI with and/or without gadolinium which shows clumping without compression of the lumbosacral nerve roots within the thecal sac. Patients with chronic adhesive spinal arachnoiditis (see Figure 7.1) should not undergo any intervention, including surgery or spinal injection therapy. Their deficits can stabilize. Improvement is uncommon.

Cauda equina syndrome secondary to long-standing ankylosing spondylitis is a rare syndrome that occurs in patients with long-standing, usually burned out ankylosing spondylitis. The cauda equina syndrome in these patients is characterized by roughly symmetric, slowly progressive deficits which include motor and sensory loss in the fifth lumbar and sacral nerve roots, including prominent urinary and rectal sphincter disturbance. These patients can also develop fleeting or persistent pains in the rectum and/or lower limbs which respond to carbamazepine or gabapentin. Imaging in patients with cauda equina syndrome secondary to long-standing ankylosing spondylitis shows characteristic enlargement of the caudal sac including a capacious bony canal with dorsal arachnoid diverticula that erode into the laminae and spinous processes. The nerve damage and expansion of the caudal sac are thought to be due to increased cerebrospinal fluid (CSF) pulse pressure, which in turn is related to paraspinal soft tissue fibrosis caused by the long-standing ankylosing spondylitis. The rigid soft tissues do not allow for the normal dampening of transmitted CSF pulse pressure. Surgery in these patients is technically difficult and often associated with post-operative worsening. Lumboperitoneal shunting to reduce transmitted CSF pulse pressure is sometimes utilized but is of uncertain benefit. The course is only slowly progressive, and almost all patients retain the ability to walk. In general, patients with cauda equina syndrome secondary to long-standing ankylosing spondylitis do not need to be referred to a spine surgeon.

Lumbar spinal stenosis

Lumbar spinal stenosis (LSS) is defined as narrowing of the lumbar spinal canal, its lateral recesses, and neural foramina which can cause compression of the lumbosacral nerve roots. The stenosis can be symptomatic or asymptomatic. Although precise incidence and prevalence figures are not available, the occurrence of LSS increases with advancing age. Probably because of advancing age of the population, increased recognition of the clinical syndrome, increased availability and diagnostic capability of imaging studies, and increased desire for optimal quality of life, there has been a marked increase in the number of operations performed for LSS over time. Men and women are affected about equally. While disability and pain control issues are much less frequent with LSS than with acute and chronic low back pain, the impact on quality of life is about the same.

Lumbar spinal stenosis can be the result of congenital or acquired causes. Frequently, they are combined. Congenital stenosis is due to the following factors in decreasing order of significance: short pedicles, relatively large laminae and facet joint structures, a narrower horizontal interpedicular distance, and a more sagittal than coronal orientation of the facet joints. Congenital stenosis of the lumbar spine is often associated with stenosis of the thoracic and/or cervical levels. Patients with congenital LSS usually do not develop symptomatic disease until they acquire additional, superimposed degenerative changes. As a rule, patients with congenital stenosis present at a younger age than patients with LSS due purely to acquired causes.

Any of the structures that surround the lumbar spinal canal can hypertrophy and lead to narrowing. Facet joint hypertrophy is the leading cause of LSS with contributions from disk degeneration and protrusion, vertebral body hypertrophy, thickening and bulging of the ligamentum flavum, and degenerative spondylolisthesis. In descending order, the most commonly affected levels are L4–L5, L3–L4, L2–L3, L5–S1, and L1–L2. Most patients have narrowing at more than one level. Degenerative spondylolisthesis is present in one-third of patients, often at L4–L5, and is typically due to facet joint degeneration and instability. Disk degeneration with a resulting decrease in disk height can reduce the height of the intervertebral foramina at the same level.

In addition to static narrowing, there is a dynamic component which helps to account for the postural relationship of symptoms (see Figure 4.9). When seated or supine, the lumbosacral spine is relatively straight, but when standing or walking, individuals develop increased lumbar lordosis due to extension of the lower spine. With extension, the inferior articular processes and facets slide downward and backward on the superior articular processes and facets of the vertebra immediately below, the lumbar disks and posterior longitudinal ligament bulge posteriorly, and the ligamentum flavum buckles forward, all of which narrow the lumbar vertebral canal and intervertebral foramina and can compress the lumbosacral nerve roots. Most authors favor mechanical compression of the lumbosacral nerve roots rather than compromised circulation as the mechanism for the characteristic symptoms and frequent persistent neurologic findings.

Due to bulging of the lumbar disks and the slight outward flare of the vertebral bodies adjacent to the disk, LSS virtually always occurs at the level of the intervertebral disk.

Spinal canal narrowing can be asymmetric or only affect the lateral recess or neural foramen on one side and produce asymmetric or unilateral symptoms.

About 70% of patients with LSS report a remote history of episodic low back pain, and 20% or more have had sciatica in the past. In general, LSS is a chronic and gradually progressive condition so that over time patients note that their tolerance for standing and walking declines. Occasional patients report spontaneous improvement. The cardinal feature of symptomatic LSS is neurogenic claudication also called pseudoclaudication. Patients report pain, numbness, tingling, and/or weakness in the lower limbs typically brought on by standing and walking and relieved by sitting or flexing forward at the waist. Occasionally patients with LSS will report unsteadiness after standing and walking instead of or in addition to pain, numbness, or weakness. Postures which maintain or increase lumbar flexion (walking behind a cart or lawn mower, using a stationary bicycle, or leaning against an object) help to prevent or relieve pseudoclaudication. Conversely, factors that increase lumbar lordosis such as wearing higher-heeled shoes or walking down an incline can increase symptoms. In advanced cases, patients may experience symptoms when recumbent, especially if lying prone. Typically, the pseudoclaudication affects the entire lower limb, usually the posterior aspect, but can affect the thigh alone or leg alone. Patients report that their pseudoclaudication symptoms are often variable. Some report that they do better in the morning and worse in the afternoon, while other patients report just the opposite. Some patients report that their symptoms are more easily provoked when they walk on certain surfaces, especially very hard floors. Some patients report that their symptoms only occur with standing,

77

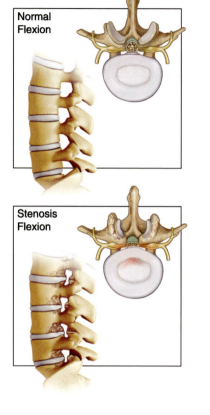

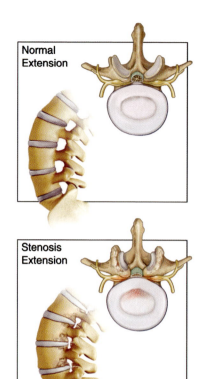

Figure 4.9. The upper two boxes show lateral and axial views of a normal lumbar spine in flexion (on the left) and extension (on the right). The lower two boxes show the same views of a stenotic lumbar canal in flexion and extension. Lumbar extension is associated with standing and walking. With lumbar extension, there is movement of the articular facet joint surfaces which narrows the posterolateral canal, the lumbar disks and posterior longitudinal ligament bulge backward into the canal, and the ligamentum flavum buckles forward. In the normal spine the degree of narrowing that occurs with extension is modest and easily accommodated, but in the stenotic lumbar spine the nerve roots can be compressed in the vertebral canal and intervertebral foramina and cause pseudoclaudication.

and some only with walking. About two-thirds of patients have accompanying, usually mild to moderate, low back pain which can occur with or be aggravated by the same postures that cause their lower limb symptoms.

There are relatively few physical signs on examination; none are diagnostic. Deep tendon reflexes are reduced or absent at the ankle in about 50% of patients and at the knee in about 20%. Vibration sense is often reduced or absent in the feet, but this is a common finding in older individuals. Mild unilateral or bilateral weakness and/or sensory loss in an L5 and/or S1 distribution are found in up to one-third of patients. The deficits are typically mild but can be more severe especially if the patient has a concomitant peripheral neuropathy. Straight leg raise (SLR) testing is typically negative.

Differential diagnosis

The differential diagnosis of pseudoclaudication is vascular claudication, osteoarthritis of the hips and/or knees, lumbar disk protrusion with radiculopathy, and other neurologic disorders such as multiple sclerosis,

intraspinal mass lesion, arteriovenous malformation of the spinal cord, peripheral neuropathy, and, rarely, communicating hydrocephalus (see Table 4.9). Differentiating between vascular and neurogenic claudication can be difficult; the main differences between these two conditions are outlined in Table 4.1. Older patients can have both conditions, and some patients are diagnosed as having LSS (or vascular claudication) only after the other condition has been treated surgically without helping the patient's symptoms.

Investigation

If the diagnosis of LSS is clear and the provider and patient concur that no intervention is indicated at this time, additional investigation can be deferred. Vascular laboratory evaluation can help confirm or exclude lower limb atherosclerotic occlusive disease. Plain X-rays of the lumbosacral spine are nondiagnostic but can show dense bony structures, one or more degenerated disks, facet joint arthritis, and degenerative spondylolisthesis, typically L4 on L5. Plain X-rays of the hips and/or knees can help determine if arthritis of these joints is contributing to symptoms.

Table 4.9. Differential diagnosis of lumbar stenosis

Vascular claudication – usually due to atherosclerotic disease

Osteoarthritis of hips and/or knees

Lumbar disk protrusion with nerve root compression

Unrecognized neurologic disease

   Multiple sclerosis

   Intraspinal tumor

   Arteriovenous malformation of spinal cord

   Peripheral neuropathy

   Rarely, communicating hydrocephalus

Electromyography can show neurogenic changes consistent with lumbosacral nerve root injury in as many as 90% of patients. EMG can also exclude peripheral neuropathy and plexopathy. Muscles supplied by the L5 and S1 nerve roots are most often affected. A normal EMG does not exclude LSS.

If there is a need to confirm the clinical diagnosis, to exclude an alternative condition, or if surgery is being considered, MRI is the imaging study of choice (see Figure 4.10). Compared to CT, MRI provides superior delineation of the soft tissue elements of the spinal canal, and use of the contrast agent gadolinium can help to identify tumors and scar tissue. CT scanning better demonstrates bony pathology including fractures and shows if calcification of disks or ligaments is present (see Figure 4.11). Myelography, usually with CT scanning, can also confirm LSS and exclude other mass lesions and, when compared to MRI, has the advantage of more easily examining the patient with their spine in extension (see Figure 4.11). Surgery can be performed on the basis of MRI alone. Plain CT can be used as a screening test in patients who are unable to undergo MRI.

If doubt remains about whether the pain is coming from the spine or the lower limbs, intra-articular injection of local anesthetic can help determine the hip or knee joint's contribution to the patient's symptoms. Response to an epidural injection can help determine if spinal stenosis is responsible for the patient's symptoms. Up to 10% of patients with LSS may have co-existing cervical spinal stenosis with associated symptoms or, more likely, asymptomatic neurologic signs (hyperreflexia and Babinski and/or Chaddock signs).

Because LSS symptoms are typically present when the patient is standing and absent when they are supine, vertical MRI machines and MRI with simulated weight-bearing have been promoted as helpful diagnostic studies. The vertical MRI machines use a low field strength magnet which compromises image quality. While the degree of LSS may increase modestly with erect posture, most patients have significant narrowing of their lumbar spinal canal when imaged in a supine position.

Treatment

Treatment options include physical, pharmacologic, and surgical methods (see Table 4.10). Exercises which strengthen the abdominal muscles and reduce lumbar lordosis can be beneficial. Use of a short cane or walker allows the patient to stand for longer and walk farther. A four-wheeled rolling walker with hand brakes, seat, and basket is recommended instead of a walker with two wheels or no wheels. Corsets and braces may help to reduce lumbar lordosis when the patient is standing and walking and delay the onset of symptoms. In obese patients, much of the excess weight is carried in their abdomen, which forces them to extend their lumbar spine in order to maintain their balance when standing. Very substantial weight loss can help to relieve LSS symptoms by reducing the degree of lumbar lordosis needed to stand erect and by also reducing the axial load borne by the lumbar spine. However, such weight loss is exceedingly difficult to achieve.

Analgesics are not very helpful, because the patient's pain is intermittent and can be relieved by changing posture. NSAIDs and acetaminophen are preferred over opioid analgesics. Muscle relaxants are of no benefit. Epidural steroid injections do not provide lasting benefit, but they can provide welcome temporary pain relief. Injections are sometimes difficult to perform because of the accompanying degenerative changes and canal stenosis.

The mainstay of effective treatment of LSS is surgical decompression which may need to be coupled with fusion if there is pre-operative or the potential for post-operative spondylolisthesis and/or instability. Because LSS can be present on imaging studies without clinical accompaniment, surgery should only be considered in patients with a compatible clinical history. Because LSS is frequently a multi-level process, the majority of patients require decompression of more than one spinal level. Foraminotomies for lateral recess or intervertebral foraminal stenosis may be needed, and part or all of one or more facet joints on one or both sides may need to be removed. Simultaneous fusion, especially if performed with

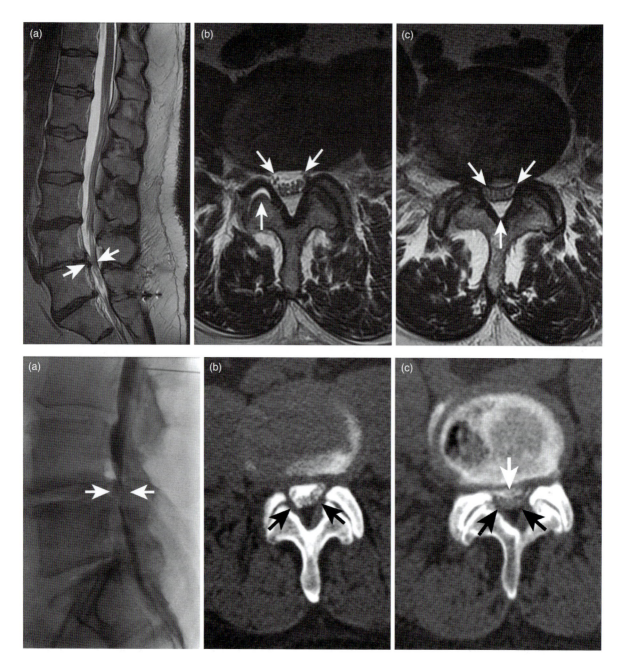

Figures 4.10 and 4.11. Lumbar spinal stenosis. Figures 4.10 and 4.11 show comparable images from T$_2$-weighted MRI (4.10) and CT myelogram (4.11) in the same patient with L4–L5 lumbar spinal stenosis. Figures 4.10 (a) and 4.11 (a) are sagittal views with arrows showing the stenosis. Figures 4.10 (b) and 4.11 (b) are axial views at the L3–L4 interspace where there is no significant stenosis (diagonal arrows), and Figures 4.10 (c) and 4.11 (c) are axial views at L4–L5, the level of stenosis, with absence of cerebrospinal fluid (CSF) or contrast surrounding the nerve roots (diagonal arrows). In 4.10 (b), note the fluid in the right facet joint (upward pointing arrow). In 4.10 (c), note the triangle of epidural fat posterior to the thecal sac (upward pointing arrow). In 4.11 (c), note the calcification just anterior to the thecal sac (white arrow) indicating calcified disk or osteophyte rather than soft disk.

instrumentation, increases the cost and complication rate without necessarily improving clinical outcomes.

With surgery, about three-fourths of patients have good to excellent relief of their lower limb symptoms for one to several years. Low back pain, even if it is postural and accompanies the pseudoclaudication symptoms, may or may not improve after surgery. In general, surgery is not recommended for patients

Table 4.10. Treatment options for lumbar spinal stenosis

Physical

    Activity modification

    Exercises

    Corsets and braces

    Short cane or walker

    Very substantial weight loss

Pharmacologic

    Analgesics

    Epidural steroid injections

Surgical

    Decompression alone

    Decompression with fusion

    X-Stop

with postural low back pain alone associated with a stenosed lumbar canal if they do not also have postural pseudoclaudication symptoms affecting their lower limbs. When compared to nonoperated patients, LSS patients who undergo decompressive surgery report significantly better pain relief and functional status which declines over time.

Complications from surgery are reported in up to 10%–15% of patients. Factors associated with complications and disappointing results from surgery for LSS include inappropriate indications, inadequate decompression, performing fusion with decompression, increase in mechanical low back pain after surgery, and "co-morbidities." By co-morbidities, we mean additional medical problems that increase the risk of operating and limit the patient's functional ability and survival. Because of recurrent back and lower limb symptoms, about 20% of patients who have LSS surgery will undergo another operation over time.

Because of the risk of complications, the unpredictable outcome of the surgery, and the intermittency of symptoms, surgery for LSS is elective. In general, surgery should not be considered during the first 3 months of symptoms because of potential spontaneous reversibility. Surgery should only be undertaken if the patient's symptoms interfere enough with their daily activities, they are otherwise in good health, and they choose surgery with a full understanding of the potential risks and hoped-for benefits.

In 2005, the U.S. Food and Drug Administration (FDA) approved the X-Stop interspinous implant for the treatment of LSS. This is a short titanium rod or spacer that is placed between the posteriorly protruding spinous processes of one or two lumbar levels associated with symptomatic LSS. The X-Stop is designed to limit extension of the lumbar spine at the implanted level(s) and to relieve symptoms of LSS. The X-Stop can be implanted on an outpatient basis under local anesthesia.

The X-Stop should not be used in patients with allergy to titanium, neurogenic bowel and bladder dysfunction, severe osteoporosis, active systemic or local infection, recent steroid use, or spinal anatomy that would prevent implantation of the device or result in instability of the device after implantation such as instability of the lumbar spine itself, fusion at the affected level(s), acute fracture of the spinous process or pars interarticularis, or significant lumbar scoliosis. The device is theoretically attractive and described in further detail in Chapter 12.

Acute and chronic low back pain

Acute and chronic low back pain without sciatica or spinal stenosis is very common. More than two-thirds of all people will experience low back pain during their lifetime. It is estimated that 10%–15% of the population will experience a bout of significant low back pain each year. Acute low back pain is variably described as less than 6 weeks or 3 months in duration, and chronic low back pain as lasting longer than 6 weeks or 3 months. Although the vast majority of patients with chronic low back pain start with episodes of acute low back pain, the causes and treatments are not the same for acute as for chronic low back pain. This section will cover both acute and chronic low back pain pointing out the similarities and differences between the two.

Low back pain is not a single disorder and can be caused by multiple pathophysiologic mechanisms affecting the region of the lower spine and surrounding structures. Most patients with acute and chronic low back pain are thought to have an underlying musculoskeletal cause. Despite extensive investigation which is often inappropriate and unnecessary, especially in patients with acute low back pain who are likely to improve, a large percentage of the patients with low back pain alone, perhaps 85%, cannot be given a precise pathoanatomic diagnosis.

The more common condition of acute low back pain is often provoked by a single action such as lifting or bending or twisting, or similar repetitive movements, overactivity, or an injury. For acute low back pain without sciatica and without systemic signs or symptoms, the prognosis is very good; most patients improve in days to weeks. However, recurrences of acute low back pain are common, affecting perhaps half of patients within 1 year of their first bout. Many patients with a history of acute low back pain are left with lingering fluctuating or intermittent low back pain. A minority develop significant chronic low back pain which may begin after an initial, single bout of acute low back pain, after a series of bouts, or with a gradual onset. Risk factors for developing low back pain include heavy lifting and twisting, body vibration, obesity, and deconditioning. Chronic disabling low back pain is more likely in patients with an increased fear of pain, psychological distress, job dissatisfaction, medical-legal claims, or involvement in a workers' compensation system. Smoking is a weak, but definite risk factor for disk degeneration and low back pain. While patients with chronic low back pain account for less than 5% of the total patients with low back pain, they account for >60% of the costs for the care of all low back conditions in the United States.

Differential diagnosis

Major sources of low back pain are listed in Table 4.11. The large majority of patients with both acute and chronic low back pain will have a primary spondylotic (from the spine) cause. Likely possibilities include the paraspinal muscles, degeneration and herniation of lumbar disks, facet joint disease, spinal stenosis, and spondylolisthesis. Much less likely possibilities include fracture, tumors, infection, inflammatory arthritis, and spondyloarthropathy, Scheuermann disease, Paget disease and other bony conditions, pain arising from visceral structures, and, rarely, psychogenic pain.

Investigation

Because most patients with acute low back pain will improve on their own over time, and most patients with chronic low back pain remain stable and have no underlying significant medical condition, the job of clinicians is to make sure that there are no worrisome symptoms or findings that should prompt early, additional investigation and, if there are none, to treat patients conservatively while watching for the emergence of these symptoms and findings. The same previously noted red flags (see Table 4.5) should be sought in the patient with acute and chronic low back pain. In their presence, additional investigation is warranted and in their absence, additional conservative treatment can be safely continued. In the patient

Table 4.11. Major sources of low back pain

Musculoskeletal structures of the spine, pelvis, and proximal lower limbs

    Joint (e.g., facet including synovial cyst, sacroiliac, hip)

    Disk (e.g., herniation, degeneration)

    Bone (e.g., osteoporotic or traumatic fracture, metabolic bone disease)

    Muscle (e.g., acute strain or chronic muscle-origin pain)

    Ligament, tendon, bursa, and other soft tissue

    Congenital or acquired deformity, often with superimposed degenerative changes (e.g., spondylolysis, spondylolisthesis, kyphosis, scoliosis)

    Lumbar spinal stenosis

Rheumatologic

    Ankylosing spondylitis and other spondyloarthropathies

    Rheumatoid arthritis

    Polymyalgia rheumatica

Trauma

    Fractures and dislocations

    Sprains

    Soft tissue injuries

Nonmusculoskeletal spinal conditions

    Tumors (e.g., primary and metastatic to bone, primary and metastatic to nervous system)

    Infection (e.g., bone, disk, epidural, or intraspinal)

    Neurologic (e.g., lower spinal cord, cauda equina, nerve root, meninges, plexus)

Referred from visceral structures

    Pancreas (e.g., tumor or pancreatitis)

    Upper gastrointestinal tract (e.g., penetrating duodenal ulcer)

    Lower gastrointestinal tract (e.g., diverticulitis)

    Kidney (e.g., kidney stone, pyelonephritis)

    Ureter (e.g., kidney stone)

    Bladder (e.g., infection or stone)

    Prostate (e.g., prostatitis)

    Ovary (e.g., tumor or cyst)

    Ectopic pregnancy

    Uterus (e.g., pregnancy, infection, tumor)

    Pelvic inflammatory disease

    Abdominal aortic aneurysm

Psychogenic

    With an additional source of pain

    Rarely, without an additional source of pain

Malingering

with chronic low back pain alone, a progressively worsening course should prompt investigation.

Imaging study recommendations for low back pain alone are similar to those for radiculopathy. Plain X-rays should probably be limited to patients with signs or symptoms indicative of infection, tumor, a history of trauma, or risk factors for spontaneous compression fracture including the older patient with known or suspected osteoporosis. Plain X-rays can also be used to screen for spondylolisthesis. MRI is the best imaging study to uncover all of the serious underlying causes of low back pain of spinal origin. Plain CT or CT myelography is recommended in patients who cannot undergo MRI. Plain CT is useful in looking for fractures and spondylolysis. CT and MRI have similar sensitivities for herniated lumbar disks and lumbar spinal stenosis, but MRI is more sensitive for infections, tumors, and nerve root impingement. Many patients with chronic low back pain undergo both plain radiography and MRI.

Degeneration of the lumbar disks and facet joints is very common in the aging population. It has been estimated that one-third or more of asymptomatic adults undergoing MRI will have at least one herniated lumbar disk, and 5% will have lumbar spinal stenosis. Given the commonness of these changes in asymptomatic adults, how do we know that pain experienced by the acute or chronic low back pain patient is coming from the abnormalities seen on their MRI? In an effort to try to answer this question, techniques have been developed to search for "pain generators." Two such techniques are provocative discography and injections of local anesthetics. Provocative discography involves introducing needles into the suspect lumbar disk and at least two adjacent disks under X-ray guidance from a posterolateral approach. Iodinated contrast material is injected into one disk at a time in increments such that the intradiscal pressure increases. The degree and character of pain provoked at each disk level injected is determined in an effort to find one level where the pain is "concordant" with the patient's typical low back pain. Plain X-rays and post-discography CT scanning provide information about the internal structure of the disks studied. Positive results from discography are thought to help identify the disk that is the patient's pain generator due to "internal disk disruption" which can then, presumably, be addressed directly such as with intradiscal electrothermal therapy (IDET), fusion, or placement of an artificial disk.

There will be more on discography in Chapter 5, "Diagnostic testing in the patient with spine and limb pain."

The other technique involves injection of facet joints and/or the medial branches of the dorsal rami of the spinal nerves that innervate the facet joints with local anesthetics of differing durations of action and a placebo under X-ray control. If the patient's typical pain is helped for the expected length of time, then that facet joint is thought to contribute to the patient's pain. Identification of one or more facet joints as pain generators might then lead to neuroablation procedures directed at the medial branches. There is more about this technique in Chapter 5. Discography and medial branch blocks are best left to experienced spine specialists where consideration is being given to more invasive treatment.

For the patient with low back pain and no lower extremity pain, electromyography and nerve conduction studies have basically no role.

Depending upon the patient's age, gender, the presence of red flags, and other medical conditions, one could consider obtaining blood tests such as blood count, sedimentation rate, prostate-specific antigen, serum protein electrophoresis, and rheumatoid factor. Radionuclide scanning can help diagnose infection. The abdomen and pelvis may need to be imaged in order to exclude pain referred to the spine from the abdominal aorta, kidney, gastrointestinal tract, and genitourinary structures.

Treatment

The treatment of acute low back pain is similar but not identical to that of chronic low back pain. As noted, the dividing line between acute and chronic low back pain is variable; some use 6 weeks, and some use 12 weeks. Episodes of acute back pain often recur. Most patients with acute back pain improve to the point where they have no spine pain or minor low back pain that does not require any treatment. The available treatments for acute and chronic low back pain are summarized in Table 4.12.

Patient education and reassurance can be helpful, especially for the patient with acute low back pain. If the initial assessment finds no hint of an underlying serious condition, the patient can be reassured of this and informed that their acute pain should rapidly recover. Patients with chronic low back pain, sometimes after investigation, can also usually be reassured that there is no serious underlying cause, that they can

83

Table 4.12. Evidence of usefulness of common therapies for acute and chronic low back pain

	Treatment	Acute low back pain	Chronic low back pain
Self-care	Patient education	Yes	Yes
	Avoid aggravating activity	Yes	Yes
	Heat	Yes	Only if helpful
Pharmacologic therapy	Acetaminophen	Yes	Yes
	NSAIDs	Yes	Yes
	Muscle relaxants	Yes	Probably no
	Opioid analgesics including tramadol	Yes	Controversial, maybe
	Tricyclic antidepressants	No	Yes
	Herbal medications (devil's claw and white willow bark)	Yes	No
	Epidural injections	No	No
	Botulinum toxin injections	No	Uncertain
Nonpharmacologic therapy	Exercise therapy	No	Yes
	Spinal manipulation	Yes	Yes
	Interdisciplinary rehabilitation	No	Yes
	Cognitive-behavioral therapy	No	Yes
	Functional restoration	No	Yes
	Acupuncture	No	Yes
	Massage	No	Yes
	Yoga (vini yoga)	No	Yes
	Bed rest	No	No
	Lumbar support	No	No
	Back schools	No	Yes
	Transcutaneous electrical nerve stimulation	No	No
	Ultrasound	No	No
	Diathermy	No	No
	Traction	No	No
	Inferential therapy	No	No
Invasive treatments	Medial branch lesioning	NA	Probably no
	Intradiscal electrothermal therapy	NA	Probably no
	Fusion	NA	Yes for spondylolisthesis Possibly for DJDD
	Placement of artificial disk	NA	Possibly for DJDD
	Spinal cord stimulation	NA	Yes for FBSS and CRPS
	Intrathecal pain pump	NA	Probably yes for FBSS

Notes:
DJDD, degenerative joint and disk disease; FBSS, failed back surgery syndrome; CRPS, complex regional pain syndrome; NA, not appropriate.

pursue most normal activities, and that treatment options are available. Brochures and additional educational materials may be of help for patients with both types of low back pain.

Bed rest is not advised for patients with acute or chronic low back pain. In the acute phase, patients with low back pain should be told to be as active as their pain will allow and avoid any activities or exercises that increase their pain or are known to increase mechanical stress on the spine such as unsupported sitting, heavy lifting, body vibration, and bending or twisting the back. Patients with chronic low back pain should also avoid activities that put undue stress on the back or aggravate their pain insofar as possible. Otherwise, they can be advised to gradually resume their normal lifestyle.

Medications whether given by mouth, by patch, or by injection are best viewed as comfort control measures. Nonsteroidal anti-inflammatory drugs (NSAIDs) can be recommended for acute and chronic low back pain. Acetaminophen has been little studied but can also be recommended for acute and chronic low back pain. Cyclo-oxygenase-2 (COX-2) inhibitors may be of some help for chronic low back pain, but the benefit is modest and this class of drug is associated with cardiovascular side-effects. There is one report that tramadol is helpful for chronic low back pain.

Muscle relaxants are helpful for acute low back pain. Different types of muscle relaxants are probably equally effective. Muscle relaxants have more side-effects than NSAIDs. Muscle relaxants are probably no more effective than NSAIDs, and there may be no additional benefit obtained by adding a muscle relaxant to an NSAID in the treatment of acute low back pain. There is limited evidence for the effectiveness of muscle relaxants for chronic low back pain.

Opioid analgesics are our strongest pain relievers. They can be used for acute, severe low back pain on a time-limited basis. While most authors recommend against the use of opioid analgesics for chronic low back pain, there are reports that a small minority of patients may benefit despite the risk of substantial side-effects. Pros include the fact that opioid analgesics are our most effective pain-relieving drugs, there is no ceiling effect on the dosage, there is no organ damage caused by these medications such as occurs with acetaminophen (liver) or NSAIDs (kidneys), and our obligation to provide effective pain relief for our patients. Cons of opioid analgesic therapy for chronic low back pain include the multiple side-effects (altered mental status, nausea, itching, constipation, hypogonadism, and swelling), the need for dose escalation, dependence on the medication, rare cases of addiction, occasional illicit diversion of drugs, regulatory scrutiny, the need to closely follow and monitor patients on opioids, and patient, family, physician, and societal disdain for this class of medications.

Tricyclic and tetracyclic antidepressants, but not serotonin reuptake inhibitor-type antidepressants,

provide modest benefit for patients with chronic low back pain and this is more likely to be true if they have an accompanying radicular pain component.

Injections of corticosteroids and local anesthetics into the lumbar facet joints, epidural space, and trigger points are commonly given, but there is little evidence to support their use in the treatment of acute or chronic low back pain without radicular pain. While more study is needed, botulinum toxin injections may be of some help for patients with chronic low back pain.

Some physical therapies can be helpful to the patient with acute and chronic low back pain. For patients with acute pain, local application of heat more likely than ice can be recommended for home use. Other physical modalities such as acupuncture, massage, diathermy, ultrasound, biofeedback, traction, and transcutaneous electrical nerve stimulation have no proven benefit for the patient with acute low back pain but are safe. Spinal manipulation, generally practiced by chiropractors and osteopaths, is safe and effective for patients with acute low back pain. Short-term use of a lumbar corset for patients with acute low back pain has no proven benefit but may help individual patients prevent movements which could aggravate their pain. For acute low back pain, heat has the best evidence for efficacy of any physical therapy.

For patients with low back pain of at least 1 month's duration, cognitive-behavioral therapy, exercise therapy, spinal manipulation, and interdisciplinary rehabilitation are more effective than acupuncture, massage therapy, yoga, and functional restoration (work hardening), which are more effective than placebo or sham therapy. The following treatments have not been shown to be of definite help for patients with chronic low back pain: lumbar supports, traction, ultrasound, diathermy, transcutaneous electrical nerve stimulation, and inferential therapy. The treatments with good evidence of moderate efficacy for chronic low back pain include cognitive-behavioral therapy, exercise therapy, spinal manipulation, and interdisciplinary rehabilitation. No one type of exercise program has been shown to be clearly superior.

Invasive treatments for low back pain include neuroablation procedures, percutaneous treatments directed at the intervertebral disk or vertebral body, fusion of two or more levels, replacement of a degenerated disk with an artificial disk, implantation of a spinal cord stimulator, and placement of an intrathecal drug delivery system. Because of the self-limited duration of symptoms in patients with acute low back pain, these procedures should only be considered in patients with chronic low back pain that is significant and has failed to respond to more conservative measures. How long should more conservative measures be tried before considering invasive low back therapy? Probably for 1 year or longer.

Radiofrequency lesioning of the medial branches which supply the lumbar facet joints is used to help chronic low back pain that has been determined to be on the basis of facet joint disease using injections of local anesthetics as described above. If one or more facet joints is thought to be responsible for the patient's pain, radiofrequency lesioning of the medial branches of the dorsal rami of the spinal nerves at and above each suspect facet joint is performed. This treatment is probably ineffective for most patients with chronic low back pain but may be of benefit in an extremely small subgroup of patients who respond favorably and consistently to placebo-controlled anesthetic blocks.

Intradiscal electrothermal therapy (IDET) is used to treat patients whose chronic low back pain is thought to be due to internal disk disruption or degeneration, which in turn is typically determined by provocative discography. IDET involves placement of a flexible, steerable electrothermal catheter into the abnormal intervertebral disk via a needle introduced through a posterolateral approach under local anesthesia and fluoroscopic control. The electrode is advanced so that it bends around circumferentially just inside the posterior annulus fibrosus, ensuring coverage of the posterior annulus. The electrode is then heated to 90°C, which presumably coagulates collagen and nociceptive nerve fibers. IDET is of uncertain benefit for chronic discogenic low back pain and its use is on the decline. There is more on IDET in Chapter 12.

Vertebroplasty or kyphoplasty can reduce the pain and suffering of acute and subacute vertebral compression fractures due to osteoporosis, significant trauma, malignant tumors, or vertebral hemangiomas. Patients with chronic pain (for more than 6 months) due to compression fracture are not usually candidates for this form of treatment.

Surgical treatment for chronic low back pain consists of lumbar fusion using various approaches and techniques (see Chapter 11) and more recently, placement of an artificial disk (see Chapter 13). Spinal fusion should be considered for patients with chronic low back pain and demonstrated spondylolisthesis who have had severe low back pain with or without sciatica associated with significant functional impairment that persists for a year or longer. Patients with spondylolisthesis and significant or progressive neurologic deficits are also candidates for fusion. Fusion for low back pain secondary to degenerative disk and facet joint disease alone is controversial and usually unnecessary, but is a consideration. Several recent controlled trials of various fusion techniques versus conservative management for patients with significant lumbar spondylosis without spondylolisthesis have been reported. Results of four recently reported trials suggest that surgery (fusion) may be more effective than unstructured nonsurgical care for chronic low back pain secondary to lumbar spondylosis without spondylolisthesis or nerve root impingement, but that fusion is not more effective than structured cognitive-behavioral therapy.

Since 2004 in the United States, and before this elsewhere, placement of an artificial disk has been an alternative to lumbar fusion for patients with lumbar spondylosis without spondylolisthesis. Artificial disk surgery requires an anterior approach with removal of the degenerated native disk and placement of an artificial disk. In October, 2004, the United States FDA approved the Charité artificial lumbar disk. In August, 2006, the FDA approved a second artificial lumbar disk, the ProDisc-L. Both have upper and lower metal plates sandwiching a piece of high-density polyethylene. Indications for total disk arthroplasty are reported to include a mature skeleton with degenerative disk disease usually at just one level, which is often L4–L5 or L5–S1. The patient should have significant discogenic pain confirmed by radiographic studies which often include discography. They should have failed at least 6 months of conservative therapy. Contraindications include facet joint arthrosis, spinal instability or spondylolisthesis of greater than 3 mm or grade 1, altered posterior elements due to prior surgery such as laminectomy and facetectomy, prior fusion, significant scoliosis or lumbar spinal stenosis, nerve root compression, infection, metabolic disease such as osteoporosis, morbid obesity, "too many" levels, acute fracture, tumor, a large Schmorl node (a protrusion of an intervertebral disk upward or downward into the bone of the adjacent vertebral body), and allergy or sensitivity to the implanted materials. Artificial disk placement has been compared to fusion with comparable or slightly better results. Durability of the artificial disks is uncertain, and re-operation on an implanted artificial disk can be difficult and requires an additional anterior approach procedure.

Spinal cord stimulation is used in the treatment of refractory chronic pain. Slender wire leads can be implanted percutaneously, or a "paddle" lead can be implanted via a small laminotomy. Both lead types have multiple electrodes. They are placed epidurally over the dorsal surface of the spinal cord. If trials of stimulation are successful, the electrodes are permanently implanted and powered through an external radiofrequency transmitter or, more commonly, an implanted battery. Spinal cord stimulation is especially useful for patients with failed back surgery syndrome and complex regional pain syndrome. Statistically significant pain reduction has been shown, but probably only half of patients experience truly meaningful improvement. Limb pain is helped more than axial spine pain, and benefit typically wanes over the course of several years.

Intrathecal drug delivery systems (intrathecal pain pumps) are used for patients with chronic, severe, refractory low back pain with or without lower extremity pain. Morphine is the most commonly infused analgesic. A potential side-effect is intrathecal granuloma formation around the catheter tip which can be associated with neurologic deficits. These systems should probably not be placed in patients with suspected chronic adhesive spinal arachnoiditis. Intrathecal drug delivery systems can be considered as a very last resort for severe chronic low back pain.

Chronic low back pain is a complex and debilitating disorder which affects the individual patient in many ways, and a single therapy is unlikely to relieve their pain. Intensive multidisciplinary pain rehabilitation programs have been developed for patients with severe chronic low back and other intractable pains. Such programs typically last for several weeks and combine specific and general physical exercises, biofeedback and relaxation training, stress management, behavioral modification, and cognitive restructuring. Medications are reduced and eliminated if possible. The goals of this type of program are to improve patients' quality of life and restore their ability to function normally. Intensive multidisciplinary pain rehabilitation programs can be tried before rather than after some of the more invasive treatments described above. Unfortunately, many patients who might benefit decline to consider this type of approach.

Further reading

1. Ahn UM, Ahn NU, Buchowski JM, et al. Cauda equina syndrome secondary to lumbar disk herniation: a meta-analysis of surgical outcomes (literature review). *Spine* 2000; **25**(12):1515–1522.

2. Armon C, Argoff CE, Samuels J, Backonja MM. Assessment: use of epidural steroid injections to treat radicular lumbosacral pain: report of the Therapeutics and Technology Assessment Subcommittee of the American Academy of Neurology. *Neurology* 2007; **68**(10):723–729.

3. Borenstein DG, Wiesel SW, Boden SD. *Low Back and Neck Pain: Comprehensive Diagnosis and Management*, Third Edition. Philadelphia, PA: Elsevier Inc. 2004.

4. Bruske-Hohlfeld I, Merritt JL, Onofrio BM, et al. Incidence of lumbar disk surgery: a population-based study in Olmsted County, Minnesota, 1950–1979. *Spine* 1990; **15**(1):31–35.

5. Carragee EJ. Persistent low back pain. *New Engl J Med* 2005; **352**:1891–1898.

6. Carragee E. Surgical treatment of lumbar disk disorders. *J Am Med Assoc* 2006; **296**(20):2485–2487.

7. Chou R, Huffman LH. Nonpharmacologic therapies for acute and chronic low back pain: a review of the evidence for an American Pain Society/American College of Physicians Clinical Practice Guideline. *Ann Intern Med* 2007; **147**:492–504.

8. Chou R, Huffman LH. Medications for acute and chronic low back pain: a review of the evidence for an American Pain Society/American College of Physicians Clinical Practice Guideline. *Ann Intern Med* 2007; **147**:505–514.

9. Chou R, Qaseem A, Snow V, et al. Diagnosis and treatment of low back pain: a joint Clinical Practice Guideline from the American College of Physicians and the American Pain Society. *Ann Intern Med* 2007; **147**:478–491.

10. Crisostomo RA, Schmidt JE, Hooten WM, et al. Withdrawal of analgesic medication for chronic low-back pain patients: improvement in outcomes of multidisciplinary rehabilitation regardless of surgical history. *Am J Physical Med Rehabil* 2008; **87**:527–536.

11. Dagenais S, Haldeman S, eds. Special issue on evidence-informed management of chronic low back pain without surgery. *Spine J* 2008; **8**(1):1–278.

12. DeJong RN. *The Neurologic Examination: Incorporating the Fundamentals of Neuroanatomy and Neurophysiology*, 4th edn. Hagerstown, MD: Harper & Row, 1979.

13. Deyo RA, Weinstein JN. Low back pain. *New Engl J Med* 2001; **344**(5):363–370.

14. Deyo RA, Rainville J, Kent DL. What can the history and physical examination tell us about low back pain? *J Am Med Assoc* 1992; **268**(6):760–765.

15. Freeman BJC, Fraser RD, Cain CMJ, et al. A randomized, double-blind, controlled trial: intradiscal electrothermal therapy versus placebo for the treatment of chronic discogenic low back pain. *Spine* 2005; **30**:2369–2377.

16. Katz JN, Harris MB. Lumbar spinal stenosis. *New Engl J Med* 2008; **358**(8):818–825.

17. Mirza SK, Deyo RA. Systematic review of randomized trials comparing lumbar fusion surgery to nonoperative care for treatment of chronic back pain. *Spine* 2007; **32**(7):816–823.

18. Nachemson AL, Jonsson E, eds. *Neck and Back Pain: The Scientific Evidence of Causes, Diagnosis, and Treatment*. Philadelphia, PA: Lippincott Williams & Wilkins, 2000.

19. Peul WC, van Houwelingen HC, van den Hout WB, et al. Surgery versus prolonged conservative treatment for sciatica. *New Engl J Med* 2007; **356**:2245–2256.

20. Rathmell JP. A 50-year-old man with chronic low back pain. *J Am Med Assoc* 2008; **299**(17):2066–2077.

21. Slipman CW, Derby R, Simeone FA, Mayer TG. *Interventional Spine: An Algorithmic Approach*. Philadelphia, PA: Saunders, 2008.

22. Waddell G, McCulloch JA, Kummel E, Venner RM. Nonorganic physical signs in low-back pain. *Spine* 1980; **5**(2):117–125.

23. Weinstein JN, Lurie JD, Olson PR, et al. United States' trends and regional variations in lumbar spine surgery: 1992–2003. *Spine* 2006; **31**(23):2707–2714.

24. Weinstein JN, Tosteson TD, Lurie JD, et al. Surgical versus nonoperative treatment for lumbar disk herniation: the Spine Patient Outcomes Research Trial (SPORT): a randomized trial. *J Am Med Assoc* 2006; **296**(20):2441–2450.

25. Weinstein JN, Lurie JD, Tosteson TD, et al. Surgical versus nonoperative treatment for lumbar disk herniation: the Spine Patient Outcomes Research Trial (SPORT): observational cohort. *J Am Med Assoc* 2006; **296**(20):2451–2459.

26. Weinstein JN, Lurie JD, Tosteson TD, et al. Surgical versus nonsurgical treatment of lumbar degenerative spondylolisthesis. *New Engl J Med* 2007; **356**(22):2257–2270.

27. Weinstein JN, Tosteson TD, Lurie JD, et al. Surgical versus nonsurgical therapy for lumbar spinal stenosis. *New Engl J Med* 2008; **358**(8):794–810.

28. Wong DA, Transfeldt E. *Macnab's Backache*, Fourth Edition. Philadelphia, Pennsylvania: Lippincott Williams & Wilkins, 2007.

5 Diagnostic testing in the patient with spine and limb pain

Introduction

This chapter will address the diagnostic tests that are used to evaluate patients with spine and limb pain. All attempts to diagnose the patient with spine and limb pain must start with the patient. The decision on whether or not to conduct any tests and, if so, which ones is dependent upon the patient's symptoms and examination as outlined in the previous three chapters. Diagnostic testing should only be undertaken in two circumstances: (1) to confirm the presence of a suspected condition which will require additional intervention if found; and (2) in the patient with significant signs and/or symptoms where the diagnosis is uncertain, testing is obtained in order to achieve a diagnosis which may or may not lead to intervention and also to exclude more sinister conditions which would lead to intervention.

Testing every patient with spine and/or limb pain is not appropriate. This is especially true if they have had symptoms for only a short period of time. The tests to be described are very expensive, and some are associated with risk. Because many asymptomatic adults will demonstrate significant incidental findings, especially on imaging studies, there is a substantial risk that inappropriate diagnostic studies will show abnormalities which will be followed by more diagnostic testing and, worse yet, unnecessary treatment. The additional investigation and possible therapy would be associated with more expense, discomfort, and risk. While a normal inappropriate diagnostic study might reassure the provider, patient, and family, finding asymptomatic, incidental abnormalities is likely to cause the patient and their provider undue worry. Even in the patient who merits diagnostic testing, the results must be interpreted in light of the patient's symptoms and physical and neurologic findings. One must be alert to the possibility of and disregard incidental findings on diagnostic studies if they do not explain the patient's clinical situation.

The diagnostic tests covered in this chapter include imaging studies, physiologic studies, provocative studies (mostly injections aimed at improving or aggravating symptoms as an aid to diagnosis), and other tests (mostly blood tests). This order is the author's rough estimation of the utility of diagnostic studies in descending order. For the imaging and physiologic categories, the tests will also be presented in order of decreasing utility. Table 5.1 estimates the ability of the history, musculoskeletal and neurologic examinations, and diagnostic tests to detect anatomic and physiologic abnormalities and their risk of providing misleading information.

Imaging studies
Magnetic resonance imaging (MRI)
Introduction

While it is the most expensive imaging test, MRI is the best imaging tool we have for spine conditions and, in fact, it is the best test overall for evaluating the spine. Studies which have been done comparing MRI with myelography, computed tomography (CT) myelography, and plain CT were performed ten or more, and in many cases twenty or more, years ago. They showed that MRI was the same as or slightly better than CT myelography and better than plain CT. But, MRI has improved over time and unquestionably shows better soft tissue detail than does CT myelography or plain CT. In particular, the nervous tissue including the spinal cord, nerve roots, and dorsal root ganglia are seen much better with MRI than CT. For most patients, MRI can obviate the need for any additional imaging studies and, by itself, can serve as the basis for operative intervention.

Full explanation of how MRI works is beyond the scope of this book. Suffice it to say that the body is placed into a very strong magnetic field which causes atoms, especially hydrogen atoms which are found in various concentrations in all body tissues, to line up because of their magnetic moment or dipole.

Table 5.1. Estimated ability of history, examination, and diagnostic tests to determine anatomic and physiologic abnormalities

	Anatomic abnormality	Physiologic abnormality	Risk of being misled
History	+	++	++
Musculoskeletal examination	+	++	++
Neurologic examination	++	+++	+
Blood and urine tests	0	++	++
EMG/NCS	++	+++	+
Radionuclide scan	++	+++	+
Plain X-rays	+	0	+
CT	+++	0	+
CT myelography	+++	0	++
MRI	++++	0	++
Discography	++	+	++

Notes:
0, no help; ++++, maximally helpful; EMG, electromyography; NCS, nerve conduction studies.
Sources: Adapted from Bigos et al. (1994), *Quick Reference Guide for Clinicians, No. 14.*

A radiofrequency pulse is transmitted to the part of the body under study using a coil which may be built into the MRI machine. The transmitted energy is specific to the hydrogen atom protons causing some of them to spin or process in a different direction. When the radiofrequency pulse is turned off, the hydrogen atom protons return to their normal alignment within the magnetic field and release energy imparted by the radiofrequency waves. These signals are picked up by a receiver coil and analyzed by computer; images are generated similar to CT methodology. MRI contrast agents work by altering the local magnetic field. MRI can look at a slice of any part of the body in any orientation.

How the study is performed
The patient removes all metal-containing objects and clothing and they are placed into the scanner, which is usually a cylinder. Patients with ferromagnetic aneurysm clips, pieces of metal in critical areas within the body (such as near the eye or optic nerve), and those with implanted wires (pacemakers, defibrillators, spinal cord stimulators, most cochlear implants, etc.) cannot undergo MRI. Patients with metallic artificial joints can undergo MRI. The apertures of the MRI machines into which the patient is placed have gotten somewhat larger over time, and the length of the gantry has also gotten somewhat shorter. Nonetheless, there are some patients who are simply too big to fit into the aperture of standard MRI machines. In addition, there are patients who find the claustrophobia of an MRI machine intolerable,

and these patients either need to take a tranquilizer beforehand or need conscious sedation in order to undergo the procedure. To help accommodate patients with claustrophobia (about 3% of the population), so-called open MRI machines are made that are C-shaped and open on one side. The open MRI machines to date have required use of a smaller magnet, and the images are not as good as with an enclosed MRI. There is a loud hammering noise that occurs during an MRI that can bother some patients.

Magnetic resonance images can be obtained of the cervical, thoracic, and/or lumbar spine. The usual images are sagittal slices with T_1- and T_2-weighting and axial slices with T_1- and T_2-weighting. T_1 and T_2 are relaxation times related to molecular behavior in longitudinal and transverse electromagnetic field directions, respectively. Differences in the images generated for specific tissues depend on their proton density (usually hydrogen atoms in water), T_1 and T_2 characteristics, and how the magnetic fields are manipulated in the MRI machine. Additional imaging sequences can be obtained. While not necessary, imaging can also be performed after the administration of a paramagnetic contrast agent, usually gadolinium. Paramagnetic contrast agents can detect breakdown in the spinal cord–blood barrier or nerve–blood barrier, and can reveal infectious and noninfectious inflammation in nervous and nonnervous tissues. Examples include epidural fibrosis following surgery, in tissue surrounding a disk herniation, in disk space infection, and with spinal cord demyelination. Gadolinium contrast enhancement

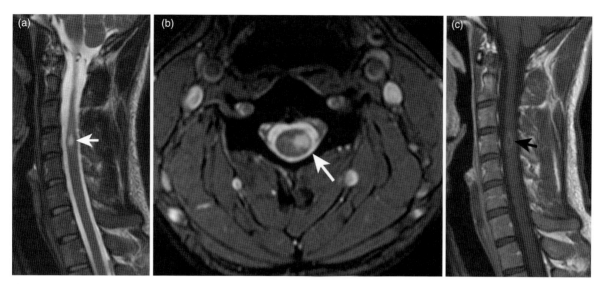

Figure 5.1. MRI showing multiple sclerosis affecting the spinal cord. (a) Sagittal and (b) axial T_2-weighted views show an area of increased T_2 signal in the left side of the spinal cord at C4 (arrows). There is mild enlargement of the left side of the spinal cord as well. (c) Sagittal T_1-weighted image after gadolinium demonstrates some peripheral enhancement (arrow). This 33-year-old physician presented with a 2-week history of altered sensation and sensitivity on his right side from the neck down. Examination showed only that pin and touch felt different on his right side. MRI showed one additional abnormality in the thoracic spinal cord and two in the brain leading to a diagnosis of multiple sclerosis (MS) after MS mimics were excluded.

imaging is not routinely performed in the spine patient who has not undergone surgery and in whom there is no strong suspicion of tumor, infection, or a vascular malformation.

Helpful aspects

Magnetic resonance imaging is an excellent technique for viewing the spinal cord and pathologic processes therein such as syringomyelia, infarction, tumors, multiple sclerosis, transverse myelitis, intrinsic cord signal abnormality due to external compression, and arteriovenous malformations (see Figure 5.1). MRI is also excellent for imaging the exiting nerve roots in the cervical and thoracic spine and for imaging the nerve roots within and exiting from the lumbar spine. MRI is superb for demonstrating pathologic processes outside of the dura including tumors, disk protrusions, synovial cysts, spinal stenosis, disk space infection, epidural abscess, and abnormalities within the bony spine and paraspinal muscles (see Figure 5.2).

Magnetic resonance imaging is especially helpful in the evaluation of spinal spondylosis. MRI can show loss of water content within the intervertebral disks, a common accompaniment of degeneration. Disk tears and bulges, enlargement of the facet joints, bulging ligaments, synovial cysts, and narrowing of the vertebral canal and intervertebral foramina can all be

readily detected with MRI. In addition, degenerative marrow changes within vertebral bodies adjacent to the intervertebral disks are also revealed with MRI. Type 1 Modic changes in the vertebrae are accompanied by decreased T_1 and increased T_2 signal and are thought to represent granulation tissue or edema, can be associated with an acute process, and enhance with gadolinium. Type 2 changes, the most common type, represent fatty degeneration of the marrow, show increased signal on T_1- and T_2-weighted images, and may or may not enhance. Type 3 changes show decreased signal intensity on T_1- and T_2-weighted images, are associated with bony sclerosis, and do not enhance. Type 1 changes especially can be associated with low back pain, but many patients have low back pain without bony vertebral abnormalities on MRI.

Less helpful aspects

Magnetic resonance imaging is not as good for acute trauma but can detect ligamentous injury which is not seen well with other modalities. The amount of edema within a compression fracture on MRI can help judge its age: the more edema, the more recent the fracture. MRI cannot easily differentiate between soft disk protrusion and bony osteophytic spur formation. In the first 6 weeks after spine surgery, MRI has difficulty differentiating between post-operative scar and

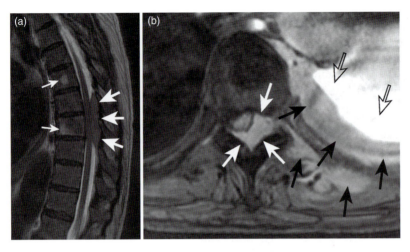

Figure 5.2. MRI demonstrating epidural lymphoma. (a) Sagittal T_2-weighted image shows a posterior extradural soft tissue mass (large arrows) extending from T7 to T9 with compression of the spinal cord immediately in front of the tumor. Areas of bone marrow replacement (small arrows) suggest skeletal metastases. (b) Axial T_2-weighted image shows intraspinal tumor (white arrows) which shifts the spinal cord to the patient's right. The tumor extends through the left T8 neural foramen into the left paraspinal tissues and left posterior pleural space (black arrows) where there is an associated pleural effusion (hollow black arrows). This 61-year-old man presented with a 9-month history of increasing left mid thoracic pain radiating to his upper abdomen. Neurologic examination showed only decreased touch and pin perception in the left mid thoracic dermatomes. Pathology from several sites showed low-grade follicular lymphoma.

recurrent primary disease (usually disk). Caution should be exercised in interpreting MRI within 6 weeks of surgery. During this interval, MRI is helpful in evaluating for hemorrhage, pseudomeningocele, and discitis, but evaluation for recurrent disk and even for post-operative discitis can be a problem. After 6 weeks, MRI is very helpful in distinguishing between scar tissue and recurrent disk herniation.

Magnetic resonance images are almost always obtained with the patient supine. However, for patients with lumbar more often than cervical spinal stenosis, the degree of spinal canal narrowing varies with the patient's posture and is greater when the spine is in extension and, in the case of the lumbar level, the patient is standing. Vertical MRI machines are available, but image quality is not as good as with horizontal MRI machines. Axial loading of a patient in the supine position can also be performed. This technique simulates the effect of standing weight-bearing and allows imaging in a standard MRI machine.

Risks

The risks of MRI include the risk of migration of internal metal objects which have not been recognized and generation of a current in an implanted wire electrode. There is some risk to the patient if sedation or general anesthesia is required to perform the MRI. The safety of MRI in pregnancy has not been established. It is good practice to try to avoid MRI during pregnancy, especially during the first trimester, but MRI is preferable to any studies using ionizing radiation in this situation. Intravenous gadolinium does cross the placenta into the fetal circulation where it has an unknown effect. Intravenous gadolinium should only be used in pregnant women if absolutely essential.

Intravenous gadolinium can cause mild side-effects such as headache, nausea, injection site pain, and, rarely, low blood pressure or light-headedness. Very rarely patients can prove allergic to gadolinium. In recent years, a serious side-effect of gadolinium administration has been recognized. Initially termed nephrogenic fibrosing dermopathy, the condition is more commonly called nephrogenic systemic fibrosis (NSF). The illness develops over a period of weeks following administration of gadolinium to patients with reduced renal function. This debilitating and potentially fatal illness is characterized initially by pain, redness, swelling, and itching in the lower then upper limbs followed by thickening and hardening of the skin similar to scleroderma which can result in severe contractures and reduced mobility. Internal organs such as muscle, heart, liver, kidney, and lung can be affected. There is evidence of deposition of gadolinium in the tissues which sustain damage.

Use of the specific gadolinium-containing contrast agent gadodiamide (Omniscan) is reported to be associated with a higher risk of developing NSF.

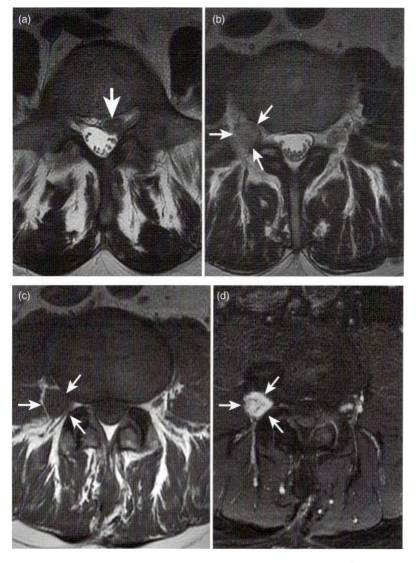

Figure 5.3. MRI demonstrating asymptomatic tumor. (a) Axial T_2-weighted image which shows this patient's expected left L4–L5 disk extrusion (arrow). (b) Axial T_2-weighted, (c) unenhanced T_1-weighted, and (d) gadolinium-enhanced T_1-weighted images of the L3–L4 level show an apparent round, enhancing tumor lying within and beyond the right L3–L4 neural foramen (arrows). This 55-year-old man presented with a 2-week history of low back and left lower limb pain and severe left L5 distribution weakness. Discectomy relieved his symptoms. We are observing the asymptomatic probable nerve sheath tumor (schwannoma). A 1-year follow-up MRI showed no interval change.

A higher dose of gadolinium-based contrast agent or repeated administrations may increase the risk of NSF. NSF occurs in patients with significantly reduced renal function and a glomerular filtration rate (GFR) of $<30\,\mathrm{ml} \cdot \mathrm{min}^{-1} \cdot 1.73\,\mathrm{m}^{-2}$ and is very unlikely to occur if the GFR is $>60\,\mathrm{ml} \cdot \mathrm{min}^{-1} \cdot 1.73\,\mathrm{m}^{-2}$. Patients who will be receiving gadolinium should have their renal function checked beforehand. In many settings, this can be done at the point of care by the radiologist.

There is no effective treatment for NSF. Intensive physical therapy is recommended. Phototherapy and extracorporeal photopheresis may be of help. Very prompt, same day hemodialysis after the administration of a gadolinium-based contrast agent may help to prevent NSF in patients with chronic renal failure.

Depending on the age of the group studied, somewhere between one-third and two-thirds or more of asymptomatic adults undergoing an MRI scan of the lumbar spine will be found to have significant abnormalities. In the cervical spine, the range of significant abnormalities is from 15% of patients in their 20s to 60% of those more than age 40, and more than 85% of patients over the age of 60. The most serious side-effects arising from a diagnostic MRI of the spine are more invasive diagnostic studies and the risks of surgical intervention on what turn out to be asymptomatic MRI findings (see Figure 5.3).

Additional MRI techniques

Magnetic resonance angiography of the spine can be used to confirm the presence of and plan treatment for arteriovenous malformations and can sometimes demonstrate large vessel arterial occlusive disease. MR myelography without the use of intrathecal contrast material is in limited use. Finally, MR neurography can be used to look at the nerve roots within the spinal canal, and MR can be used to examine nerves outside of the spine. When the differential diagnosis includes lesions of the brachial plexus, lumbosacral plexus, or peripheral nerves (especially the sciatic nerve), MRI can be utilized to examine these structures and provide an alternative, extra-spinal diagnosis for a patient's spine and limb pain.

Magnetic resonance imaging does not utilize ionizing radiation. Exposure to high-strength magnetic fields and radiofrequency waves is not thought to be harmful to human tissues.

Myelography and CT myelography
Introduction

Conventional myelography utilizing air and then various liquid contrast materials has a long history, but currently is almost always performed with additional CT imaging. Myelography with CT is infrequently used as an initial procedure, having been replaced by MRI. Myelography and myelography with CT require the instillation of contrast material intrathecally, usually in the lumbar spine, utilizing a midline interspinous process puncture but occasionally at the C1–C2 level from a lateral approach. The contrast material is denser than cerebrospinal fluid (CSF) and by tilting head-down gravity is used to allow the contrast material to reach the cervical region after instillation into the lumbar thecal sac. Currently, the main uses of CT myelography are: (1) for patients who have contraindications to or are intolerant of MRI; (2) to complement an MRI study where the findings are equivocal or inconclusive; (3) to study a patient who has previously had an instrumented procedure where the level of interest is at or near the level of the implanted hardware and the implanted metal interferes with MR image quality; and (4) occasionally when the MRI is negative but the index of suspicion of a structural lesion is high. The individual CT images can be obtained in a matter of seconds. The CT machine has the configuration of a doughnut rather than a tube or tunnel, and claustrophobia is almost never a concern.

How is the procedure performed?

Lumbar puncture is performed in the prone or lateral decubitus position, usually with fluoroscopic guidance. Spinal fluid can be withdrawn for analysis. Water-soluble, iodinated contrast material is injected into the thecal sac; more may be needed if the cervical level needs to be imaged. Plain radiographs can be taken after the instillation of contrast material (this is a myelogram), and CT scans are taken at the spinal levels of interest (the CT myelogram) (see Figure 4.11). Patients should not eat for at least 4 hours before the procedure. Afterward, they should not lay flat for several hours to prevent too much contrast material from reaching the intracranial subarachnoid space too rapidly where it can rarely cause seizures. There is no need to remove the water-soluble contrast material, which eventually enters the blood stream and is excreted in the urine. Myelography and CT myelography are usually performed on an outpatient basis.

Helpful aspects

Myelography alone shows defects in the column of contrast material that can be created by extradural (outside the dura), intradural extramedullary (inside the dura but outside the spinal cord), and intramedullary (within the spinal cord) processes. The addition of CT shows bony structures to good advantage and gives some information about the soft tissues in and around the spine and within the dura (the nerve roots and spinal cord). CT myelography is good for studying nerve root and spinal cord compression and can help differentiate between "soft" disk material and osteophytic spurring (see Figure 4.11). Somewhat more easily than for MRI, patients can be standing to some extent during a CT myelogram to look for positional foraminal and central canal stenosis. CT myelography is also useful for demonstrating CSF leaks.

Less helpful aspects

Imaging with CT myelography may be incomplete if there is a complete block to the flow of contrast material. Soft tissues are not shown as well as with MRI. The use of intravenous contrast to look for enhancement is typically not performed with CT myelography. In order to image the cervical spine, a larger amount of contrast material must be given intrathecally in the lumbar region, or a C1–C2 puncture must be performed.

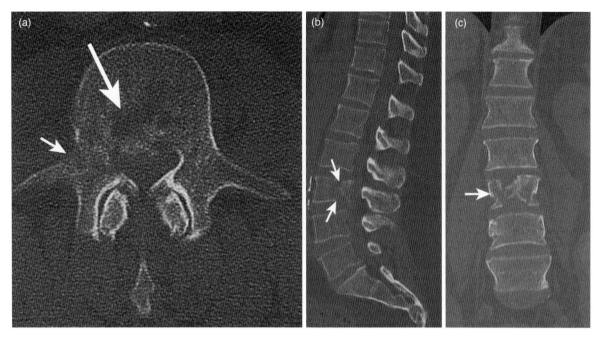

Figure 5.4. Metastasis to L3 vertebral body on CT. (a), (b), and (c) are axial, sagittal, and coronal views respectively of an unenhanced CT scan and demonstrate a destructive process of the L3 vertebral body (arrows). There is a pathologic fracture with posterior displacement of bone backward into the spinal canal on the sagittal view. Soft tissue setting images showed abnormal epidural tissue filling the spinal canal at the L3 level which was better seen with MRI. This 50-year-old man reported a 3-month history of progressive, severe low back pain after lifting a heavy object and a ten-day history of possible cauda equina syndrome. On examination, there was decreased sensation in the right buttock and lower limb and in the left leg and foot with an absent right ankle reflex. Evaluation led to a diagnosis of metastatic grade 3 of 4 adenocarcinoma of the rectum.

Risks

Myelography and CT myelography expose the patient to ionizing radiation and should not be used in pregnancy. The newer, nonionic water-soluble contrast materials such as iohexol (Omnipaque) have fewer side-effects than their predecessors, but can cause headache, neck ache and stiffness, nausea and vomiting, and rare seizures. Because patients undergo lumbar puncture, they can experience a post-lumbar-puncture headache. C1–C2 puncture can result in puncture of, or injection of contrast media into, the upper cervical spinal cord or vertebral artery, the risks of which are minimized with use of fluoroscopic guidance.

Plain CT of the spine

Plain CT of the spine is a fast and cost-effective method for assessing the central spinal canal, lateral recesses, intervertebral foramina, and the bones of the spine. When compared to MRI, plain CT does not have the same ability to discriminate between different kinds of soft tissue including fluid such as the spinal fluid. As a result, it is insensitive to intradural and intramedullary (spinal cord) disease.

How the test is performed

The patient is placed in the CT scanner, and individual regions of the spine can be examined, sometimes as fast as in seconds and with slices as thin as 0.6 mm. The administration of intravenous contrast is an option to look for enhancement which might be seen with inflammation including post-operative scarring or tumors.

Helpful aspects

Plain CT is very good for the assessment of spinal trauma and bony lesions (see Figure 5.4). When CT is performed with and without the use of iodinated contrast material, it may be helpful in the diagnosis of bone tumors and in differentiating between recurrent disk protrusion and scarring in the patient who has undergone recent spine surgery. Because the images can be rapidly obtained, CT may be a better screening test than MRI for some patients who cannot tolerate the supine position for more than a few minutes. Plain CT can be obtained with the patient in different positions to look for postural effects on stenosis.

Risks

Computed tomography does expose the patient to ionizing radiation and should be avoided in pregnancy. Administration of intravenous iodinated contrast material can result in symptoms that include urticaria, nausea, vomiting, bronchospasm, cardiac arrhythmias, hypotension, and syncope. In addition, the iodinated contrast material can be toxic to the kidneys. Contrast agent-related nephropathy is more often temporary than persistent and more likely to occur in patients with pre-existing renal insufficiency. Delayed, chiefly flu-like symptoms can occur up to seven days following the injection of iodinated contrast material.

Plain X-rays
Introduction

Plain X-rays are often the starting point for any spine-related imaging assessment. The cost is low. They will often show some abnormalities, but the findings may not be germane to the patient's symptoms.

How is the procedure performed?

In the cervical spine, anteroposterior and lateral views are the routine nontrauma films that are obtained; open-mouth odontoid, right and left oblique films, flexion and extension views, and a "swimmer's view," which is a lateral image of the cervicothoracic junction, can be added. In the thoracic spine, the routine views are anteroposterior and lateral views only. In the lumbar spine, the routine images are an anteroposterior view, a lateral view, and a focused lateral view of the lumbosacral interspace. Additional lumbar views include right and left oblique and flexion and extension images. The additional views of the cervical and lumbar spine increase the expense and exposure to radiation and may not add significant information; they should not be routinely obtained.

Helpful aspects

Plain X-rays of the spine show alignment, evidence of degenerative disk and joint disease, integrity of cortical bone, congenital bony anomalies, scoliosis, kyphosis, possible compression fracture and/or osteoporosis, and enumeration of vertebral segments at the level imaged. Accurate numbering is critical, especially if surgery is planned, and particularly in the

thoracic and lumbar levels where there can be one too many or one too few vertebrae.

Risks

Plain imaging exposes the patient to ionizing radiation and should be avoided in the pregnant woman if at all possible. Plain X-rays are the least sensitive of the imaging modalities in terms of determining the cause of the patient's symptoms. As is the case with other imaging techniques, plain imaging can suggest false leads and is more likely to provide false reassurance.

Radionuclide imaging
Introduction

There are three radioisotopes that are used in scanning the spine: technetium-99 m (^{99m}Tc) is used most commonly; gallium-67 (^{67}Ga); and occasionally radioisotope-labelled white blood cells, often with indium-111 (^{111}In). Radionuclide imaging is a good technique for detecting bone and some soft tissue abnormalities. Interruption of blood flow or reduced metabolic activity can result in decreased activity on a bone scan, while increased metabolic bone or inflammatory processes can increase uptake and scan activity. ^{99m}Tc and ^{67}Ga can both identify tumors and areas of active inflammation including infection. Routine radionuclide studies record the images in anterior and posterior views only. Imaging can focus on a single part of the patient's anatomy or their entire body. Single photon emission computed tomography (SPECT) uses CT methodology to take sliced images of a specific region in axial (transverse), sagittal, and/or coronal planes. SPECT imaging can be obtained using ^{99m}Tc or ^{67}Ga isotopes.

Positron emission tomography (PET) is a nuclear medicine study that usually uses the glucose analog fluorodeoxyglucose labeled with the radioactive isotope ^{18}F to detect cancer throughout the body and can be used to look for bone abnormalities in patients with unexplained spine pain, especially in patients with a history of cancer.

How is the procedure performed?

The radionuclide is given by intravenous infusion. Immediate imaging (a radionuclide angiogram), imaging after several minutes, and again 2–4 hours after injection is termed a "three-phase study." Occasionally, images are obtained 18–24 hours after injection. There is no preparation, but the patient does receive a small dose of radiation internally. Radionuclide imaging of pregnant women is not advised.

Helpful aspects

Radionuclide imaging of the spine is very helpful in diagnosing primary metastatic tumors (with the exception of multiple myeloma), infection, fractures (especially stress fractures and fractures of complex structures), arthritis, generalized bone disease associated with metabolic abnormalities (but not osteoporosis), and other conditions such as Paget disease of bone, sickle cell disease, and osteonecrosis due to bone infarction. ^{99m}Tc SPECT imaging is especially useful in the detection of pars interarticularis fractures resulting in spondylolysis, and a positive SPECT scan can help determine if radiographic spondylolysis is symptomatic (see Figure 5.5). A positive radionuclide bone scan in compression fracture can help to predict a beneficial response to vertebroplasty. Radionuclide scans are helpful in diagnosing disk space infection with a sensitivity of greater than 90%. Additional ^{67}Ga imaging may increase the specificity of a positive ^{99m}Tc scan in discitis. Osteomyelitis is more likely if ^{67}Ga activity is greater than that of ^{99m}Tc. ^{99m}Tc activity occurs earlier than plain X-ray abnormalities in many conditions such as metastatic tumors, osteomyelitis, arthritis, and bone trauma including stress fracture.

Less helpful aspects

Radionuclide studies are very sensitive but often non-specific. They do not provide the pathoanatomic detail of MRI and CT. Nevertheless, radionuclide imaging may show abnormalities before other imaging techniques, especially those that are X-ray-based, reveal them. In general, if the radionuclide study is positive, additional testing or correlation with other imaging studies is needed in order to reach a diagnosis. Radionuclide studies can also be used to follow inflammatory, infectious, traumatic, metabolic, and neoplastic bone disease. Radionuclide scans are not helpful for osteoporosis in the absence of fracture.

Spinal angiography
Introduction

Transfemoral selective angiography of the spinal cord blood supply can be performed.

How is the procedure performed?

Transfemoral catheterization under local anesthesia and mild sedation allows for selective angiography of a vertebral artery and the upper (cephalad) formation of the anterior spinal artery or, more commonly, the major supply to the lower end of the vessel through the aorta and artery of Adamkiewicz.

Helpful aspects

Spinal angiography can aid materially in establishing the mechanism of spinal cord infarction and in the diagnosis of and planning for surgical treatment of spinal cord vascular malformations including dural arteriovenous fistulas.

Risks

The main complications are local bleeding in the groin, rare instances of thrombosis of the femoral artery, and infarctions in the territories being examined with the angiogram, in this instance the spinal cord.

Physiologic testing
Electromyography (EMG) and nerve conduction studies (NCS)
Introduction

The most serious problems in the spine and the ones that most frequently require intervention are those related to compression of the spinal cord, cauda equina, or individual spinal nerve roots. It is important to know how these nervous structures are functioning. The history and especially the neurologic examination tell us a lot about how these structures are functioning, but electrophysiologic testing can enhance our understanding. Electromyography (EMG) and nerve conduction studies (NCS) can inform us about the status of the anterior horn cells, spinal nerve roots, spinal nerves, plexi, and peripheral nerves. Somatosensory evoked potentials and motor evoked potentials help to assess the central nervous system, especially the spinal cord. Some of the findings, especially those on EMG, are delayed in their onset, and interpretation of the findings is dependent on the expertise and thoroughness of the person performing the study. Nonetheless, neurophysiologic testing can be very helpful by providing objective information about the presence of, extent and severity of, and prognosis for neurologic deficits.

Electromyography

Electromyography and NCS are typically performed together but in the evaluation of radiculopathy the EMG part of the exam is generally more helpful. EMG consists of placing a needle electrode into skeletal muscle and asking the patient to contract their

97

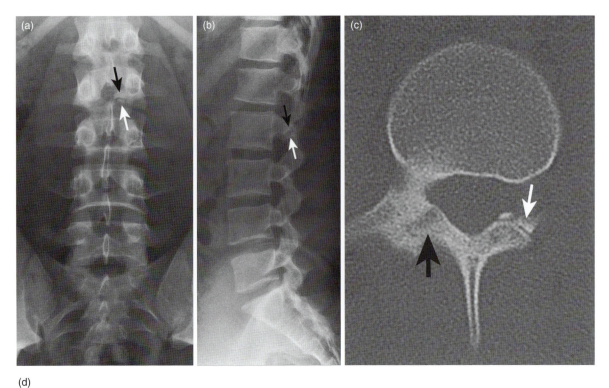

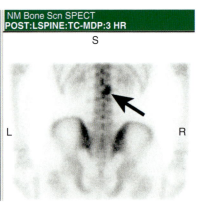

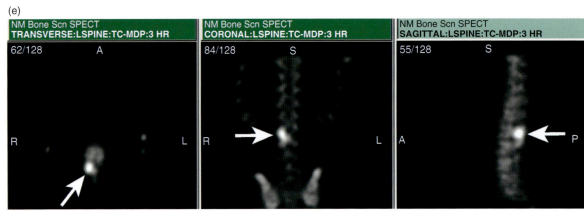

Figure 5.5.

muscle and poking the needle electrode into the muscle when it is at rest. The resulting electrical activity is displayed on a monitor and the audible signal of the activity is played over a loudspeaker to assist in the interpretation by the electromyographer. With increasing levels of contraction, individual motor units fire more rapidly and then additional motor units are recruited. The combination of multiple motor units firing at an acceptable rate in a sustained fashion results in a normal electrophysiologic pattern. Abnormalities in the duration, amplitude, shape, and recruitment of motor unit action potentials can help to determine if there is lower motor neuron or primary muscle disease. The EMG can also help determine if the nerve damage is chronic or recovering.

Characteristic changes of denervation

Typically, normal muscle is silent at rest. Fibrillation potentials are spontaneous discharges of individual muscle cells seen with muscle denervation, usually due to conditions affecting the lower motor neuron; they can also be seen with some muscle diseases, especially inflammatory muscle disease (myositis). Fasciculations represent the spontaneous discharge and contraction of individual motor units; they can be seen with abnormalities of the lower motor neuron but can also be seen in patients without any associated disease. In normal muscle, the insertion and movement of the needle electrode causes only very brief electrical activity. Prolonged insertional activity or the presence of specific electrical activity such as positive waves can be seen in denervated muscles and in some muscle conditions, much like fibrillation potentials. Reduced or absent insertional activity may occur in severely atrophied muscles. EMG evidence of denervation (particularly fibrillation potentials) may take 2–4 weeks to develop. Therefore, EMG is best performed 3–4 weeks after the onset of symptoms to allow these electrophysiologic changes in muscle to develop.

In radiculopathy, fibrillations usually appear first in more proximal muscles, such as the paraspinals, and later in limb muscles. Reinnervation occurs in a similar proximal to distal sequence. The diagnosis of radiculopathy by EMG requires the presence of neurogenic findings in two or more muscles innervated by the same nerve root but different peripheral nerves. Involvement of the paraspinal muscles in addition to the limb muscles (or intercostal or abdominal muscles in the case of thoracic radiculopathy) helps to confirm that the pathologic process is occurring at the level of the spinal nerve root or spinal nerve and before the spinal nerve has divided into ventral and dorsal rami. Previous spine surgery itself can cause neurogenic EMG changes in paraspinal muscles so they cannot be reliably used to test for evidence of denervation and are therefore typically not sampled in the patient with prior back surgery at the segmental level of prior surgery. Some EMG changes, such as fibrillation potentials, may disappear as reinnervation occurs, while chronic neurogenic motor unit action potentials may persist indefinitely. Lack of complete reinnervation and chronic neurogenic changes despite apparent reinnervation make the interpretation of subsequent EMG testing for radiculopathy more challenging. Also, fibrillation potentials can occasionally be seen in lumbar and less commonly in cervical paraspinal muscles in asymptomatic, older people, in patients with localized spine disease (e.g., facet arthropathy) and in other conditions such as myositis. Paraspinal fibrillation potentials may not necessarily be present in all cases of documented radiculopathy possibly due to technical issues, sampling error, and sometimes because of early reinnervation. Also, because of overlapping levels of segmental innervation, paraspinal muscle abnormalities cannot be localized to a single spinal level. For these reasons, EMG testing of the paraspinal muscles is less helpful than testing the limb muscles.

Nerve conduction studies

Motor and sensory nerve conduction studies are performed by stimulating a nerve at one or more different points and recording the response over a

Caption for Figure 5.5. Left L2 spondylolysis and right L2 pars interarticularis stress reaction. (a) Anteroposterior and (b) lateral plain X-rays show left L2 spondylolysis with sclerotic margins suggesting chronicity (arrows). (c) Axial CT image shows spondylolysis of the left L2 pars interarticularis (small white arrow) and sclerosis and subtle lucency suggesting spondylolysis of the right L2 pars interarticularis (large black arrow). (d) Anteroposterior (left) and posteroanterior (right) ^{99m}Tc bone scan images reveal intense delayed uptake in the right posterior element of the L2 vertebral body (arrow). (e) Three SPECT images show radiotracer uptake on axial (transverse), coronal, and sagittal views (arrows). This 17-year-old military recruit developed right upper lumbar pain after a long run with a 50-pound pack. He was diagnosed as having an acute right L2 pars interarticularis stress reaction that could evolve into spondylosis such as he already has on the left side at this level. He did well with activity modification, exercises, and temporary use of a lumbar corset.

distal muscle or proximal or distal nerve. A conduction velocity is calculated by dividing the distance between two stimulation points along the same nerve by the difference in time it takes for the two stimuli to reach a common end point. A distal motor latency represents the time for terminal conduction through nerve, neuromuscular junction, and muscle from a fixed distance; since the conduction times through these structures are not uniform, this cannot accurately be expressed as a conduction velocity. Sensory conduction can be measured as a conduction velocity or latency; since conduction is relatively uniform in sensory nerves, a single point of stimulation can be used for measuring both. The amplitude of motor (compound motor action potential or CMAP) and sensory (sensory nerve action potential or SNAP) responses are measured and compared to data from controls as well as the patient's contralateral side. Changes in CMAP are uncommon in radiculopathy unless the motor deficit is severe. The SNAPs are even less likely to be affected in radiculopathy. Only rarely when the dorsal root ganglion is compressed will the amplitude of the SNAP be reduced.

Additional tests which are sometimes utilized in electrodiagnostic testing include the H-reflex and the F-wave, so-called late responses. The H-reflex is the electrodiagnostic equivalent of a deep tendon reflex; for all practical purposes, its utility is limited to the S1 segment. However, the H-reflex may be absent in normal individuals. An F-wave assesses single motor axons conducting antidromically to the anterior horn cell and then orthodromically back down the nerve to the muscle. F waves can help assess proximal nerve fiber function more commonly in diffuse polyradiculopathies than in compressive lesions of single roots. Finally, repetitive nerve stimulation can be used to look for defects in neuromuscular transmission such as myasthenia gravis and myasthenic syndrome.

In sum, with radiculopathy, CMAP is infrequently reduced in the affected myotome. While the H-reflex may be abnormal and is frequently absent in S1 segment lesions, it adds little because it is the equivalent of the ankle reflex. Otherwise, motor and sensory conduction studies are generally normal in radiculopathy and spinal cord compression.

How is the procedure performed?

There is no preparation for EMG and NCS. The test is somewhat painful. Young children may need sedation. The needle EMG testing can cause minor bleeding and caution is urged in the testing of patients on anticoagulants. Patients who are on warfarin should have their prothrombin time checked; needle examination is usually deferred in patients with International Normalized Ratio (INR) >3 and limited to some extent in patients with a therapeutic INR of 2–3 (e.g., certain muscles such as paraspinal muscles are typically not examined).

Helpful aspects

Electrodiagnostic testing can be very helpful in the patient with undiagnosed limb pain where there is a suspicion of cervical or lumbar radiculopathy. In this circumstance, EMG and NCS may confirm the presence of radiculopathy, establish the level or levels of involvement, help judge the severity of the radiculopathy, estimate its age, help determine if reinnervation is taking place, and, most importantly, exclude other peripheral nerve and myopathic conditions which could explain the patient's symptoms and mimic nerve root, spinal cord, or cauda equina compression. In the patient with axial spine pain alone, EMG and NCS are unlikely to be helpful and may provide misleading information. In the patient who has had symptoms for 2 or 3 weeks or less, EMG is often best deferred. However, NCS can show evidence of a generalized peripheral neuropathy or a focal neuropathy (for example, peripheral entrapment neuropathies or mononeuritis multiplex). Early testing can also establish pre-existing EMG changes which can be particularly helpful in medical-legal situations. Electrodiagnostic testing may also be helpful in the patient who cannot undergo MRI or in whom imaging studies are normal, inconclusive, or show multiple findings. Based on the presence and distribution of neurogenic EMG changes, the absence of myopathic abnormalities, and normal nerve conduction velocity testing, the person performing EMG and NCS can often determine if the patient has a radiculopathy and which nerve root is involved. Although electrodiagnostic testing can identify the location and severity of such nerve injury, it cannot determine its cause.

Less helpful aspects

Similar to the imaging studies described above, EMG and NCS can provide misleading data. The studies will be normal when the patient's symptoms of pain and numbness reflect injury of sensory structures proximal to the dorsal root ganglion only. The studies may also show abnormalities due to prior disease (e.g., old radiculopathy) or concurrent conditions which, though present, are not necessarily responsible for the patient's symptoms (e.g., asymptomatic carpal tunnel syndrome). EMG findings of denervation will only be present if the nerve root is sufficiently compressed to cause denervation. EMG and NCS are very much dependent on the person conducting the study. The electromyographer decides what muscles and nerves to test, and the EMG findings are subject to interpretation. Unlike the situation with an MRI or CT, where one can review the images and make one's own judgment, the ordering provider is dependent on the electromyographer's report of the findings and interpretation of the EMG more so than NCS. EMG tends to be a lagging indicator of nerve function. Notwithstanding these caveats, electrodiagnostic testing can be very helpful in diagnosing acute and subacute radiculopathy. EMG can also be helpful in the diagnosis of lumbar spinal stenosis if it shows evidence of chronic neurogenic changes in multiple lumbosacral nerve roots, usually bilaterally.

Risks
Aside from pain and minor local bleeding from the needle EMG examination, there are no risks.

Somatosensory evoked potentials (SSEPs) and motor evoked potentials (MEPs)
Introduction
Somatosensory evoked potentials can be used in awake patients for assessment of central conduction of large sensory fibers that travel in the posterior columns to the brain. They can help to determine if there is a disturbance of posterior column function in the spinal cord or brain, but their ability to localize is limited and dependent on the ability of the peripheral nervous system to transmit sensory information to the central nervous system. SSEPs are not particularly helpful in diagnosing radiculopathy. SSEPs can be abnormal in the presence of focal spinal cord disease (e.g., tumors, spondylotic myelopathy) and diffuse spinal cord damage (e.g., hereditary ataxias, subacute combined degeneration). SSEPs are used to help determine prognosis in post-ischemic encephalopathy where absence of a cortical response to median nerve stimulation predicts an outcome no better than a persistent vegetative state. MEPs have no utility in diagnosing

radiculopathy, but can be helpful in documenting spinal cord dysfunction in multiple sclerosis, cervical spondylotic myelopathy, following trauma, and other conditions.

How is the procedure performed?
Somatosensory evoked potentials are performed by repetitively stimulating the median or ulnar nerve in the upper limb or posterior tibial or common peroneal nerve in the lower extremity while recording over proximal nerves or plexi, spine, and scalp. Evoked potentials from these stimuli are very small and must be averaged to improve the signal to noise ratio and allow the responses to be clearly identified. The procedure causes patients some discomfort. MEPs are produced by electrical stimulation through a cutaneous electrode or by using surface magnetic stimulation, which is much less painful. Either the motor cortex or the cervical spinal cord can be stimulated. With both techniques multiple descending motor pathways are stimulated. MEPs are recorded from surface or needle electrodes in target muscles or over the distal spinal cord. Prolonged latency of the evoked potential is more significant than reduced amplitude and can indicate myelopathy but does not indicate its cause.

Helpful aspects
Somatosensory evoked potentials and MEPs have very limited utility in the diagnostic work-up of the patient presenting with myelopathy. They can confirm the presence of spinal cord dysfunction which is usually evident on neurologic examination. They are sometimes used in the patient with suspected multiple sclerosis to look for evidence of myelopathy when none is present on examination or MRI. They have a greater role in the intraoperative monitoring of patients undergoing spinal surgery. In this role, the two studies are complementary.

Risks
Aside from discomfort, there are essentially no risks associated with MEPs or SSEPs. MEPs can rarely provoke seizures in seizure-prone individuals. Magnetic stimulation generates heat in the stimulating coil, which can cause local skin problems.

Visual evoked potentials (VEPs) and brain stem auditory evoked potentials (BAEPs)
Visual evoked potentials and BAEPs assess physiologic function of the visual and auditory pathways in

or without a local anesthetic. Even when spinal injections are performed mostly for therapeutic purposes (with the use of a corticosteroid), there is a strong and understandable temptation to use the patient's response as a diagnostic aid. Ideally, the injections should be given in a double-blind, controlled fashion, but this is rarely done. It is difficult to use local anesthetics in a blinded fashion because the active drug causes local or regional numbness. One can use different local anesthetics with different durations of action in a blinded fashion. In this situation, the patient's pain relief should be longer for longer-lasting local anesthetics and shorter for those with shorter durations of action. Again, this is rarely done. In general, the use of diagnostic/therapeutic injections is more established for use in the lumbar than cervical than thoracic levels. Injections into the spine should be performed with X-ray guidance and typically with instillation of contrast material to ensure the accuracy of needle placement and to ensure injected material does not disappear, indicating that the needle tip is in a vein. In general, spine imaging, usually with MRI, is a prerequisite to performing these injections. This is done to ensure that there is no serious structural problem including tumor or infection where placement of a needle and injection might be hazardous. The need to perform an MRI before injecting the spine means that our best diagnostic study has been obtained before the diagnostic/therapeutic injection. As a result, if we feel the patient might benefit from an injection now, we must obtain the MRI (or other imaging study) before it is indicated or truly necessary. Such premature imaging carries with it the risks of finding a problem (think big disk) which explains the patient's symptoms but would have resolved on its own with conservative treatment, or discovering an incidental, asymptomatic, possibly significant abnormality. Because the MRI has already been obtained, when injections are used only for diagnostic purposes they are usually performed in patients with multiple findings, equivocal findings, or a paucity of findings on their MRI.

Localization of the patient's pain generator with the use of local anesthetics and corticosteroid injections is complicated by the fact that locally placed corticosteroids can have regional and systemic effects. A genuine placebo effect can confound interpretation. Finally, it is important to keep in mind that blocking a nerve may relieve pain from a more distant site or structure. For example, epidural anesthetics are used to relieve the pain of childbirth, but no one believes that this pain is coming from the spine.

Structures and areas that can be injected for diagnostic purposes include the epidural space adjacent to individual spinal nerves, more widespread epidural injections, the spinal joints (facet and sacroiliac joints), the medial branches of dorsal rami that innervate the facet joints, and trigger points of pain usually within muscle. In general, the risk of these various injections is relatively low and includes local pain, inadvertent puncture of the dura with postspinal headache, a small risk of infection, a low risk of nerve root injury, and transient systemic effects of injected corticosteroids. Facet blocks will be discussed in further detail.

Facet joint interventions

The spinal facet joints are richly innervated, subject to degenerative joint disease, and are a significant potential source of spine pain. Some have estimated that 15% of younger and 40% of older patients have low back pain of facet joint origin. However, the existence and clinical characteristics of a facet joint syndrome are uncertain.

Injections can be made directly into the facet joints themselves or near the medial branches of the dorsal rami of the spinal nerves at and above one or more facet joints on one or both sides. Each facet joint receives sensory innervation from the medial branch of the spinal level at and one above the joint. If these injections are temporarily beneficial, radiofrequency lesioning of the appropriate nerves is performed at a later date.

How is the procedure performed?

With the patient prone and under fluoroscopic X-ray guidance and sterile conditions, the spinal needle is placed into a facet joint or the predicted position of the appropriate medial branches. Administration of contrast is utilized to confirm accurate needle placement and exclude venous uptake. While not always utilized, control blocks (placebo versus local anesthetic) and/or comparative local anesthetic blocks (comparing the patient's response to the expected duration of benefit from different injected local anesthetics) can be employed. Whether based on the patient's benefit from the facet joint or medial branch diagnostic blocks, a similar procedure directed at the appropriate medial branches is performed, but instead of injection, a radiofrequency neurotomy is performed utilizing an electrical current at the tip of a needle electrode. The patient should be conscious for all of these procedures.

Helpful aspects

Radiofrequency neurotomy of the medial branches of the dorsal rami may be helpful for patients with chronic, very significant axial spine pain who have failed other treatments. In the cervical spine, the treatment may be especially helpful for pain after whiplash-type injury. If obtained, benefits are typically not permanent; these are short nerves that can regenerate. Authors stress the need to carefully select patients who undergo this procedure. Control and/or comparative blocks prior to radiofrequency lesioning of nerves are strongly encouraged to winnow out placebo responders. The medial branches also supply some paraspinal muscles in addition to the facet joints, and it is not clear that facet joint denervation is the mechanism of benefit. Radiofrequency lesioning of the medial branches of the dorsal rami is controversial; there is no other joint in the body that is denervated in an effort to provide pain relief. There is at least some theoretical reason not to denervate joints; joints that have lost their sensory nerve supply are subject to accelerated, neuropathic degeneration (Charcot joint).

Risks

Temporary and more permanent lesioning of medial branch nerves can cause local pain, infection, rare damage to more important nerve structures, and rare skin burns.

Other diagnostic studies

Bone densitometry

Plain X-rays give some unreliable information about bone density. There are several methods for measuring bone density more precisely. The methods include dual-energy X-ray absorptiometry (DXA), single-energy X-ray absorptiometry, quantitative computed tomography (QCT), and ultrasound which measure how bone attenuates different forms of energy. DXA more often than QCT is the most commonly used. QCT may provide more information and have better predictive value for spine fracture, but costs more and exposes the patient to much more radiation. Hip and lumbar spine are usually tested, although any bone can be used. Results are compared to age- and sex-matched normative data and can be repeated over time. Hypertrophic degenerative changes in the spine

can lead to falsely increased bone density determinations at that site. Nonetheless, bone densitometry testing of the spine can be helpful to the spine surgeon in deciding if there is sufficient bone mass to support metallic implants or an artificial disk. Osteoporosis in and of itself does not cause spine pain, but can lead to fracture. If osteoporosis is discovered, additional testing may be indicated to determine if there is an underlying cause (see Table 1.5). The procedures are noninvasive; all but ultrasound expose the patient to a small amount of radiation.

Noninvasive lower limb arterial testing

Exercise assessment of lower extremity circulation is a noninvasive test that can help determine whether or not a patient's walking-induced lower limb symptoms are due to true vascular claudication or pseudoclaudication due to lumbar spinal stenosis. If the patient is unable to exercise on a treadmill because of symptoms, they can be tested using a sitting or recumbent bicycle, which allows their lumbar spine to be in flexion and reduces the likelihood of provoking spinal stenosis-related symptoms.

Blood tests

Blood tests such as white blood count, sedimentation rate, and C-reactive protein can serve as nonspecific indicators of underlying inflammatory disease. Rheumatoid factor and HLA-B27 antigen determination can help in the diagnosis of rheumatoid arthritis and spondyloarthropathy respectively. Vitamin B_{12}, folate, NMO immune globulin G antibodies (for neuromyelitis optica), HTLV-1 serology, HIV serology, serum copper, vitamin E, very long chain fatty acid determination, angiotensin-converting enzyme level (for sarcoidosis), tests for systemic autoimmune diseases (antinuclear, anti-double-stranded DNA, extractable nuclear, and anti-ribonucleoprotein antibodies), paraneoplastic antibodies (for remote effect of occult malignancy), syphilis serology, and Lyme and ehrlichiosis serologies can be obtained, looking for metabolic and infectious causes of myelopathy and radiculopathy. Enzyme and genetic tests are available for some hereditary diseases that affect the spinal cord such as for several spinocerebellar ataxia syndromes. Tumor markers can be helpful if metastatic tumor is suspected.

Cerebrospinal fluid (CSF) examination

Cerebrospinal fluid analysis is helpful in the diagnosis of multiple sclerosis, infectious diseases, chronic inflammatory demyelinating polyradiculoneuropathy, malignancy that invades the meninges, and other conditions. Testing includes CSF cell count, protein, glucose (and its comparison to a concomitant blood sugar), gamma globulin determination, oligoclonal bands, cultures, antibody testing, polymerase chain reaction (PCR) testing for infectious agents, and cytologic examination.

Biopsy of the spine

Imaging guidance allows for safe needle biopsy or aspiration of suspicious tissue and fluid in and around the spine. Culture material can be obtained via closed biopsy and infections confirmed and sensitivities to antibiotics determined. Biopsy of suspicious mass lesions in or near the spine can provide a diagnosis and either obviate the need for an open procedure or help plan an open operation. Bone biopsy, such as of the posterior iliac crest, can be performed in order to assess generalized bone disease. Percutaneous biopsy should be performed with caution on vertebral lesions with extensive destruction (where collapse or instability could ensue) or if there is a risk of uncontrolled bleeding such as with a very vascular lesion or in a patient who is anticoagulated.

How is the procedure performed?

Patients should not eat before the procedure. They can be given a sedative and an analgesic. Local anesthesia down to the periosteum of the bone to be sampled is given. The patient is usually prone and imaging guidance is employed to ensure the lesion is sampled and no critical structures encountered. The patient is observed for some hours after the procedure to ensure no complications occur. Pain, local infection, bleeding, bony collapse, and, theoretically, spread of infection or tumor can occur. Of course, needle biopsy or aspiration of the spine would be unnecessary if a more easily accessible lesion were available for sampling.

Urine and urologic tests

Urinalysis can be helpful if a genitourinary cause for the patient's pain is suspected. Protein analysis of the urine can be helpful in patients with multiple myeloma. Urodynamic study of the bladder can help determine if there is upper motor neuron, lower motor neuron, sensory, or sphincter dysfunction. Postvoid residual can be measured by catheterization

or ultrasound of the just-emptied bladder. Inability to completely empty the bladder can be due to neurogenic changes or outlet obstruction.

Spinal cord and/or nerve root biopsy

Biopsy of one of the intradural nerve roots, the exiting spinal nerves, or the spinal cord can be performed. Such biopsies are infrequently needed. While sometimes associated with indeterminate pathology, the results can be diagnostic. These biopsies are discussed further in Chapter 10.

Further reading

1. Bigos S, Bowyer O, Braen G, et al. *Acute Low Back Problems in Adults: Clinical Practice Guideline No. 14.* AHCPR Publication No. 95-0642. Rockville, Maryland: Agency for Health Care Policy and Research, Public Health Service, U.S. Department of Health and Human Services. December 1994.

2. Bigos S, Bowyer O, Braen G, et al. *Acute Low Back Problems in Adults: Clinical Practice Guideline, Quick Reference Guide Number 14.* AHCPR Pub. No. 95-0643. Rockville, Maryland: Agency for Health Care Policy and Research, Public Health Service, U.S. Department of Health and Human Services. December 1994.

3. Bolton CF, Cascino GD, Daube JR, Sharbrough FW. *Electrodiagnosis in Clinical Neurology,* Fifth Edition. Philadelphia, Pennsylvania: Elsevier Churchill-Livingstone, 2005.

4. Borenstein DG, Wiesel SW, Boden SD. *Low Back and Neck Pain: Comprehensive Diagnosis and Management*, Third Edition. Philadelphia, Pennsylvania: Elsevier Inc., 2004.

5. Carragee EJ, Lincoln T, Parmar VS, Alamin T. A gold standard evaluation of the "discogenic pain" diagnosis as determined by provocative discography. *Spine* 2006; **31**(18):2115–2123.

6. Castillo M. *Neuroradiology Companion: Methods, Guidelines, and Imaging Fundamentals.* Philadelphia, Pennsylvania: Lippincott Williams & Wilkins, 2006.

7. Daube, JR. *Clinical Neurophysiology*, Second Edition. New York: Oxford University Press, Inc, 2002.

8. Kumar N, ed. Spinal cord, root, and plexus disorders. *Continuum Lifelong Learning Neurol* 2008; **14**(3):1–271.

9. Mettler FA, Guiberteau MJ. *Essentials of Nuclear Medicine Imaging*, Fifth Edition. Philadelphia, PA: Saunders Elsevier, 2006.

10. Prince MR, Zhang H, Morris M, et al. Incidence of nephrogenic systemic fibrosis at two large medical centers. *Radiology* 2008; **248**:807–816.

11. Rydahl C, Thomsen HS, Marckmann P. High prevalence of nephrogenic systemic fibrosis in chronic renal failure patients exposed to gadodiamide, a gadolinium-containing magnetic resonance contrast agent. *Invest Radiol* 2008; **43**(2):141–144.

12. Thomsen HS. ESUR Guideline: gadolinium-based contrast media and nephrogenic systemic fibrosis. *Eur Radiol* 2007; **17**:2692–2696.

13. Van Goethem JWM, van den Hauwe L, Parizel PM. *Spinal Imaging: Diagnostic Imaging of the Spine and Spinal Cord.* New York: Springer, 2007.

Chapter 6

When and to whom to refer your patients for spine surgery

Introduction

Occasionally, surgery on the spine is lifesaving. Much more frequently, surgery on the spine preserves or restores quality of life. Thus, a decision to operate on the spine and the surgery itself can be life-changing. On the other hand, in many situations, surgery on the spine is unlikely to help the patient and subjects the patient to possible worsening of their condition, a decline in their quality of life, and sometimes death. Whether or not to operate on a spine patient, what operation to perform, and when to perform it are critically important decisions. These decisions are just as important if not more important than the surgeon's skill in determining the patient's outcome. This chapter will summarize the indications for surgery that have been described in Chapters 2, 3, and 4 regarding the cervical, thoracic, and lumbar spine and constitute the "when to refer your patients for spine surgery."

Some patients clearly should be strongly considered for spine surgery, and for others spine surgery is clearly best avoided. There is a large gray zone of patients in whom surgery on the spine is elective or of uncertain benefit. All patients need to be fully informed about the risks, hoped-for benefits, and likely outcomes before they actually undergo spine surgery. For most spine operations, the patient has a deciding vote about whether or not to undergo surgery and, if so, when the operation should be performed. Just as important as when to operate on your patient is to whom you should refer the patient for possible surgery. The judgment of the surgeon about which patient should have surgery, what operation they should have, and the surgeon's skill in operating are critical to a successful outcome. This chapter will suggest criteria for selecting a surgeon to whom to refer your patient for possible surgery on the spine.

The indications for surgery and to whom to refer your patients for spine surgery are arguably the most important topics covered in this entire book. The main focus of this chapter is to whom to refer your patients for possible spine surgery. The fact that this

chapter is one of the shortest illustrates the fact that it is very difficult to determine who is the best surgeon to decide if surgery is needed and perform the best operation for an individual patient. In fact, the surgeon who is the best judge of the need for surgery may be different from the surgeon with the best operative technique. For all intents and purposes we refer our patients to a single surgeon for both purposes. There is precious little information to guide us in determining who the best surgeons are for specific operations. There is only a little more information on outcomes based on the hospital where the spine surgery is performed. However, the best surgeon may or may not operate at the best hospital, and some spine operations are now being performed as same-day surgery on an outpatient basis in ambulatory surgical centers, and, in general, we have fewer data regarding outpatient facilities.

If you are a surgeon, you might be tempted to skip this chapter, but the questions posed are ones you should be asked and will be expected to answer, preferably with data rather than anecdotes. Whether you are a surgeon or a nonsurgical provider, these are questions that patients need to ask us.

When to refer your patients for spine surgery

For some spine conditions, it is obvious that a patient needs the help of a surgeon, but for many conditions that affect the spine, surgery is either elective or controversial. This section will present general considerations about when to refer your patient for spine surgery, then specific indications for surgical referral based on the information presented in Chapters 2, 3, and 4.

General considerations

There are three main situations when you need to obtain surgical consultation. The first is if you believe an operation is indicated or think one might be and need input from and action by a surgical colleague. The second situation is when you do not believe an operation is indicated, but you feel a need to have a spine surgeon confirm your advice (e.g., because you sense that the patient or perhaps their family thinks that an operation is needed). A third situation is when you do not believe that an operation is indicated, but you, the patient, their family, or sometimes their employer requests a surgical opinion. In both the second and third situations, you should choose a surgeon who, in your experience, thinks like you do and will reinforce your recommendation not to have an operation. There is a fourth situation in which you might want to refer a patient to a spine surgeon and that is for their help in diagnosis. In many practice settings, spine surgeons are very knowledgeable about the diagnosis of spine and limb pain, and referral to a spine surgeon who is experienced in the diagnosis and nonoperative and operative treatment of spine patients for a second opinion can be very helpful to you and your patient.

Nonspondylotic conditions that can occur at any spinal level

In the course of evaluating patients with spine and limb pain, you will surely discover patients with infection such as an epidural abscess, or more likely a disk space infection. These patients require urgent culture and possible drainage. Any level of the spine can be affected. Disk space infection and/or osteomyelitis requires culture which can be performed by a spine surgeon or an interventional radiologist. Such cultures are often acquired using CT guidance. An abscess may require surgical drainage and is often performed on an urgent or emergent basis. Usually, time is of the essence in these situations, and accessibility is more important than the individual to whom you refer the patient. Often in this setting, the patient is referred to a hospital for triage, consultation, diagnostic testing, and treatment, which is frequently undertaken on an inpatient basis.

In the course of evaluating patients with spine and limb pain and neurologic symptoms, you will undoubtedly diagnose tumors and tumor-like conditions affecting the spinal cord, nerve roots, meninges, and adjacent musculoskeletal structures. Expanding mass lesions usually require biopsy and/or removal which will, in many instances, require referral to a spine surgeon, more often a neurosurgeon. Some patients such as those with primary or metastatic spinal canal tumors and a rapid downhill course may require urgent or emergent consultation with a spine surgeon. Some tumors such as vertebral body and paravertebral primary and metastatic tumors can be diagnosed by needle biopsy performed by an interventional radiologist using imaging guidance, usually with CT. Some conditions, such as leptomeningeal carcinomatosis or lymphomatosis, can be diagnosed with spinal fluid examination and do not require referral to a spine surgeon.

Fractures, especially compression fractures and occasionally fracture dislocations, are discovered by nonsurgeons. If there is neural compression or significant deformity, the patient will likely require referral to a spine surgeon, sometimes urgently and, in this instance, an orthopedic surgeon might be favored. Many benign compression fractures improve with conservative treatment and do not require surgical intervention. New techniques for treating thoracolumbar compression fractures with persistent pain and, to a lesser extent, kyphotic deformity (vertebroplasty and kyphoplasty) are available and can provide significant and prompt symptomatic benefit. These percutaneous injections of polymethylmethacrylate are usually performed by interventional radiologists but are sometimes performed by spine surgeons.

Specific indications for spine surgery and referral to a spine surgeon

The common indications for spine surgery (and referral to a spine surgeon) for cervical radiculopathy, myelopathy, and neck pain alone are included in this chapter in brief tabular form (see Tables 6.1, 6.2, and 6.3). Similarly, indications for surgery and surgical referral for the thoracic spine for radiculopathy, myelopathy, and mid back pain alone are shown in Tables 6.4, 6.5, and 6.6. Indications for surgery and possible referral to a spine surgeon for lumbar radiculopathy, lumbar spinal stenosis, cauda equina syndrome, and low back pain alone are presented in Tables 6.7, 6.8, 6.9, and 6.10. Uncommon conditions that may require surgery are not included in these tables. For some indications such as tumor and abscess, biopsy or culture may lead to nonoperative treatment.

To whom to refer your patients for spine surgery

Both orthopedic surgeons and neurosurgeons operate on the spine. Practice patterns vary from one community to another and between surgeons. As a rule,

Table 6.1. Indications for surgery for cervical radiculopathy

Tumor or abscess compressing cervical nerve root(s)

Fracture with demonstrated cervical root impingement and significant symptoms

For cervical spondylosis:

 Severe or progressive weakness of important upper limb muscles

 Persistent, significant upper limb pain with:

  Strong evidence for physiologic dysfunction of a specific cervical nerve root

 One of the above with confirmation of root compression on an imaging study

  Imaging study is usually an MRI

  Alternatively, CT myelogram or occasionally plain CT

Factors that can influence decision to operate:

 Concomitant spinal cord compression

 Large disk on imaging study

 Profound radicular pain

 Weakness is critical to patient's vocation or avocation

 Patient preference

 Weakness can be minimally symptomatic or asymptomatic

 Pain can lessen as root compression worsens

Table 6.2. Indications for surgery for cervical myelopathy

Tumor, abscess, or fracture compressing cervical spinal cord

For cervical spondylosis:

 Definitely for

  Moderate to severe neurologic deficits

  Documented progressive neurologic deficits

 Possibly for

  Mild signs and symptoms of myelopathy

 One of the above with evidence of compression of cervical spinal cord

  Imaging study is usually an MRI

  Alternatively, CT myelogram

Factors that can influence decision to operate:

 Young age

 Frequent falls

 Significant pain

 Increased T_2 signal in spinal cord on MRI

 Degree of cord compression

 Involvement of bowel and bladder

Table 6.3. Indications for surgery for neck pain alone

Tumor or abscess involving cervical spine

 Kyphoplasty and vertebroplasty can be used for benign and malignant bone lesions

Instability of cervical spine, for example due to trauma with fracture or spontaneous craniocervical or C1–C2 subluxation related to rheumatoid arthritis or ankylosing spondylitis

Fracture associated with imminent or potential neural compression

Questionably for cervical spondylosis alone (cervical disk, spondylosis, or cervical spinal stenosis without neurologic findings)

 Severity of imaging findings may influence decision

Options include fusion from anterior or posterior approach with or without instrumentation

Table 6.4. Indications for surgery for thoracic radiculopathy

Tumor or abscess compressing thoracic nerve root(s)

Fracture with demonstrated thoracic root impingement and persistent significant symptoms

For thoracic spondylosis:

 Persistent, significant radicular thoracic pain

  Unresponsive to nonsurgical treatment

  At least 4–6 weeks' duration

  At least moderately severe if not severe pain

 With evidence of significant compression of a thoracic nerve root usually by a large disk or possibly by osteophytic spur

  Imaging study is usually an MRI

  Alternatively, CT myelogram

Factors that can influence decision to operate:

 Thoracic myelopathy

 Spinal cord compression without myelopathy

Table 6.5. Indications for surgery for thoracic myelopathy

Tumor or abscess compressing thoracic spinal cord

Fractures including compression or burst fracture compressing thoracic spinal cord

Dural arteriovenous fistula and other arteriovenous malformations with myelopathy

For thoracic spondylosis:

 Persistent moderate to severe neurologic deficits

 Progressive neurologic deficits

 One of the above with evidence of compression of thoracic spinal cord

  Imaging study is usually an MRI

  Alternatively, CT myelogram

For fracture, X-rays and plain CT are useful

For dural arteriovenous fistulas, conventional and MR angiography can be helpful in addition to MRI or CT myelogram

Factors that can influence decision to operate:

Young age

Significant pain

Degree of cord compression

Involvement of bowel and bladder

Table 6.6. Indications for surgery for thoracic spine pain alone

Tumor or abscess involving thoracic spine

Kyphoplasty and vertebroplasty can be used for benign and malignant bone lesions

Severe or progressive scoliosis or kyphosis

Fracture including compression or burst fracture

Surgery may be required if there is instability or imminent neural compression

Consider vertebroplasty and kyphoplasty for compression fracture due to osteoporosis or another cause

Surgery for thoracic spondylosis and mid back pain alone is best avoided

Imaging confirmation of severe/progressive scoliosis or kyphosis, instability, or fracture

Plain films and CT can be used

MRI or CT myelogram used to exclude spinal cord compression

Table 6.7. Indications for surgery for lumbar radiculopathy

Tumor or abscess compressing lumbosacral root(s)

Fracture with demonstrated lumbosacral root impingement and significant symptoms

For lumbar spondylosis:

Severe or progressive weakness of important lower limb muscles

Persistent, significant sciatica usually with neurologic symptoms, if not signs

Pain and/or neurologic deficits persist for greater than 4–6 weeks

Pain and/or deficits progress

One of the above with confirmation of nerve root compression on an imaging study

Imaging study is usually an MRI

Alternatively, CT myelogram or occasionally plain CT

Factors than can influence decision to operate:

Evidence of cauda equina syndrome (CES)

Large disk on imaging study

Profound radicular pain

Involvement of two lumbosacral roots

Weakness is critical to patient's vocation or avocation

Patient preference

Weakness can be minimally symptomatic

Pain can lessen as root compression worsens

Table 6.8. Indications for surgery for lumbar spinal stenosis

Tumor causing lumbar spinal canal narrowing and symptoms

For spondylotic lumbar spinal stenosis:

Presence of pseudoclaudication symptoms for greater than 3 months

Pseudoclaudication symptoms significantly interfere with work or leisure activities and/or progressive neurologic deficits in the distribution of one or more lumbosacral nerve roots

Both of the above with imaging study showing evidence of significant lumbar spinal stenosis at one or more levels

Imaging study is usually an MRI

Alternatively, CT myelogram or occasionally plain CT

Patient is otherwise in good health

Patient elects surgical intervention with a full understanding of risks and hoped-for benefits which do not occur in all patients

Surgery for lumbar spinal stenosis for low back pain alone is generally not indicated

Table 6.9. Indications for surgery for cauda equina syndrome (CES)

Tumor or abscess affecting cauda equina

Fracture including compression or burst fracture with neural compression

Spondylolisthesis with CES

Lumbar spinal stenosis with CES

Synovial cyst with CES

Large lumbar disk herniation with CES

One of the above with imaging study confirming diagnosis

Imaging study is usually an MRI

Alternatively, CT myelogram or occasionally plain CT

Surgery is indicated for mild or worse and for progressive neurologic symptoms and signs

Urgent if not emergent surgery is appropriate if the CES is recent in onset or progressive or both

Table 6.10. Indications for surgery for low back pain alone

Tumor or abscess affecting lumbosacral spine and felt to be responsible for pain

> Kyphoplasty and vertebroplasty can be used for benign and malignant bone lesions

Fracture including compression or burst fracture

> Surgery may be required if there is instability or imminent neural compression

> Vertebroplasty or kyphoplasty can be considered for compression fracture due to osteoporosis or another cause

For spondylolisthesis

> Severe or progressive weakness

> Severe low back pain and/or sciatica for greater than 1 year

> Instability

Possibly for severe lumbar spondylosis alone limited to one or two levels

> Persistent, significant pain for greater than 1 year

> All other conservative measures have failed

One of the above with imaging studies confirming the diagnosis

> Imaging studies can include plain X-rays, MRI, CT myelogram or plain CT

Options include fusion with or without instrumentation for fracture, spondylolisthesis, and severe spondylosis and placement of an artificial disk for severe spondylosis alone

orthopedic surgeons are more apt to perform fusions, and neurosurgeons are more apt to perform decompressions. Also, as a rule, neurosurgeons are more likely to operate on patients with spine tumors.

What kind of a surgeon to choose

It is very helpful to have more than one surgical referral option. This includes having the option to refer to both an orthopedic surgeon and a neurosurgeon and to have more than one surgeon within each category. Your knowledge of the individual surgeon's practice and preferences is very useful. Some surgeons are more aggressive, and others are more conservative. As a rule, older surgeons tend to be somewhat more conservative than younger ones. Experience seems to make surgeons less likely to operate on patients with an equivocal indication for surgery.

It is very useful to have at least one more aggressive surgeon and one more conservative surgeon to whom to refer your patients. In the situation where you think that an operation is needed but the indication is soft, you might refer them to the more aggressive individual. Conversely, in the situation where you think the patient does not need surgery but you need to refer them to a spine surgeon for one or more of the reasons listed earlier in this chapter, you should choose a more conservative individual who will, hopefully, reinforce your recommendation to continue with medical management. Some surgeons are capable of performing instrumented fusions and placement of artificial disks, and others are not. Among surgeons who are capable of performing fusion, some have a tendency to perform more fusions, and some use fusion more judiciously. Your judgment about what kind of operation the patient should have can influence your referral choice based on the surgeon's ability and/or tendency to perform spinal fusion or placement of an artificial cervical or lumbar disk. If you feel the patient should be considered for a fusion or placement of an artificial disk, refer them to a surgeon who is capable of performing these operations and performs a lot of them. Conversely, if you feel that the patient would be better served by having decompression alone (or no surgery), refer them to a surgeon who either does not perform fusions or place artificial disks at all or disdains their use.

Of course, in some practice settings, your choice of a spine surgeon may be limited because there are not that many available, or restricted because you need to refer the patient to a colleague within your group practice or university or other healthcare system.

As mentioned above, there are situations where you do not think an operation is needed, but you need to refer the patient for a surgical consultation anyway. This may be because of patient and/or family pressure, or because of an imaging finding such as a large disk that does not need surgery, but you need to convince the patient and their family of this fact. You need to refer these patients to a conservative spine surgeon who will support your recommendation to continue observation with medical therapy and follow-up alone.

Objective criteria for selecting a spine surgeon

There are a number of criteria which are helpful in the selection of a spine surgeon for your patient or yourself! These include the surgeon's training: Where did they train? What is their specialty? Did they have subspecialty training in spine surgery that usually consists of at least 1 year of additional training dedicated to spine surgery? How long have they been in practice? Some would suggest that surgeons can be too young or too old. A surgeon who has just finished their training may be up to date on the most recent techniques but may be too eager to operate. A surgeon who has been in practice for 20 years or more may have greater wisdom and exercise better judgment. On the other hand, the older spine surgeon may not be up-to-date on new techniques and may have developed bad surgical habits or medical problems of their own. In the USA is the surgeon board eligible (if they are just out of training) or board certified in their surgical specialty (neurosurgery or orthopedic surgery)? Specialty Board eligibility and certification are important to verify that the surgeon has had appropriate training in spine surgery. You can check on a surgeon's specialty certification status by accessing the American Board of Medical Specialties' website at www.abms.org. How much of the surgeon's practice is devoted to spine surgery? Some authorities suggest that more spine work, especially if at least half of the surgeon's operating room time is spent on spine work, is preferable. What operations is the surgeon capable of performing? This information should be available from the surgeon and/or their office. More importantly, how many spine procedures of what type do they perform per year? How many operations of the kind that your patient needs do they perform per year? For every operative procedure examined in the USA, surgeon volume was inversely related to operative mortality. Other outcomes are less frequently studied. Unfortunately, outcomes from spine surgery have not been specifically examined even though they are frequently performed, especially in the USA. There is also evidence that high-volume hospitals have better outcomes above and beyond the contribution from high individual surgeon volumes. The effect of higher surgeon and hospital volume on outcomes is probably modest beyond an uncertain threshold. With regard to spine surgery, high volumes could indicate that the surgeon is performing too many unnecessary operations.

There are "who's who" publications that tout individual physicians in all different specialties. These listings are often based more on patient and peer opinion than on factual data. As a rule, very few surgeons are listed per geographic area. Listing in such a publication is an indication of respect and soft evidence in favor of current surgical expertise.

There is some other objective evidence that you may be able to obtain of a negative sort. Has the surgeon frequently relocated? This can be a red flag that the surgeon has run into problems with colleagues, clinics, hospitals, or state medical boards in previous practice settings. Have there been actions against them by their state medical boards in the state they now practice in or in states where they have practiced before? Some of this information can be obtained through websites run by the Federation of State Medical Boards. Through their main website (www.fsmb.org) or directly at www.docinfo.org, the Federation of State Medical Boards provides professional information on physicians and some physician assistants licensed in the USA. This includes information on disciplinary sanctions, education, medical specialty, licensure history, and practice locations. For a fee of $9.95 per profile ordered, the general public can determine if any state medical or osteopathic board in the USA has reported taking disciplinary action now or in the past against a specific physician. This includes their current and previous practice locations throughout the USA. Both websites also provide a list of and links to all state medical boards. Most state medical boards' websites allow the visitor to verify current licensure for individual physicians and provide some information about current and sometimes previous state board actions taken against the licensee. An additional website run by the Federation of State Medical Boards is available at their main website or directly at www.drdata.org. The so-called Federation Physician Data Center is a central repository for formal actions taken against physicians by state licensing and disciplinary boards, Canadian licensing authorities, the U.S. Armed Forces, the U.S. Department of Health and Human Services, and other national and international regulatory bodies. These data are used in credentialing of physicians and pre-employment background checks, but are only available to the agencies listed and private agencies and organizations involved in the employment and/or credentialing of physicians and therefore have limited access. The hospital(s) where the surgeon operates may also have a registry of complaints against the surgeon which might be difficult to access even if you are a physician on the staff of the same hospital!

Other information

Subjecting an individual's name to a search on a search engine such as Google on the Internet can provide useful information. The results are not vetted or screened in any way. The results might not even pertain to the person you or the patient is "Googling."

Some of the results may be favorable to the surgeon, which is helpful. There can be negative search results which may be very useful. For example, a claim or lawsuit may have been covered by a local newspaper but did not prompt action by the State Medical Board.

The surgeon's outcomes

The data that you would really like to have about your patient's surgeon (or your own surgeon) are what are their outcomes for the operation that is being considered? What are the length of stay, peri-operative morbidity and mortality, post-operative convalescence, satisfaction, and short- and long-term outcomes? Is pain reduced or eliminated? Is function improved or fully restored? This very important information is almost never available. There are many reasons why it is difficult to obtain this information, chief among them the fact that it is expensive to collect. Even if outcomes data are collected, to be relevant they must be risk adjusted, and there must be comparable data available for other possible surgical referral options. Even if all of these conditions are met, surgeons and hospitals are quite reluctant to share their data. If you are a provider, think about your own practice. Do you collect outcomes data on your patients? What kind of data? For how long? If you collect these data, are they risk adjusted? Do you have any ability to compare your outcomes to data from local, regional, and national peers? If this information were available, how willing would you be to share these data? Would you share them with your colleagues, your competitors, your referral sources, your patients, the hospitals where you work, and insurance companies? Would you worry that the risk adjustment did not reflect the fact that you see more difficult and sicker patients? Would you worry that other physicians gamed the system to make their data look better? Obtaining useful, valid, comparable data is very difficult; sharing them with others is even more difficult.

Your experience with a surgeon

While it is extremely difficult for a healthcare provider or a patient and their family to determine the operative outcomes and complications of an individual spine surgeon's practice, your personal experience as a colleague and referrer should be considered when sending future patients to a specific spine surgeon. These are probably the best data you are going to get and should be utilized. What is your experience with an individual surgeon? In general, do they agree with you about the need for surgery in most patients? Do they agree with you about the kind of surgery the patient should have? Do they perform too many fusions? Do they place too many artificial disks? Are they too aggressive? Or, are they too conservative, in your opinion? Do they too quickly incorporate new techniques into their practice, or do they stick with old techniques for too long in your estimation? What are the outcomes from the operations performed on your patients by this surgeon? Do they get along with the patients and their families that you have referred to them? Are they willing to answer multiple questions from patients and their families? Do they get along with you and other physicians? Is there good communication between the surgeon and the patient and their families and with you? Do you and the surgeon agree about who will follow the patient subsequently, both after a "no surgery" opinion and post-operatively? If requested by the patient and/or their family, are they open to a second surgical opinion?

Personality issues

In any line of work or walk of life, some people are better at getting along with their fellow human beings than others. This also applies to physicians and surgeons. Patients' interpersonal relationships are also quite variable. There are some personality characteristics that most people would agree are desirable in a surgeon. Some of these were mentioned in the preceding paragraph, and some are mentioned at the end of this chapter. These include affability, attentiveness, kindness, compassion, responsiveness, patience, and confidence. In addition, there may be specific personality characteristics of a surgeon that are better suited to some patients than others. For example, patients who are indecisive may do better with a surgeon who is emphatic in their recommendations. Conversely, some patients want to know about and study all possible treatment options, and they might do better with a surgeon who offers the patient more choice of options. Like surgeons, some patients are more aggressive and some more conservative regarding their own care. It is probably better to match aggressive patients with aggressive surgeons and conservative patients with conservative surgeons.

Ideally, we should refer the "right" patient to the "right" surgeon based on a good fit between their personalities. Unfortunately, matchmaking of this sort is very difficult. Physicians are not always good judges of their patients' or their colleagues' personalities, and it is not easy to predict which patient (and family) will hit it off with which surgeon. Nonetheless, the patients' and surgeons' personalities and emotional traits should be kept in mind when referring patients for possible spine surgery.

Patient/family/employer/third party payer input

The patient and/or their family may also weigh in with a strong preference for a specific spine surgeon to whom they wish to be referred. This can be based on the family's experience, word of mouth from friends, or the surgeon's reputation. Sometimes a family member works in a nearby medical center and has strong feelings about the surgeon to whom Mom or Dad should be referred or the hospital where the surgery should be performed. In general, the family's request should be honored unless the surgeon chosen does not perform the type of surgery the patient needs. The patient's employer or, more likely, their insurance plan is likely to restrict your choice of surgeon and, in some cases, mandate referral to a specific individual, group, or practice setting.

The surgeon's practice setting

The surgeon could practice in one of several different settings. They may be a solo practitioner or work in a small group practice restricted to one or two specialties (e.g., neurology and neurosurgery). They could be part of a large multispecialty group, or they could practice in a university setting. Distance from the patient's location to the surgeon also needs to be considered. The different practice settings and locations can influence your referral decision and/or the patient's choice. If you refer the patient to a solo or small specialty practice, it is very likely that the surgeon to whom you refer the patient will actually perform the operation that is recommended, and this might be an important consideration. Of course, it is also possible that the surgeon could fall ill or have a planned absence and turn the patient over to a colleague. Even with a large multispecialty group practice, if you refer your patient to a specific surgeon, it is likely that surgeon will see the patient and perform any agreed-upon surgery. You may have less control if you refer the patient to a university practice setting where the surgical care is more likely to be shared among staff physicians and with trainees. Nonetheless, many university practices provide truly excellent surgical spine care.

The location of the patient and the surgeon and his or her practice can greatly influence patients and families. Some patients are more and others much less willing to travel any distance to obtain surgical consultation and care. Finally, beware of itinerant surgeons, especially when it comes to spine care. Patients occasionally need the presence and intervention of their spine surgeon in the post-operative period.

The practice setting itself

While the surgeon is the key determinant of whether and what kind of operation is performed and is largely responsible for its outcome, surgeons do not work in a vacuum. Spine procedures are performed in hospitals or ambulatory surgical centers. The setting in which the surgery is performed and where aftercare is provided contributes greatly to the outcome of spine surgery. Facilities do vary; some have more and some have less "state-of-the-art" equipment. Even more important than physical structure and technical capability of the hospital or ambulatory surgical center are the people who work there. A surgical procedure is a team effort with contributions from nursing, anesthesia, pharmacy services, laboratory and imaging services, physical therapists, and aides of all sorts. These other nonsurgeon healthcare providers contribute significantly to surgical results.

It is difficult to judge a hospital's or ambulatory surgical center's expertise. We may have some personal experience based on where we work, where our patients have had surgery, or where our family members have had surgery. While hospitals and ambulatory surgical centers generally have similar quality across "product lines," there could be differences between, for example, spine surgery and cardiac surgery. An additional consideration is the "brand name" and reputation of a hospital and medical center. National rankings of hospitals and medical centers such as those published by *U.S. News and World Report* annually can be of some help. However, the criteria for ranking medical centers can be obscure and are sometimes based more on opinion than factual data.

Overall, hospital expertise or expertise in one kind of surgery (e.g., cardiac) does not guarantee expertise in another kind of care (e.g., spine disease).

Hospitals and most ambulatory surgical centers are reviewed by outside agencies including the Joint Commission, and state departments of health. Some limited information about hospitals and ambulatory surgical centers is available at www.jointcommission.org/ and from some individual state departments of health. The Joint Commission has a Disease-Specific Care Certification for healthcare organizations that can be granted for spine care.

Important questions for you and the surgeon

It is quite difficult to obtain the important surgeon-specific information described above. Some of the data can be sought directly from the surgeon. Patients, their family members, or other advocates for the patient should be encouraged to ask pertinent questions from the list below. In some instances, referring providers can ask the surgeon these questions on behalf of the patient. Unfortunately, there is a natural reticence for all of us to ask these sometimes personal questions of our surgeons. Truth be told, many surgeons will not be able to provide answers to many of the questions, especially specifics about outcomes, complication rates, and how their performance compares to that of their peers. Certain surgeons will take offense at being asked many of these questions. However, a competent, confident surgeon should not get angry with the patient or family when asked these questions. To help deflect such umbrage, it may be helpful for the patient or their family to inform the surgeon that the patient has a list of questions that have been recommended to them and state beforehand that they mean no harm in asking them.

Patients and families should consider asking the following questions:

1. What do you think is causing my symptoms?
2. What type of spine surgery are you recommending?
3. What are the anticipated benefits of having the operation?
4. What are your results with this operation?
5. Are there other surgical treatments that should be considered?
6. Are there medical alternatives to surgery that have not been tried?
7. What if I elect not to have this operation?
8. Do you perform this operation frequently?
9. How often do you perform this operation?
10. Exactly what does this operation entail?
11. If a fusion is performed, will you use my bone, bone from a cadaver, or BMP (bone morphogenetic protein)?
12. If a fusion is performed, will metal pieces be implanted, and if so, how many and what type?
13. Will you be performing the surgery yourself?
14. Will others be assisting you and, if so, who and to what extent?
15. What are the risks associated with this operation?
16. What is the rate of these different complications in your hands?
17. Where will the operation be performed?
18. What kind of anesthesia is usually given for this operation?
19. Are there any other options for anesthesia?
20. Is it likely I will need a transfusion because of the surgery?
21. If so, can I donate my own blood beforehand?
22. How long will I be in the hospital?
23. How long will it take me to recover from the operation?
24. How soon can I resume my normal activities?
25. How soon can I return to work?
26. When can I expect to be fully recovered from surgery?
27. How much does the operation and hospitalization cost?
28. What will I need to know when I go home after surgery?
29. Will I need physical therapy after the operation?
30. Will I need any other ongoing treatments post-operatively?
31. When will I next see you?
32. When will I see you following surgery?
33. Are you board certified in orthopedic surgery or neurosurgery?
34. Did you receive additional training in spine surgery (sometimes called a spine fellowship)?
35. How long was your subspecialty training in spine surgery?
36. Do you have any health problems that would affect your ability to perform this surgery on me?
37. When can you perform the operation on me?
38. Is it possible to talk to some of your patients who have had this operation?
39. If I have more questions, what is the best way for me to contact you?
40. From whom could I get a second opinion?

This is a daunting list of questions, but none is out of line. Dr. T. R. Russell, Executive Director, American College of Surgeons recommends many of these questions and, in fact, many others to patients and their families in the recently published, *I Need an Operation . . . Now What?* Additional lists of appropriate questions can be found on the Agency for Healthcare Research and Quality website at www.ahrq.gov and at www.spineuniverse.com which is affiliated with some spine-related professional associations.

Whether we are surgeons or not, how would each of us respond if we were asked all 40 of these questions? While we shouldn't, I am afraid to say that many of us might become irritated. Every provider feels that they are doing a great job, that their outcomes are better than those of their peers, and that they have only the patient's best interest at heart even when unnecessary testing and treatment is undertaken. It is natural for us to feel this way even though we lack objective data about our complication rates and outcomes. Our strongly held beliefs often lead to less than honest answers. Competent, caring providers must be ready and willing to answer all of the patient's and family's questions. It is our responsibility to explain as honestly and openly as we can the reasons for the therapy we recommend, the details of that treatment, the anticipated outcomes, our results, potential complications and their rates in our hands, the specifics of follow-up, how soon patients can return to work, and our credentials. No questions should be off the table. We should answer any questions posed as honestly as possible.

Patients are well advised to avoid the rushed, distracted, unresponsive provider who gives answers that are self-serving or glib or who doesn't answer them at all. Patients and families who do not feel that they have their questions answered adequately, who do not feel that the surgeon or nonsurgeon spent enough time with them, or who do not feel that their perspective has been understood should seek a second opinion on their own. These same feelings increase the likelihood that the patient or their family will complain or take legal action against a provider.

Second opinions

If the patient and/or their family is not satisfied with the initial surgical consultation or if you, the referring provider, strongly disagree with the advice that has been given or sense that the patient is upset, a second opinion should be obtained. There is some small risk that the first surgeon may be offended. There is also risk that the patient will receive conflicting advice regarding operative intervention and what kind of surgery should be performed. This conflicting advice can be very unsettling to patients and may necessitate a third opinion! The Agency for Healthcare Research and Quality endorses second opinions as a very good way to make certain that having the recommended operation is the best choice for the patient.

Reference

Russell TR. *I Need an Operation . . . Now What?* Chicago, Illinois: American College of Surgeons, 2008.

Websites

Agency for Healthcare Research and Quality
www.ahrq.gov, accessed 2 January 2009
American Board of Medical Specialties
www.abms.org, accessed 2 January 2009
Federation of State Medical Boards
www.docinfo.org, accessed 2 January 2009
Federation of State Medical Boards – Federation Physician Data Center
www.drdata.org, accessed 2 January 2009
Spine Universe
www.spineuniverse.com, accessed 2 January 2009
The Joint Commission
www.jointcommission.org/, accessed 2 January 2009
U.S. News and World Report
http://health.usnews.com/sections/health/best-hospitals, accessed 2 January 2009

Chapter

7 What to do when the patient has persistent or new symptoms following surgery

Introduction

Only 1%–2% of all patients with back problems come to surgery on their spine. Of those who do, somewhere between 70% and 90% of patients have an excellent outcome from their spine operation. However, 10%–30% of patients are not helped by surgery and another 10% or more develop recurrent spine and/or limb pain in the months and years following a beneficial spine operation. Repeat surgery in the patients who fail their initial operation is only helpful in about 50%. While surgery, we hope, makes the patient better, surgery does not make the spine normal. It is extremely frustrating for the patient, the patient's family, their employer, the surgeon, and the patient's other medical providers when a patient has persistent symptoms post-operatively or worse yet, if they develop new symptoms or progression of their previous symptoms following operative intervention.

The possibilities can be broadly divided into persistent symptoms post-operatively and worsening after surgery. Persistent symptoms are generally due to pre-operative factors or intra-operative errors. The pre-operative factors which lead to persistent symptoms can be divided into choosing the wrong patient, reaching the wrong diagnosis, choosing to perform the wrong operation, or performing the surgery at the wrong time (either too soon or too late). Unrealistic patient expectations can also be considered a pre-operative factor. Intra-operative errors which can lead to persistent symptoms include operating at the wrong level, deciding to perform the wrong procedure in the operating room, and performing incomplete surgery. In addition to complications indirectly related to the operation, post-operative worsening can be due to intra-operative errors such as excessive surgery, early complications, delayed complications of surgery including arachnoiditis, progression of underlying disease, and new disease including reoccurrence of the patient's original problem (e.g., recurrent disk herniation at the same level)

(see Table 7.1). Lack of improvement and post-operative worsening can also be divided into those occurring after decompression procedures (relieving pressure on neural structures) and after operations directed at the intervertebral disk without neural compression (fusion and placement of an artificial cervical or lumbar disk). The same categories can be further subdivided into the level of spine which was operated upon (cervical, thoracic, or lumbar). The possible causes for persistent symptoms and post-operative worsening will be reviewed, and strategies for evaluating and treating the patient who has done poorly after surgery will be presented.

Persistent symptoms post-operatively
Pre-operative errors
The wrong patient

You have no doubt heard the phrase, "It's the singer, not the song." When evaluating the patient with low back pain, we must look at the whole individual including their previous medical and surgical history, the outcomes from previous interventions, and psychosocial factors. Does the patient have a true physical impairment or are there historical features or examination findings that suggest a nonorganic component to the patient's presentation? There are tremendous pressures placed on the patient to get better. There are also pressures on providers to help, if not cure, patients. A sense of desperation on the part of the patient, the family, the employer, and the providers can lead to operative intervention on individuals who, in hindsight, were unlikely to improve with surgery. All of us have some "functional reaction" in response to physical illness. Determining which patients have a lot more or a lot less of this functional component is difficult. Factors including the patient's personality, psychologic state, other medical problems, past history of pain, past history of multiple previous surgical interventions, past history of lack of response to medical and surgical treatment,

Table 7.1. Reasons for spine surgery failure

Persistent symptoms post-operatively

Pre-operative errors

    Wrong patient

    Wrong diagnosis

    Choosing to perform the wrong operation

    Wrong time

    Unrealistic expectations

Intra-operative errors

    Wrong level

    Performing the wrong operation at surgery

    Incomplete surgery

Worsening of pre-operative or new symptoms after surgery

Complications

    Indirectly related to surgery

    Directly related to surgery

        Excessive surgery

        Early

        Delayed

            Arachnoiditis (scarring)

Worsening of original disease

New disease

Persistent, worsening, or new symptoms according to type of surgery

Following encroachment (decompression) surgery

Following fusion

Following total disk arthroplasty (placement of artificial disk)

Subdivide according to level of spine

Cervical

Lumbar

Thoracic

Table 7.2. Psychosocial risk factors for poor outcomes and the development of chronic pain

Belief that pain and physical activity are harmful

"Sickness behaviors" such as extended rest and fear-avoidance behavior

Depressed or down mood, social withdrawal, distress, or anxiety

Treatment that has been excessive, unsatisfying, and unhelpful

Claims and compensation issues including lack of financial incentive to return to work

History of previous pain problems with time off from work or previous claims

Problems at work including low job satisfaction and stress at work

Physically demanding work, long hours, wrong hours, and shift work

Overprotective family or lack of support from family

legal entanglements, and reimbursement issues can suggest the probability of a less-than-optimal outcome from pending spine surgery. The wrong patient can undergo surgery for decompression or fusion. In general, patients with axial spine pain are less likely to do well after surgical intervention. Thus, fusions on the lumbar, thoracic, and cervical spine performed for midline spine pain alone have poorer outcomes as a rule than operations for single nerve root, cauda equina, or spinal cord compression. Outcomes from placement of an artificial disk are probably comparable to those from fusion.

It is much better to identify "the wrong patient" before rather than after their first spine operation, but there is no foolproof way of making this determination. Signs suggestive of a nonorganic component to the patient's low back pain are listed in Table 4.4. There are a number of psychosocial risk factors that predict poor outcomes from any treatment and increase the likelihood of developing chronic pain (see Table 7.2). A number of tools have been developed to help measure the presence and severity of psychosocial risk factors as well as pain and functional status (see Table 7.3). Cigarette smoking is a risk factor for fusion failure. The presence of psychosocial risk factors can be helpful, but sometimes the factors are only recognized in retrospect. In fact, a poor outcome from surgery could cause the development of worrisome beliefs, behaviors, claims, and other problems. One is left to wonder whether the psychosocial factors were present beforehand and promoted a bad surgical outcome or whether the surgical outcome truly caused the anxiety, depression, sickness behaviors, etc. Even if a patient manifests some of these psychosocial risk factors before surgery, it does not mean that they do not have underlying organic disease with bona fide nerve root compression. The most challenging patient is the one with psychosocial risk factors and organic disease.

The wrong diagnosis

While we hope we are never party to reaching a wrong diagnosis, this can and does happen, probably much more than we are willing to admit. The wrong diagnosis can lead to choosing the wrong operation, performing an unnecessary operation, or occasionally no operation when one should have been performed

Table 7.3. Tools to assess patients with spine pain (many of the tools evaluate more than one category)

Psychosocial tools

    Waddell nonorganic signs

    Pain drawing

    DSM-IV-TR Diagnostic Criteria for Depression

    CAGE screening test for alcoholism

    Beck Depression Inventory

    Hamilton Rating Scale for Depression

    Minnesota Multiphasic Personality Inventory

    SF-36 Health Survey

    Acute Low Back Pain Screening Questionnaire (Linton and Hallden)

    Zung Self-Rating Depression Scale

    Geriatric Depression Scale

Pain tools

    Numerical (0 to 10) pain scale

    Visual analog pain scales

    Faces pain scale

    McGill Pain Questionnaire

    The Brief Pain Inventory

    Pain drawing

    Oswestry Low Back Pain Disability Questionnaire

    Roland–Morris Disability Questionnaire

    Quebec Back Pain Disability Scale

    Neck disability index

Functional status and pain tools

    SF-36 Health Survey

    Acute Low Back Pain Screening Questionnaire (Linton and Hallden)

    Oswestry Low Back Pain Disability Questionnaire

    Roland–Morris Disability Questionnaire

    Quebec Back Pain Disability Scale

    Neck disability index

or offered. The biggest error that is made in spine disease is reaching a definite diagnosis when the facts do not warrant this conclusion. Hubris, desperation, and gallantry – I know what is wrong with this patient, I have to help this patient, and I will fix it – can lead to unnecessary or inappropriate surgery. So can ignorance. So can avarice. While we cannot be right when we say we do not know what is wrong with the patient, we cannot be wrong either. The ability of magnetic resonance imaging (MRI) to show abnormalities in the spine in almost every adult, even those

who are asymptomatic, is very seductive and often leads to a wrong diagnosis. The patient has back pain, and there is an abnormality in the spine on their MRI. The two have to be related, don't they? We must remember that there are many asymptomatic abnormalities on modern imaging studies, and there are many causes of spine pain that do not show up on these studies. Attribution of the patient's spine-related complaint to the findings on the imaging study is not always possible. The admission of uncertainty can be very helpful in avoiding unnecessary spine surgery.

Choosing to perform the wrong operation

The wrong operation could be a pre-operative error or it could be a mistake made at the time of surgery. Spine surgery includes decompression for nerve root or spinal cord impingement by disk or bone, fusion to eliminate painful motion of a vertebral segment, and the recently approved total disk arthroplasty for the cervical and lumbar levels. Some patients need both decompression and fusion performed simultaneously. Did we identify the correct syndrome pre-operatively? Did the patient need both decompression and fusion? Was the disk the primary pain generator? There are many types of lumbar fusions. Was the correct type of lumbar fusion performed for the patient's problem (if there is one correct type)? Was the best approach (anterior versus posterior) used? In the lumbar spine, most operations are performed from a posterior approach, while some fusions and all artificial disk replacements are performed from an anterior approach. At the cervical level, one can operate from an anterior or posterior approach for decompression of nerve root(s), decompression of the spinal cord, and/or to accomplish fusion, while artificial disk replacement is performed from an anterior approach.

The wrong time

It is possible to perform the right operation for the right diagnosis but at the wrong time. If a patient was going to improve with conservative treatment, operative intervention, even if successful, would be unnecessary. In this situation, any ensuing complications would be especially troublesome. Alternatively, the operation could be delayed too long with resultant irreversible damage to a nerve root, the cauda equina, or the cervical or thoracic spinal cord. For lumbar radiculopathy, there is some anecdotal evidence that surgery should be performed within 3–4 months of onset of symptoms to avert irreparable nerve damage. Even this interval may be too long in some patients.

Unrealistic expectations

Some patients who have clearly been helped by their spine surgery report continuing symptoms which trouble them. Most commonly, this is pain, but it could be their neurologic deficit. Some of these patients may have harbored unrealistic expectations before surgery was performed. Despite clearly explaining the limitations of surgery and the expected outcomes, some patients and/or their families believe that surgery will eliminate all of their spine-related symptoms. Some patients focus excessively on their residual symptoms. Other patients, while reporting resolution or marked improvement in their radicular pain and deficits, complain of new spine pain that is related to their surgery and which was not present pre-operatively. This, too, represents an unrealistic expectation if we explained to the patient before surgery that operating on their spine can cause some post-operative back pain. Patients who do not feel they have been helped enough may need additional evaluation, but their desire to be completely free of symptoms should not force additional, inappropriate surgery. Most of these patients should be treated conservatively and observed for worsening. It has been said that back pain is part of the aging process, and we do not have a cure for aging. The patient's providers, especially the surgeon, can promote unrealistic expectations by implying that surgery is certain to relieve their symptoms and minimizing or neglecting to describe potential complications. Painting too rosy a picture of the outcome of surgery can certainly lead to patient disappointment. On the other hand, some patients and families only remember "the good news" from pre-operative discussions.

Intra-operative errors

The wrong operation can be performed because: (1) we selected the wrong level for surgery pre-operatively (really a wrong diagnosis), (2) at the time of surgery, operated on the wrong level (really a technical mistake), (3) the wrong surgical procedure was chosen pre-operatively (another form of wrong diagnosis) or at the time of surgery, or (4) there were technical errors of omission or commission during the operation.

The wrong level

Despite the advances in pre-operative imaging (chiefly MRI) and the availability of intra-operative imaging, it is possible for the surgeon to operate on the wrong level. Multi-level pathology is especially likely to predispose to a pre-operative decision to operate at the wrong level, which is really a wrong diagnosis. Congenital anomalies of the lumbosacral spine are also likely to lead to problems with pre-operative or intra-operative localization. The surgeon should know what pathology they are likely to encounter and, if they do not find what they expect, they should suspect that they may be operating at the wrong level. Pre-operative plain films of the level of interest reduce the likelihood of a vertebral counting error. When in doubt, intra-operative X-rays can help to confirm the level of intervention. It is helpful to have similar pre-operative X-rays for comparison.

Performing the wrong operation at surgery

The surgeon has a definite plan of what he or she intends to do during the patient's spine operation. However, some decisions are made at the time of surgery. Based on the intra-operative findings, the surgeon may decide that they have found a sufficient explanation for the patient's nerve root impingement, and they do not need to look further out along the root or higher or lower in the spine. Irrespective of the pre-operative decision, the surgeon could make a judgment during the operation that more or less needs to be done and change plans accordingly. For example, the surgeon may decide that a fusion is or is not needed or that one more or one less level needs fusion than was originally planned. These "game time" decisions, like all others in medicine, are subject to error. As a rule, persistent, unchanged symptoms are more likely to occur if the surgeon does less, and post-operative worsening is more likely if the surgeon does more than was planned.

Incomplete surgery

Incomplete surgery can be divided into surgery to decompress nervous tissue or "fixing" a disk either by fusion or placement of an artificial disk. Removing too little bone with resulting lack of adequate exposure can hinder the surgeon's view of pathology and could result in incomplete decompression of neural structures. For decompressive surgery, persistent symptoms can occur if not all of the offending disk material, disk fragments, or bone or bony spurs are removed. Alternatively, there could be more than one cause of nerve root compression (e.g., osteophyte and disk, or in the lumbar spine the root is compressed at more than one spinal level). A far lateral disk protrusion or extrusion is easily missed. A small disk which compresses conjoined nerve roots (two nerve roots

121

which leave the thecal sac together in a common dural sleeve, most frequently at L5–S1) can cause severe sciatica and be difficult to treat surgically. For spinal stenosis, multiple levels may need to be decompressed in the lumbar more likely than cervical spine. In addition to central spinal stenosis, there may be a need to decompress one or more roots more laterally (e.g., foraminal stenosis or a disk fragment farther out in the intervertebral foramen).

Worsening of pre-operative or the development of new symptoms after surgery

Complications

Indirectly related to surgery

Indirectly related to surgery, the patient can, rarely, die, suffer a myocardial infarction, experience deep vein thrombophlebitis with or without pulmonary embolism, develop lung atelectasis or pneumonia, develop urinary retention or a urinary tract infection, develop delirium which is more common in patients with underlying dementia, or sustain pressure palsy of a peripheral nerve or stretch injury of the brachial plexus due to improper padding and positioning.

Directly related to surgery

Excessive surgery

Excessive surgery more often leads to worsening of symptoms post-operatively than to unchanged persistence of symptoms. Patients may be subjected to decompression plus fusion when one alone would have sufficed. Perhaps more levels were decompressed or more levels were fused than was necessary. In the case of fusion, anterior and posterior procedures may be performed when only one was needed. Alternatively, at the time of surgery, the surgeon can be too aggressive in removing disk material or bone, resulting in increased pain, accelerated degenerative change, or bony spinal instability. Additionally, too much hardware can be implanted.

Early complications directly related to surgery

Local complications related to the level of surgery and occurring immediately or soon after operation are outlined below.

At the cervical level, there can be injury to the spinal cord, cervical nerve roots, dura, and vertebral arteries when operating from a posterior approach. In addition to these complications, when operating from the anterior approach, damage can occur to the carotid artery, jugular vein, esophagus, trachea, and peripheral nerves in the neck. Structural bony instability can also be created as a result of cervical spine surgery.

Similarly, in the thoracic spine, there can be injury to the spinal cord, thoracic nerve roots, and dura. Bony spinal instability can result. At the thoracic level, pulmonary complications including pneumonia, atelectasis, and pleural effusion are relatively common. Pleural tears and CSF–pleural fistulas can occur. Intercostal neuralgia is not uncommon following thoracic operations in which a rib is resected. Compromise of a unilateral radicular artery can result in spinal cord ischemia.

In the lumbar region, individual nerve roots or multiple lumbosacral nerve roots can be injured. Structural instability can also be created at the lumbar level. The dura can be injured with development of a CSF leak and/or a meningocele. Various visceral injuries, including damage to arterial and venous structures, can occur more readily from an anterior than a posterior approach. Vascular injury is more common and more easily recognized when it occurs during an anterior procedure. Post-operative sexual dysfunction in males is especially apt to occur following anterior lumbar procedures and probably more likely to occur after placement of an artificial lumbar disk than after fusion. The post-operative development of compression of multiple lumbar and sacral nerve roots (cauda equina syndrome) can present immediately post-operatively, but is more likely to occur hours or days after a lumbar spine procedure due to an expanding epidural hematoma. Frequently, a post-operative cauda equina syndrome is painless, and thus the absence of pain does not rule out this complication.

Dural tears and puncture with leakage of CSF should be repaired at surgery if discovered. Persistent CSF leakage through a dural rent can result in a post-operative low CSF pressure headache, CSF leakage through the wound, or serve as a potential entry route for infection. If not recognized at the time of surgery, the surgeon may need to go back in and repair the tear. Localized, persistent CSF collections are termed pseudomeningoceles and often do not require surgical repair.

All of the direct, specific complications arising from spine surgery are more likely to occur with more involved and more complex surgery. The more levels/sides that are decompressed or fused, the greater the risk of complications. Fusion coupled with

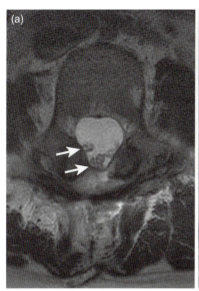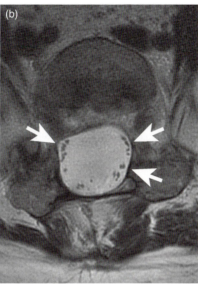

Figure 7.1. MRI scan findings in arachnoiditis. (a) and (b) Axial T$_2$-weighted images of the L4 and L5 level respectively. There is clumping of the lumbosacral nerve roots within the caudal sac at the L4 level (arrows) and clumping and peripheral dispersion of the nerve roots at the L5 level (arrows), all of which are consistent with chronic adhesive spinal arachnoiditis. The lumbosacral nerve roots did not enhance following administration of gadolinium which is often the case in arachnoiditis. The thecal sac is capacious at the L5 level secondary to a previous post-operative pseudomeningocele which required surgical repair. This 52-year-old woman had undergone three lumbar spine operations in the 1980s and had residual chronic low back and bilateral lower limb pain with evidence of right greater than left L5 and right S1 radiculopathies.

laminectomy has more complications than either procedure alone. An instrumented fusion from an anterior and a posterior approach is more likely to cause problems than an instrumented fusion from a single approach, which in turn is more likely to cause complications than an uninstrumented fusion.

Delayed complications directly related to surgery

Post-operative complications that are delayed and directly related to the surgery include disk space infections, symptoms related to further collapse of the operated segment, failure of fusion (pseudarthrosis), instability, problems related to implanted materials, and arachnoiditis. Disk space infections occur in about 0.5% of spine operations and are much more likely to occur at the lumbar level. Arachnoiditis, an inflammation of the pia-arachnoid membrane that results in adhesions between nerve roots and the pia and arachnoid membranes, is also much more common following lumbar spine surgery (see Figure 7.1). Some degree of "scarring" (usually epidural fibrosis) can be expected in most patients following lumbar spine surgery. There are many factors that can contribute to arachnoiditis, making it difficult to attribute a given patient's arachnoiditis to the most recent or only lumbar spine operation. An increased risk of arachnoiditis is associated with current or prior lumbar spine surgery; prior myelography, especially with the old oil-based contrast agent iophendylate (Pantopaque®); disk herniation; penetrating and blunt spine trauma;

spinal stenosis; previous subarachnoid hemorrhage; previous meningitis; spinal anesthesia; inadvertent intrathecal chymopapain injection; and intrathecal and epidural injections. Arachnoiditis has a slow, gradual onset which can occur weeks, months, or even years after the original injury. The patient can have back and/or leg pain, neuropathic radicular signs and symptoms, and sphincter and/or sexual dysfunction. MRI is the diagnostic study of choice and shows clumping of nerve roots, adhesion of roots to the dura giving the appearance of an empty thecal sac, and occasional focal obliteration of the subarachnoid space with blockage of CSF flow. Gadolinium contrast enhancement is an inconstant finding and is frequently absent. There is no effective primary treatment. Additional intervention on the spine should be assiduously avoided in patients who develop symptomatic chronic adhesive spinal arachnoiditis.

Worsening of original disease

Spinal spondylosis is a progressive, degenerative disease sometimes punctuated by acute signs and symptoms. Spondylosis is not always helped by surgery to decompress neural structures or stabilize the spine. In the patient who was not helped by surgery and who has slowly progressive symptoms, worsening of their underlying condition, most often spondylosis, is possible if not likely. Inflammatory arthritides might also cause progressive spine pain which is not helped by surgery. Similarly, the patient who is helped by

123

surgery to decompress neural structures or stabilize the spine for spondylosis and later experiences worsening of their previous symptoms or new symptoms referable to the same spinal level is likely to have underlying spondylosis as the cause for their recurrence.

Patients with cervical and/or lumbar spinal stenosis frequently have multi-level disease, and treatment of the current symptomatic level, be it cervical or lumbar, may provide symptomatic relief to be followed months and years later by recurrence of similar symptoms due to progression of stenosis at a level adjacent to the patient's previous surgery.

New disease

Spinal spondylosis frequently affects multiple levels in the spine. If the patient has had problems in their neck or lower back, they may later develop "new disease" at the other level due to "spread" of their underlying degenerative spondylotic disease to a new level. Alternatively, patients who have an acute disk rupture at one level who are helped by discectomy could later develop a disk herniation at the same level or a different level. While due to underlying spondylosis, this technically would be a new disk herniation and therefore could be termed new disease.

Spine complaints are very common and spine-related symptoms can be due to several different common causes. The patient with spondylotic lower back pain could later develop a compression fracture. The patient with a previous successful spine operation could later develop cancer with metastasis to the same or a different level of the spine. Especially if there has been an interval between the patient's surgery and the development of new symptoms, the possibility of an entirely new disease must be kept in mind.

Persistent, worsening, or new symptoms according to type of surgery

The problem of persistent, worsening, or new symptoms following surgery can also be subdivided by the type of surgery that was performed; namely, decompression, fusion, and placement of an artificial disk. Persistent symptom causes include the same pre-operative and intra-operative errors listed in Table 7.1 and described earlier. Worsening and new symptoms differ somewhat according to the type of surgery that was performed and will be detailed here. Causative factors can be further divided into the three spinal levels – cervical, thoracic, and lumbar.

Worsening after encroachment surgery (decompression)

Complications following encroachment surgery can be divided into increase in the patient's pre-operative spine pain, change for the worse in the limb pain soon after surgery, and relief of pain followed by recurrence of the limb pain. Relief of limb pain or other neurologic symptoms accompanied by an increase in spine pain usually relates to worsening of pre-existing instability, the development of instability which may have been promoted by encroachment surgery, or increased degenerative, spondylotic change at the operated level. This scenario may indicate that the patient should have undergone a simultaneous fusion or, at the cervical level, possibly placement of an artificial disk instead of laminectomy and discectomy. Increased degenerative change or spinal instability may relate to natural progression of the patient's underlying spine condition rather than be a consequence of the surgery performed. Disk space infection and arachnoiditis also present in this fashion.

Alternatively, the patient may note worsening of the limb pain post-operatively. This can occur as a result of immediate foraminal or central canal compromise with neural compression or direct nerve injury as a result of the surgery, retained disk material, progression of the patient's underlying spondylosis, recurrent disk herniation, or scarring. Symptoms related to the last three typically occur after a delay.

If the patient experiences complete relief of the limb pain for a varying length of time and then experiences recurrence, they likely have a recurrent disk herniation at the same level, but this can also occur with scarring, infection, foraminal or central canal narrowing, or an entirely new process. In the lower back, recurrent disk herniation most often occurs at the same level and on the same side (~75%) with less likely recurrence at a different level (~20%) or at the same level but on the opposite side (~5%).

Worsening after spinal fusion

Worsening after spinal fusion can be divided into pain arising from the fused level, pain arising from the spine above or below the fusion, and donor site pain in those patients undergoing fusion with autologous bone.

Pain arising from the fused level can be due to complications of the fusion itself, delayed complications which are outlined above (such as infection and arachnoiditis), pseudarthrosis (failure of fusion), and the development of root or spinal cord compression. If multiple lumbar levels are effectively fused, the patient can develop a flat back syndrome. Failure of fusion can also result in kyphosis, scoliosis, or increased lordosis.

Immediate complications of the fusion are usually painfully obvious. On the other hand, a fusion takes several months to heal. Failure of the fused segments to actually fuse after the expected interval is called pseudarthrosis. Pseudarthrosis may be difficult to document at the level of the fusion, especially if hardware has been used to facilitate the fusion. Importantly, pseudarthrosis need not be painful, and thus demonstration of pseudarthrosis does not necessarily mean that the cause of the patient's pain has been identified. Discography is reported to be helpful in determining if pseudarthrosis is a pain generator.

The development of signs and symptoms of nerve root injury following fusion can be due to direct injury, rupture of the disk at the level of the fusion (if it was not surgically removed), iatrogenic spinal stenosis, natural progression of the patient's spinal spondylosis, or arachnoiditis. Disk rupture beneath a solid fusion is very rare and is more likely to occur in the presence of a pseudarthrosis. Disk rupture results in rapid onset of symptoms, whereas iatrogenic or spontaneous central or foraminal spinal stenosis and arachnoiditis usually develop more gradually. Spinal or foraminal stenosis is characteristically associated with pseudoclaudication-type lower limb radicular symptoms in the lumbar spine and persistent symptoms in the cervical spine.

Pain originating from levels above or below a fusion can be related to worsening of the patient's existing spondylosis, acquired spondylolysis, disk rupture, spinal or foraminal stenosis, arachnoiditis, chronic muscle pain secondary to altered spinal biomechanics, facet joint arthritis, and spinal deformity. The spinal levels immediately adjacent to a successful fusion are subject to increased motion which can promote accelerated spondylotic change. So-called adjacent segment disease is one of the most common causes for recurrent spine pain that follows a successful fusion by a lengthy interval.

Post-operative pain originating from the bone donor site, usually the anterior or posterior iliac crest, is frequent. In a minority, perhaps 10%–15%, the pain is significant and persistent. Whether or not they have pain, 25%–50% of patients have local post-operative sensory loss or hypersensitivity. It is thought that the pain is due to injury to local nerves or cortical bone or both. Protracted, severe bone donor-site pain is probably more frequent in patients who experience a poor outcome from their spine surgery. Sacroiliac joint instability may occur if the donor site encroaches on this joint, especially if the iliolumbar ligament is sectioned. In this situation, weight-bearing on the involved extremity increases the patient's spine pain. Bone donor-site pain is difficult to treat. There has been a trend over time toward the use of bone bank bone and bone morphogenetic protein (BMP) in place of autologous bone to facilitate spinal fusion. This has been done, in part, to avoid harvesting bone usually from the iliac crest with resulting protracted bone donor-site pain.

Complications related to placement of an artificial disk

In October, 2004, the U.S. Food and Drug Administration (FDA) approved the first artificial lumbar disk, the Charité model made by DePuy Spine, a Johnson & Johnson Company, for use in the lumbar spine. In August, 2006, the FDA approved a second artificial disk, the ProDisc-L made by Synthes, Inc. In July, 2007, the FDA approved the first artificial cervical disk, the Prestige ST manufactured by Medtronics Sofamor Danek. In December 2007 the ProDisc-C made by Synthes, Inc. was the second artificial cervical disk approved for use by the FDA. More artificial disks are in the pipeline for approval in the United States. Several of these artificial disks and others have been in use in Europe and elsewhere for well over a decade.

Arthroplasty is more attractive conceptually and functionally than arthrodesis (fusion). Fusions run the risk of causing increased degenerative change at adjacent levels. We do not (usually) fuse hips or knees.

Artificial disk surgery requires an anterior approach with removal of the existing degenerated disk and placement of the artificial disk. It takes some practice for a surgeon to learn a new procedure, and this is especially true for placement of a lumbar artificial disk. It may take twenty or thirty operations for a surgeon to become skilled at performing lumbar disk replacement surgery.

Lumbar total disk arthroplasty is approved for treating pain associated with degenerative disk disease, usually limited to one level and most commonly implanted at L4–L5 or L5–S1. Cervical total disk arthroplasty is approved for treatment of cervical radiculopathy or cervical spondylotic myelopathy due to degenerative disk disease at one level from C3 to C7. Additional information regarding total disk arthroplasty is found in Chapter 13.

Complications of total disk arthroplasty at the cervical and lumbar levels include increased facet joint arthrosis at the level of surgery with increased spine pain, migration of the device out of the disk space, subsidence of the implant upward or downward into a vertebral body, injury to local nerve structures, infection, and increased spine pain. For the implanted lumbar artificial disk, there is risk of damage to abdominal and pelvic structures with local hematomas, sympathetic nerve dysfunction, and erectile dysfunction in men. At the cervical level, additional complications include local hematomas, sagittal vertebral body split fractures, paravertebral ossification, and component part wear with secondary inflammatory reaction. Because cervical total disk arthroplasty is recommended for cervical radiculopathy and cervical myelopathy, the patient is likely to have neurologic findings before surgery, and they are probably more likely to experience neurologic worsening as a result of surgery than a patient undergoing placement of an artificial lumbar disk.

Determining the cause of persistent, recurrent, or new symptoms in the previously operated spine patient

History and physical examination

As is always the case in medicine, one must start with the patient's history. While the patient might want to start the history with their recent surgery or the events that followed, it is very important to also review the patient's original spine symptoms, how they began, and how they evolved. It is also important to review pre-operative investigations and learn everything you can about what was performed at the time of surgery. The longer it has been since the patient's original surgery, the more difficult this task becomes. The patient's response to previous medical, injection, and surgical therapy should be reviewed.

What was the nature and location of their original pain? Which bothered them more, their spine pain or their limb pain? What imaging and other studies were obtained? What did they show? Are the original imaging studies available for review? Exactly what was done during the patient's spine operation? Where is their current pain? What is it like? What makes it better and worse? Is their current spine pain or their limb pain more severe? What neurologic and systemic symptoms do they have?

How long were they pain-free after their spine operation? If there was no pain-free interval, pre-operative and intra-operative errors are likely. If the initial improvement lasted less than 6 months, one should think about instability, infection, arachnoiditis, or medical causes. The longer the patient's pain-free interval, the more likely it is that they have "new disease" and might benefit from additional surgery. Thus, the patient who underwent a successful laminectomy for radicular limb pain a decade ago is likely to do well if surgery is needed for recurrent radiculopathy at the same or a different location in the spine.

If the patient's pain is only in the limb or predominantly in the limb, a neuropathic etiology is more likely. Pain that is burning or lancinating is somewhat more likely to be nerve in origin. Burning pain suggests chronic nerve root damage rather than compression.

Of course, the patient should be re-examined. It is especially helpful to compare the patient's current findings with their pre-operative examination. Change for the worse in neurologic findings suggests peri-operative or ongoing nerve root, spinal cord, or cauda equina injury. Improvement in neurologic findings suggests that the surgery was helpful to the patient. Lack of interval change on examination is less helpful.

Nerve root tension signs, range of motion, tenderness, and motion-evoked pain should be tested.

Laboratory and diagnostic imaging studies

Any and all of the diagnostic investigations that were employed initially can be used in the post-operative patient. Because original imaging studies could have been misdiagnosed by the radiologist or surgeon, pre-operative imaging studies should be personally reviewed. Possible etiologies of failed back surgery are shown in Tables 7.4 and 7.5. One picks and chooses from the following tests as appropriate to the patient's presentation:

1. Plain X-rays including flexion and extension and sometimes oblique views. Plain films can show spinal instability, pseudarthrosis, broken or misplaced hardware, wrong level surgery, and infection.

2. Blood tests including complete blood count with differential; sedimentation rate; blood chemistries

Table 7.4. Causes of persistent or new symptoms after spine surgery

For patients with predominant spine pain	For patients with predominant limb pain
Infection	Retained disk
Discitis	Recurrent disk
Osteomyelitis	Epidural hematoma
Epidural abscess	Pseudomeningocele
Soft tissue	Lateral or foraminal stenosis
Musculoskeletal injury	Central spinal stenosis
Internal disk disruption (discogenic pain)	Synovial cyst
Facet joint pain	Epidural fibrosis
Sacroiliac joint	Arachnoiditis
Instability	Nerve root injury
Pseudarthrosis	Piriformis syndrome
Spondylolysis	Iliotibial band syndrome
Spondylolisthesis	Hip or knee joint pathology
Mechanical low back pain	Complex regional pain syndrome
Problems with instrumentation	Deep vein thrombophlebitis
Foreign body	Vascular claudication
Bone donor site (iliac crest)	Tumor

Source: Adapted from Slipman et al. Etiologies of failed back surgery syndrome. *Pain Med* 2002; **3**(3):203. With permission from Blackwell Publishing.

including calcium, alkaline phosphatase, and glucose; C-reactive protein; serum protein electrophoresis; and prostate-specific antigen.

3. Radionuclide scans using ^{99m}Tc, ^{67}Ga, and radioisotope-labeled white blood cells can be used to look for tumor, infection, and other inflammatory conditions, facet and pars fractures, and pseudarthrosis. Uptake in the patient with recent surgery is likely to be nonspecific.

4. While somewhat controversial, discography can demonstrate disk pathology on the imaging component and may help identify the injected disk as a pain generator.

5. Computed tomography scanning with or without myelography. Myelography is somewhat invasive and should be used with caution in patients who have or may have arachnoiditis. Plain CT scanning is very useful for evaluation of the patient with a suspected pseudarthrosis. During the first six weeks after spinal surgery, CT scanning with myelography may be more helpful than MRI. In the patient with a contraindication to MRI and in the first six weeks after surgery, CT scanning with intravenous contrast can help differentiate between scar tissue and recurrent herniated disk. On CT and MRI, scar tissue will conform to the available epidural space, follow the plane of the previous surgery, and often retract the dura. Scar tissue will enhance on CT and MRI following intravenous contrast, whereas recurrent disk will not enhance or only enhance peripherally (see Figures 7.2 and 7.3). Additionally, recurrent disk will typically have significant mass effect and is usually adjacent to a disk space.

6. Electromyography (EMG) is useful for documenting radiculopathy and peripheral nerve injury and can also help determine if the nerve injury is new or old and whether the damage is improving, static, or active. Of course, the EMG changes can relate to pre-operative pathology and not the post-operative complication. Even if the EMG changes are due to complications of surgery, they can only confirm that nerve root injury has occurred – and not whether there is any ongoing root compression.

7. Diagnostic injections with local anesthetics (facet joints, medial branch blocks, epidural injections, root blocks, and peripheral nerve blocks) can be used to help identify and eliminate pain generators. These commonly used procedures are fraught with false-positive results and are best conducted by experienced specialists.

8. Magnetic resonance imaging with and/or without gadolinium is the best test for determining nerve root and spinal cord compression and differentiating scarring from recurrent disk herniation. Scarring is very common after lumbar spine surgery, but is frequently asymptomatic. MRI is also very good for diagnosing disk space, epidural, and soft tissue infection. MRI can also examine levels higher and lower in the spine and can be used to assess structures outside the spine such as the brachial plexus, lumbosacral plexus, and sciatic nerve.

MRI at the level of a previous fusion with instrumentation will usually provide unsatisfactory images. Additionally, MRI cannot be performed in some patients (e.g., if they have a ferromagnetic aneurysm clip, a metallic foreign body in a critical location, a cardiac pacemaker or defibrillator, a spinal cord stimulator, or a cochlear implant, or if they are too

127

Table 7.5. Causes of failed spine surgery based on time of occurrence and predominant symptoms

	Within 72 hours	Weeks to months	Months to years

Predominant spine pain	Creation of instability
	Wrong level fusion
	Bone donor-site pain
		Infection
		  Discitis
		  Osteomyelitis
		  Epidural abscess
		  Soft tissue
		Fusion failure
		  With instrumentation
		  Without instrumentation
		Instrumentation problems
		Fused too few levels
		Spondylolysis
		Spondylolisthesis
		Bone donor-site pain
		Pseudomeningocele
			Fusion failure
			  Pseudarthrosis
			  Failed instrumentation
			Painful instrumentation
			Spondylolysis
			Spondylolisthesis
			Spondylosis
			  Same level
			  Adjacent segment
			  Distant segment
			Fracture
			Tumor

Predominant limb pain	Wrong level exploration
	Insufficient exploration
	  Retained disk fragment
	Nerve root/cord/cauda equina injury
	Epidural hematoma
	  Cauda equina syndrome
		Infection
		  Epidural abscess
		Nerve root scarring
		  Epidural fibrosis
		  Arachnoiditis
		Recurrent disk herniation
		Complex regional pain syndrome
		Retained foreign body
		Pseudomeningocele
			Recurrent disk herniation
			Nerve root scarring
			  Arachnoiditis
			Central, lateral recess, or foraminal stenosis
			  Same or adjacent level
			Synovial cyst
			Osteoarthritis of limb joint

Predominant neurologic deficit	Nerve root/cord/cauda equina injury
	Epidural hematoma
	  Cauda equina syndrome
		Spinal cord compression
		Cauda equina compression
		Nerve root scarring
			Central, lateral recess, or foraminal spinal stenosis
			  Same or adjacent level
			Spinal cord compression
			Cauda equina compression
			Nerve root scarring
			  Arachnoiditis
			Tumor

big for the machine) or performed with difficulty (e.g., if they are severely claustrophobic).

During the first 6 weeks or so after spine surgery, MRI results may be misleading due to immediate post-operative reactive changes. In this setting, myelography with CT scanning or CT with and without contrast may be more helpful. MRI is useful for immediate post-operative complications such as an epidural hematoma and other causes of acute spinal cord, cauda equina, or nerve root compression.

9. Other tests may be useful in patients with selected conditions such as ultrasound of the abdominal aorta for suspected aneurysm, ultrasound of the lower limb for possible deep vein thrombophlebitis, and lower limb arterial studies to exclude vascular claudication.

What tests should you order?

Diagnostic testing must be individualized. For many patients, plain films are a useful first step. MRI is the single best imaging modality to investigate most patients with residual, recurrent, or new symptoms following spine surgery. As noted above, the usefulness of MRI may be limited in the first 6 weeks after spine surgery and can be further limited by implanted instrumentation. CT myelography is complementary to MRI and can be used as an alternative imaging study. Plain CT with and/or without contrast can also be employed. EMG can be unhelpful in the patient who has undergone previous spine surgery but should be considered.

Usual causes of persistent, recurrent, or new symptoms post-operatively
Usual causes of failed low back surgery

More low back surgery is done than cervical and thoracic procedures combined. Low back surgeries are the most likely to fail. What are the usual causes of persistent, recurrent, or new symptoms in patients who have undergone previous low back surgery? A thoughtful review of 197 such patients found that

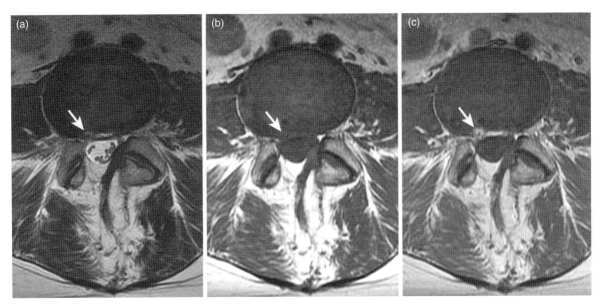

Figure 7.2. Differentiating post-operative scar from recurrent disk herniation. (a), (b), and (c) Axial T_2-weighted, unenhanced T_1-weighted, and gadolinium enhanced T_1-weighted images respectively of the L3–L4 level. Anterolaterally on the patient's right side, there is an abnormality with very subtle mass effect which enhances diffusely with gadolinium indicating that scar tissue only is present (arrows). This 55-year-old woman had previously undergone three lumbar spine operations including an L3–L4 procedure for disk protrusion 2 years earlier. She had residual right lower limb pain with a burning component which had recently worsened.

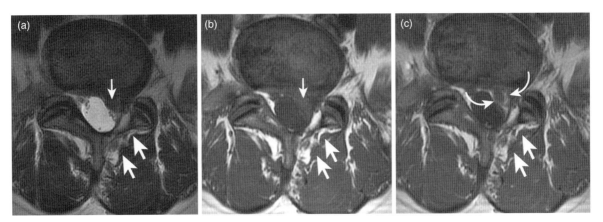

Figure 7.3. Differentiating post-operative scar from recurrent disk herniation. (a), (b), and (c) Axial T_2-weighted, unenhanced T_1-weighted, and gadolinium enhanced T_1-weighted images respectively of the L5–S1 level. On the patient's left, there is indentation of the thecal sac by an anterolateral mass which is better seen on the T_2- than T_1-weighted images (small arrows). There is evidence of a prior laminectomy at this level on the left (large arrows). On the post-gadolinium image (c) there is subtle peripheral enhancement medially and superiorly (curved arrows) but no central enhancement. The mass effect and peripheral-only enhancement help to confirm an L5–S1 disk extrusion rather than post-operative scarring. This 47-year-old man had previously undergone a successful left L5–S1 laminectomy several years beforehand. He developed severe low back and left lower limb pain consistent with sciatica after putting in a retaining wall. Examination was negative except for positive straight leg raise signs on the left and an absent left ankle reflex. After 3 months of pain he underwent this MRI. He met with a spine surgeon but eventually recovered from his left L5–S1 disk extrusion with nonoperative treatment.

stenosis, "internal disk disruption," recurrent or retained disk fragment, fibrosis (scarring), degenerative disk disease, and radiculopathy without compression were the most common diagnoses (see Table 7.6)

(see Slipman et al. 2002). The authors of this study felt that about half of patients with "failed back surgery syndrome" could be helped with additional surgery. Fifty percent seems too high to us.

129

Table 7.6. Etiologies of failed back surgery syndrome in 197 patients. The absolute number and percentage of each diagnosis

Diagnosis	Raw number	Percentage[a]
Surgical diagnoses (total = 112)		
Stenosis (total)	40	20.3
Foraminal	23	11.7
Central	11	5.6
Lateral	6	3.0
Internal disk disruption[b]	40	20.3
Recurrent/retained disk	23	11.7
Spondylolisthesis	3	1.5
Synovial cyst	2	1.0
Vascular claudication	2	1.0
Instability	1	0.5
Pseudomeningocele	1	0.5
Nonsurgical diagnoses (total = 97)		
Fibrosis (total)	28	14.2
Epidural	15	7.6
Intraneural	13	6.6
Degenerative disk disease	17	8.6
Radiculopathy	10	5.1
Radicular pain	9	4.6
Deconditioning	7	3.6
Facet syndrome	5	2.5
Battered root syndrome	3	1.5
Sacroiliac joint syndrome	3	1.5
Complex regional pain syndrome	2	1.0
Fibromyalgia	1	0.5
Discitis	1	0.5
Unknown	11	5.6

Notes:
[a]Percentage is based on number of diagnoses calculated over total number of patients, and not total number of diagnoses. Therefore, the total percentage is greater than 100%. There were 197 total patients: 186 with 198 diagnoses and 11 with an unknown etiology.
[b]Internal disk disruption syndrome refers to pain of disk origin and is included in surgical diagnoses although a nonsurgical treatment may be available and surgical intervention might not be helpful.
Adapted from Slipman et al. Etiologies of failed back surgery syndrome. *Pain Med* 2002; **3**(3):202. With permission from Blackwell Publishing.

Helpful hints in diagnosing the cause of failed spine surgery

Based on the time course and symptomatology of common causes of post-operative failure, the following key questions are suggested. Did the patient wake from surgery with symptoms unchanged? Did the patient wake with new symptoms after surgery or did they begin very soon after surgery? Did the patient have a pain-free interval after surgery and, if so, for how long were they pain free? The following guidelines can help to determine the cause of a patient's failed spine surgery:

1. Identical limb pain is usually associated with missed pathology (wrong level, incomplete surgery), wrong patient, wrong diagnosis, wrong operation, or inappropriate surgery.
2. New, significant limb pain soon after surgery is usually due to an intra-operative lesion affecting a nerve root, the cauda equina, or the spinal cord (e.g., a pedicle screw touching a root).
3. Reduced limb pain with increased neurologic deficit suggests intra-operative nerve root, cauda equina, or spinal cord injury.
4. Nonmechanical night pain of delayed onset should immediately raise a suspicion of infection.
5. The sudden onset of significant radicular pain after a pain-free interval is usually due to recurrent disk herniation.
6. A gradual onset of moderate radicular, usually lower limb pain within weeks or months of surgery after a pain-free interval is usually associated with nerve root scarring or formation of a meningocele.
7. The gradual onset of diffuse bilateral, usually lower limb pain that does not have characteristics of claudication suggests arachnoiditis.
8. The gradual and delayed onset of claudication-type lower limb symptoms is usually due to central lumbar or foraminal spinal stenosis.
9. Persistent spine pain after an attempted fusion with gradual worsening suggests a pseudarthrosis.

An approach to the patient with persistent or new symptoms following surgery

For the patient with unexplained persistent symptoms with (or for that matter without) antecedent surgery, or for the patient with progressive symptoms or new signs and symptoms post-operatively, the following suggestions are offered:

1. Go back to square one and take a new history and perform a new examination.
2. While assessing the previously operated level, keep in mind the possibility of pathologic processes higher in the nervous system and more peripherally along the spinal nerves, plexi, peripheral nerves, and non-neurologic structures.
3. Repeating tests can be helpful.
4. Ask for help from colleagues.
5. Keep in mind that spine operations are quite beneficial in only 70%–90% of patients with appropriate indications for surgery. We should expect that surgery will not help 10%–30% of patients. Failure to improve after spine surgery "happens."

Treatment of the patient with residual or new symptoms following spine surgery

Treatment of the patient with persistent or recurrent symptoms following spine surgery can be difficult. Before addressing the treatment, it is worthwhile emphasizing prevention. While spine surgery can fail in the most ideal candidate, we should do our best to avoid operating on the wrong patient, for the wrong diagnosis, choosing the wrong operation, operating at the wrong time, and ensuring as best we can that the patient and the family have realistic expectations about the outcome of the surgery performed.

Patients with recurrent symptoms or new symptoms that occur some time after surgery are more likely to be found to have disease that can be treated with another operation. Patients who have persistent, unchanging symptoms after an initial, appropriate operation are much less likely to benefit from re-operation.

Treatment obviously depends on the cause of the symptoms. The bulk of this chapter is devoted to a description of the potential reasons for persistent or new symptoms post-operatively and tests used to determine the cause. The patient with persistent, basically unchanged symptoms post-operatively in whom there was no obvious error in diagnosis, operation performed, or technical aspects of the procedure should not be subjected to re-operation. In the absence of profound or progressive neurologic deficits, most patients with persistent chronic spine and limb pain who have undergone previous spinal surgery should be treated nonoperatively. These are patients whose diagnosis may be spondylosis, internal disk disruption, "scarring," pseudomeningocele, non-compressive radicular pain, fibromyalgia, facet joint arthritis, and complex regional pain syndrome 1 and 2 among others. The occasional patient who experiences chronic, increased axial spine pain after an instrumented fusion may benefit from removal of the implanted hardware. Destructive procedures directed at the sympathetic nervous system (for complex regional pain syndrome) and the nerves supplying the facet joints (radiofrequency medial branch lesioning) may be considered in selected patients.

What can be done for patients with chronic spine and/or limb pain who have failed an initial spine operation? There are only four categories of treatment that are available for any medical problem: surgery (in this case more surgery); medications which can be given by mouth, transdermally, or by injection; physical therapies which can include modalities such as heat and ice, exercises, massage, electrical stimulation, and acupuncture; and helping people cope or live better despite a problem. In patients who have persistent symptoms after surgery and for whom additional surgery cannot be offered, we must rely on the latter three types of treatment.

The medications and injections suggested for patients with chronic spine and/or limb pain in Chapters 2–4 can be used in the patient who has failed spine surgery. These include nonsteroidal anti-inflammatory drugs, acetaminophen, tramadol, stronger opioid analgesics, and tricyclic antidepressants which can be given for axial spine pain. These same medications along with neuromodulating medications such as gabapentin and pregabalin and perhaps duloxetine can be given for radicular limb pain that may be on a nonradicular basis. Tricyclic antidepressants may be more helpful for radicular limb pain than for axial spine pain. Injections of local anesthetics and corticosteroids into the spine can also be offered but would be expected to have a limited duration of benefit.

All of the physical therapies that were mentioned in Chapters 2–4 can also be employed but must be ongoing in order to provide sustained benefit.

Patients with significant persistent pain which interferes with their ability to work and enjoy leisure activities should be considered for treatment in an intensive multidisciplinary pain rehabilitation program. As described at the end of Chapter 4, these programs often last several weeks and stress physical conditioning, biofeedback and relaxation training,

131

stress management, behavioral modification, and other techniques meant to decrease pain catastrophizing and increase functional ability while minimizing, if not eliminating, the use of medications. The objective of this type of program is not to eliminate pain but rather to enable patients to live more normally despite their pain. While this type of approach is not for everyone, it is often worth pursuing before rather than after additional surgery, implantation of a spinal cord stimulator, or placement of an intrathecal pain pump. For some patients, treatment in a multidisciplinary pain rehabilitation program should have been tried before any surgery was performed.

Spinal cord stimulation (SCS) has been used for 40 years in the treatment of refractory chronic low back and lower limb pain, especially that due to failed back surgery syndrome and complex regional pain syndrome. Individual wire leads can be implanted percutaneously into the epidural space over the lower thoracic spinal cord, or a "paddle" lead can be implanted via a small laminotomy into the epidural space. Both lead types contain multiple electrodes. Lead placement can be adjusted. A 3- to 7-day trial can be conducted with the leads coming out through the skin and connected to an external power source. Either type of lead can be permanently implanted along with a battery-operated pulse generator, or a device can be implanted and powered by an external radiofrequency transmitter through the patient's skin. Various combinations of voltage, pulse frequency and duration, and stimulus location along the multiple electrode lead can be programmed in an effort to reduce low back and lower limb pain. Epidural electrical stimulation of the dorsal sensory structures in the spinal cord is thought to inhibit transmission of chronic pain-related signals to higher levels of the nervous system and consciousness.

Spinal cord stimulation should only be employed when more conservative treatments, probably including opioid analgesic therapy, have failed. Thorough pre-implantation psychological evaluation is advised.

Contraindications include major psychiatric disorders, presence of a cardiac pacemaker or defibrillator, severe medical disease such as coagulopathy or limited life span, and drug or alcohol abuse.

The benefit appears to be moderate. Half or more of patients obtain 50% or more pain relief which typically declines over several years. Despite a 30%–40% incidence of device-related complications, there is evidence that SCS is helpful for chronic back and leg pain, failed back surgery syndrome, and complex

regional pain syndrome, types 1 and 2. SCS appears to be more effective and more cost-effective than re-operation for patients with failed back surgery syndrome.

Potential complications include spinal cord or nerve root injury, CSF leakage, bleeding, infection, electrode migration, and generation of an electric current in the implanted metal leads if the patient is exposed to an electromagnetic field.

There is less evidence to support the use of intrathecal drug delivery systems (pain pumps) for patients with chronic, very severe, refractory low back pain with or without lower limb pain. Morphine is used more commonly than other opioid analgesics and is sometimes combined with the local anesthetic bupivacaine. Alternatively, ziconotide (a non-narcotic drug derived from marine snail venom) is infused. A screening trial is conducted before a permanent delivery system is implanted. A worrisome side-effect is intrathecal granuloma formation around the catheter tip which can be associated with neurologic deficits. If there is concern that the patient has arachnoiditis, pain pumps are best avoided. The pumps are also associated with mechanical problems which can result in overdosing and underdosing the patient, for example with morphine. Intrathecal drug delivery is an accepted treatment for intractable pain due to failed back surgery syndrome.

Further reading

1. Boden SD, Bohlman HH, eds. *The Failed Spine.* Philadelphia, Pennsylvania: Lippincott Williams & Wilkins, 2003.

2. Coffey RJ, Burchiel K. Inflammatory mass lesions associated with intrathecal drug infusion catheters: report and observations on 41 patients. *Neurosurgery* 2002; **50**:78–87.

3. Deer T, Chapple I, Classen A, et al. Intrathecal drug delivery for treatment of chronic low back pain: report from the National Outcomes Registry for Low Back Pain. *Pain Med* 2004; **5**:6–13.

4. Kumar K, Taylor RS, Line J, et al. Spinal cord stimulation versus conventional medical management for neuropathic pain: a multicentre randomised controlled trial in patients with failed back surgery syndrome. *Pain* 2007; **132**:179–188.

5. Nachemson AL, Jonsson E, eds. *Neck and Back Pain: The Scientific Evidence of Causes, Diagnosis, and Treatment.* Philadelphia, Pennsylvania: Lippincott Williams & Wilkins, 2000.

6. North RB, Kidd D, Shipley J, Taylor RS. Spinal cord stimulation versus reoperation for failed back surgery

syndrome: a cost effectiveness and cost utility analysis based on a randomized, controlled trial. *Neurosurgery* 2007; **61**(2):361–369.

7. Slipman CW, Derby R, Simeone FA, Mayer TG. *Interventional Spine: An Algorithmic Approach.* Philadelphia, Pennsylvania: Saunders, 2008.

8. Slipman CW, Shin CH, Patel RK, et al. Etiologies of failed back surgery syndrome. *Pain Med* 2002; **3**(3):200–214.

9. Szpalski M, Gunzburg R, eds. *The Failed Spine.* Philadelphia, Pennsylvania: Lippincott Williams & Wilkins, 2005.

10. Turner JA, Loeser JD, Deyo RA, Sanders SB. Spinal cord stimulation for patients with failed back surgery syndrome or complex regional pain syndrome: a systematic review of effectiveness and complications. *Pain* 2004; **108**:137–147.

11. Wong DA, Transfeldt E. *Macnab's Backache*, Fourth Edition. Philadelphia, Pennsylvania: Lippincott Williams & Wilkins, 2007.

Websites

Institute for Clinical Systems Improvement (ICSI) Low Back Pain Guideline
http://www.icsi.org/index.aspx

New Zealand Acute Low Back Pain Guide
http://www.nzgg.org.nz/guidelines/0072/acc1038_col.pdf

Spinal imaging and diagnostic tests: considerations for surgical diagnosis and pre-operative planning

A variety of diagnostic imaging studies are available to assist the spine surgeon with establishing a diagnosis, deciding whether surgery would be appropriate, and determining which operation would be best for the patient. Magnetic resonance imaging (MRI) is the most widely used study; however, several other imaging studies are commonly used in surgical diagnosis and pre-operative planning.

Magnetic resonance imaging

Magnetic resonance imaging (MRI) is the imaging procedure of choice for spine disease. This modality provides superb visualization of the spinal cord, nerve roots, subarachnoid space, and paraspinal soft tissues. MRI also provides excellent bony detail, although computed tomography (CT) is superior in this regard. Another advantage of MRI is that it does not require exposure to radiation. Figure 8.1 depicts a normal MRI of the lumbar spine.

Safety issues and contraindications

Magnetic resonance imaging is widely used in the evaluation of patients with spine disorders; however, several caveats are in order. The major limitation of MRI is that there are a number of situations in which the procedure cannot be performed or is not technically feasible.

For example, MRI is contraindicated in patients with certain implanted metallic devices including cardiac pacemakers, neurostimulator devices, intrathecal drug pumps, cochlear implants, and some cerebral aneurysm clips. The potential risks of performing MRI in patients with these devices include magnetic field-induced movement, electrical or thermal injury, and impairment of device function.

Patients who have had neurostimulator devices removed may still be at risk because, in some cases, leads may not be completely removed at the time of device explantation. When placed in a strong magnetic field, a retained lead or lead fragment can act as an antenna and cause thermal injury to the surrounding tissues. These patients should therefore be carefully evaluated prior to performing an MRI study. Operative reports of the explantation procedure should be reviewed to assure the system was completely removed. If there is any question, radiographs should be obtained and reviewed for evidence of retained leads.

In some cases, it may be possible to safely perform an MRI study on a patient with a cardiac pacemaker or related device; however, this is highly dependent on both the device and the type of MRI study that is needed. Before MRI is performed in this setting, the case should be carefully reviewed with the radiologist, the implanting physician, and, in some cases, the device manufacturer.

The development of "MR safe" or "MR compatible" cardiac pacemakers and other devices is an area of active investigation; however, at the present time MRI is contraindicated for most patients with electrically, magnetically, or mechanically activated implants.

The procedure is also contraindicated in patients harboring metallic fragments in the orbit, for example related to metal work and other types of occupational exposure. The risk posed by metallic objects near the eye has been a concern since MRI was first introduced in the early 1980s. Blindness has occurred after movement of a metal object in the orbit during an MR examination. This phenomenon has also been demonstrated in animal studies.

As a result, the presence of a ferromagnetic foreign body within, or adjacent to, the orbit is now regarded as an absolute contraindication to MR imaging. In such cases, the usual clinical approach is to manage the patient without the benefit of MR imaging, and instead rely on CT scanning and other diagnostic procedures, without addressing the foreign body.

Another option is to remove the metallic foreign body to facilitate the MRI procedure. This strategy should be considered in situations where MRI is needed for optimal patient management, provided

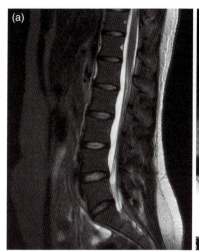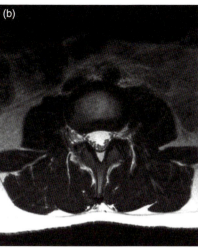

Figure 8.1. (a) Sagittal and (b) axial T$_2$-weighted lumbar MRI, depicting a normal study.

the foreign body can be localized and removed with minimal risk to the patient.

Patients have also been harmed in MRI machines by the movement of metal objects that were inadvertently left in their clothing or near the scanner during the examination.

Magnetic resonance imaging is usually not performed during pregnancy, although it has been performed in situations where the clinical benefits appeared to outweigh the risks to the fetus.

Magnetic resonance imaging can be safely performed in patients with spinal instrumentation; however, the examination may be severely compromised by susceptibility artifact from the implants. Titanium implants, more commonly used today, produce less artifact than older stainless steel implants; however, titanium devices may still degrade image quality. Figure 8.2 depicts the sagittal MRI of a patient with posterior spinal fusion with pedicle screw fixation at L3–L4. Prominent artifact at L3 and L4 on the T$_2$-weighted image with fat saturation precludes assessment of the spinal canal (Figure 8.2a). T$_2$-weighted images without fat saturation (Figure 8.2b) and T$_1$-weighted images (Figure 8.2c) produce less susceptibility artifact and provide better visualization of the spinal canal. These sequences should be used in patients with spinal instrumentation.

If metal artifact prevents satisfactory MRI, CT myelography may be required (see below).

Magnetic resonance imaging is relatively contraindicated in patients with obesity, claustrophobia, and severe pain.

Magnetic resonance imaging cannot be performed in some very large patients. Some are disqualified

because they exceed the weight limit of the scanner, while others meet the weight limit but cannot fit in the scanner because of a very large torso. MRI units typically have a weight limit in the range of 180–205 kg (400–450 pounds). This varies from one scanner to the next and should be verified with the manufacturer before attempting to scan an extremely heavy patient.

Patients with mild claustrophobia can often tolerate the examination with an oral sedative, for example, lorazepam (Xanax) 1–2 mg by mouth one hour before the examination. Individuals with more severe claustrophobia may require intravenous sedation, and in some cases general anesthesia, in order to undergo MRI.

Patients in severe pain, for example those with an acute disk herniation, tumor or vertebral compression fracture, may not be able to remain still long enough to complete the examination. In these cases, it is best to start with sagittal imaging, in the event that severe pain precludes a full examination. In some cases, e.g., vertebral compression fracture, a diagnosis can be established and treatment planned with just sagittal images, even if axial images cannot be obtained.

So-called open magnet MRI units have become increasingly popular as a way to accommodate obese and claustrophobic patients. Unfortunately, examinations performed on these scanners are often of very poor quality and are not sufficient for diagnosis or surgical planning. In these situations, the MRI often has to be repeated on a closed magnet unit, further adding to the time and expense of the investigation. Although there have been some recent technical improvements, image quality achievable on open

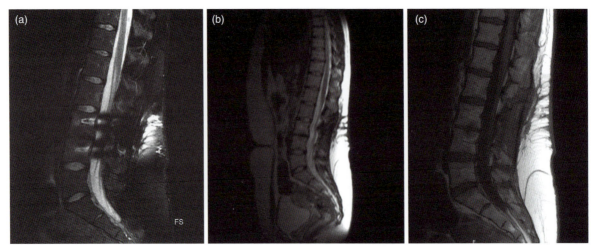

Figure 8.2. (a) Sagittal T_2-weighted lumbar MRI with fat saturation depicting susceptibility artifact related to pedicle screw construct at L3–L4. (b) Sagittal T_2-weighted MRI without fat saturation and (c) sagittal T_1-weighted MRI showing less artifact and better visualization of the spinal canal.

magnet units remains inferior to the high quality images that can be obtained on a closed magnet machine.

Pulse sequences for spinal disorders

The standard pulse sequences for an MRI examination of the spine include T_1- and T_2-weighted sagittal and axial images, supplemented with axial images using additional sequences such as fat suppression (FS), attenuation inversion recovery (FLAIR), or diffusion-weighted imaging, depending on the indication.

For patients with infectious or inflammatory disorders, neoplasms, and post-operative symptoms, the examination is often performed after intravenous injection of gadolinium contrast. In these situations, contrast enhancement improves MRI sensitivity. Lesions which are poorly defined, or even occult, on unenhanced images are often much more apparent on the contrast enhanced images.

Complications of gadolinium-based contrast agents

Gadolinium has been felt to be extremely safe, with a very low risk of allergic reaction or other complication. However, in December 2006, the FDA issued a public health advisory, which reported a new disease, known as nephrogenic systemic fibrosis or nephrogenic fibrosing dermopathy (NSF/NFD), which may occur in patients with moderate to end-stage kidney disease after MRI or magnetic resonance angiography (MRA) with a gadolinium-based contrast agent.

Patients with NSF/NFD report burning, itching, swelling, hardening, and tightening of the skin, yellow discoloration of the eyes, joint stiffness and pain, and muscle weakness. Gadolinium is identified on skin biopsy. The disease is debilitating and may be fatal.

Through the end of 2006, approximately 215 cases had been identified worldwide. Symptoms have begun anywhere from 2 days to 18 months after exposure to the contrast agent. Many, but not all, of these patients received a high dose of the contrast agent; some received only one dose. At this point, the risk of developing NSF/NFD appears to be limited to patients with moderate to end-stage renal disease.

Current FDA recommendations are for gadolinium contrast agents to be avoided in patients with moderate to end-stage renal disease whenever possible. If a contrast enhanced MRI is felt to be necessary in such a patient, prompt dialysis following the examination should be considered.

Determination of the estimated glomerular filtration rate (eGFR) may be helpful in stratifying risk. At the author's institution, the following guidelines have been instituted. If the eGFR is greater than 60, the contrast examination may be performed in the usual manner. If the eGFR is between 30 and 60 ml · min^{-1} · 1.73 m^{-2}, the examination should be performed with gadobenate dimeglumine (MultiHance®), the agent which appears to have the lowest risk of NSF/NFD, using the standard or reduced dose. If the eGFR is less than 30 ml · min^{-1} · 1.73 m^{-2}, the examination should be performed without contrast or using a reduced dose of MultiHance®.

New developments in MRI for spinal disorders: 3-T (Tesla) MRI

Since MRI was introduced in the mid 1980s, there has been a steady trend toward higher field strength magnets. The initial machines were 0.1 and 0.15 T, followed by progressively more powerful systems.

From the mid 1990s to the time of writing, the gold standard for MR imaging of the spine has been the 1.5-T unit; however, there has been ongoing interest in higher field strength magnets. 3-T MR systems are now available for clinical use, 7-T systems are emerging in research settings, and even stronger magnets are under development.

The 3-T systems have advantages and disadvantages. The main benefit is an increased signal to noise ratio (SNR), which enhances image quality. Disadvantages include increase in chemical shift, pulsatile flow, and susceptibility artifact, all of which tend to degrade image quality. Susceptibility artifact is a particular concern in patients with spinal instrumentation. It is anticipated that these challenges will be overcome by modifying imaging parameters and through other technical advances, including more efficient coil designs and high bandwidth techniques.

Preliminary experience suggests that 3-T MRI may provide better definition of intramedullary tumors and leptomeningeal disease; however 3-T does not appear to have significant advantages over 1.5-T systems in the imaging of common discogenic and degenerative processes.

The role that 3-T MRI will ultimately play in spine care will be better defined as the technology matures. One concern from a clinical standpoint is whether the 3-T magnet will increase specificity or just sensitivity. At this point, higher field strength magnets should be viewed as representing an incremental improvement in MR imaging of the spine, as opposed to a major breakthrough.

Upright magnetic resonance imaging

Until recently, virtually all MRI studies were performed with the patient in the recumbent position. For intracranial lesions, patient orientation in the scanner is not a significant issue, and the recumbent position is more than adequate.

In contrast, for some spine patients, position during the examination potentially has greater significance. It is well known that spinal deformities are often more prominent on standing radiographs than on radiographs obtained in the usual recumbent position. In addition, standing radiographs following injection of intrathecal contrast (standing myelography) often show spinal stenosis to be much more pronounced with the patient in the standing position as compared with the recumbent position.

Building on this experience with standing radiographs and myelography, fully open MRI systems have recently been developed, which allow patients to be scanned while they are sitting, standing upright, or performing flexion and extension maneuvers. These units also allow for full or partial weight-bearing. This technique is known as upright or dynamic MRI.

Early work with these new systems has shown that a number of degenerative spinal disorders may be more prominent when the patient is standing, including disk herniations, spondylolisthesis, sagittal plane imbalance, and central and foraminal stenosis. The recumbent examination may underestimate the extent of degenerative spinal pathology.

These systems may be particularly useful among patients who experience spinal symptoms only in certain positions. For example, patients with lumbar spinal stenosis and neurogenic claudication are typically symptom-free when recumbent and only become symptomatic in the standing position. The theoretical advantage of upright MRI, in these situations, is that a specific imaging abnormality might be linked to a specific position or dynamic maneuver which produces a clinical symptom. This would enable imaging findings to be correlated more precisely with the patient's symptoms and signs.

Preliminary work has also been done with scanning patients in the prone position in an effort to reproduce the effects of positioning during surgery. The goal of this is to provide the surgeon with a set of images that more precisely represent the patient's anatomy during the surgical procedure. Whether this will provide any real benefit in patient care is uncertain.

The main drawback to upright MRI is lower image quality related to the use of a lower field strength magnet, typically around 0.6 T, as compared with 1.5 T for a standard closed magnet system. Another concern regarding image quality is motion artifact. It may be difficult for a patient in the upright, weight-bearing position to remain still long enough for the scan to be performed, especially when he/she is in the anatomic position, which reproduces symptoms. Faster acquisition times may obviate this concern.

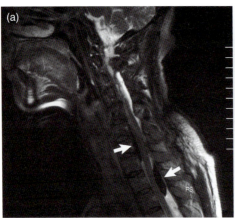
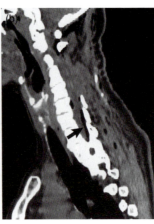

Figure 8.4. (a) Sagittal T$_2$-weighted MRI depicting decreased signal intensity ventral to the cord at C6–C7 (arrow) and dorsal to the cord at T1–T3 (arrow), which could represent acute blood and air. (b) Sagittal CT scan confirming that the abnormalities represented small collections of air related to the intradural surgical procedure (arrow).

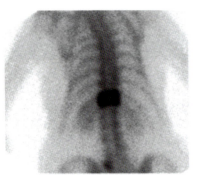

POSTERIOR

Figure 8.5. Radionuclide bone scan depicting intense radiotracer uptake at T11 and T12, consistent with acute vertebral compression fractures.

acute or subacute fracture, while the absence of uptake implies a chronic, healed fracture with no abnormal metabolic activity. This is a crucial determination because an acute fracture is often amenable to vertebral augmentation, while a chronic, healed fracture would not benefit from treatment with this technique. Figure 8.5 depicts a bone scan showing intense radiotracer uptake at T11 and T12, consistent with acute vertebral compression fractures.

Plain film radiography

Plain film radiographs are useful in evaluating spinal deformity, in surgical planning, and for postoperative assessment of spinal alignment, fusion maturation, and integrity of spinal instrumentation. Figure 8.6 depicts a post-operative radiograph of the lumbar spine showing scoliosis, pedicle screw fixation of L3–L5, intradiscal cage device, L4–L5, and posterolateral fusion mass.

Standing full torso radiographs

Standing 92-cm (36-inch) anteroposterior (AP) and lateral radiographs of the entire spinal column are very useful in selected cases. The AP view can identify coronal plane deformities (scoliosis), while the lateral view is the best means of identifying sagittal plane deformities (kyphosis). Standing radiographs may show spinal deformities much more dramatically than standard plain films, which are taken with the patient recumbent. Figure 8.7a depicts the recumbent lateral lumbar radiograph of a patient with instrumented fusion T11–L4. Note the mild kyphosis at the superior end of the fusion, measuring 19°. Figure 8.7b depicts the standing lateral radiograph of the same patient, showing a much more pronounced kyphotic deformity, measuring 45°.

Discography

Discography dates back to the 1940s and was originally used to evaluate patients with sciatica. The study was used to identify disk protrusions and to determine whether the patient's radicular pain was caused by the protrusion. In recent years, MRI and CT/myelography have replaced discography in the evaluation of radicular pain syndromes. Currently, the major role of discography is in the evaluation of patients with mechanical back pain.

Discography is a procedure which involves injection of contrast material into the lumbar disks, followed by imaging with plain films, CT, or both. The procedure has two components: first, an assessment of the radiographic appearance of the contrast-enhanced disk, and, second, the pain response elicited during the disk injection.

Disk morphology is graded from 0 (normal) to 5 (complete annular disruption, with spill of contrast

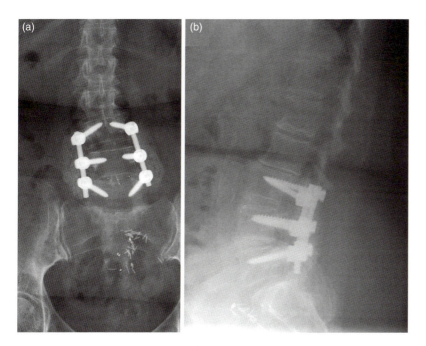

Figure 8.6. (a) Anteroposterior and (b) lateral plain radiographs of the lumbar spine depicting scoliosis and instrumented fusion, L3–L5.

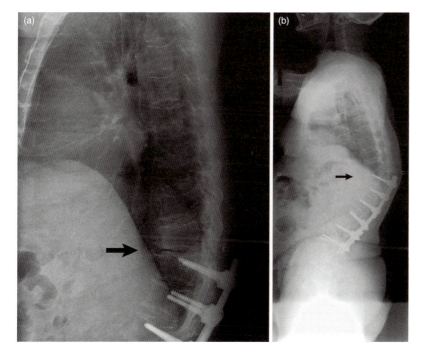

Figure 8.7. (a) Recumbent and (b) standing lateral radiograph of the lumbar spine depicting instrumented fusion T11–L4. Kyphotic deformity at the superior end of the construct is much more prominent in the standing position (arrow).

into the epidural space) using the modified Dallas discogram scale (Table 8.1). Regarding pain assessment, there are three possible responses to disc injection: (1) no pain; (2) pain which is typical of the patient's usual pain symptoms (concordant pain); and (3) pain which is not typical of the patient's usual pain (nonconcordant pain). The patient is blinded as to which disk is being injected.

Recently, some technical modifications have been introduced, including pressure and volume measurements and anesthetic injections into the disk; however, it has not yet been shown that these newer

Table 8.1. Modified Dallas discogram grading scale

Grade	
0	Contrast medium confined to a normal nucleus pulposus
1	Radial tear confined to the inner third of the annulus fibrosus
2	Radial tear extending to the middle third of the annulus fibrosus
3	Radial tear extending to the outer third of the annulus fibrosus
4	Grade 3 tear with dissection into the outer third of the annulus to involve more than 30° of the disk circumference
5	Any full-thickness tear with extra-annular leakage of contrast

refinements add to the validity and utility of the procedure.

Figure 8.8a depicts the post-discogram CT scan of a normal disk (grade 0), and Figure 8.8b depicts a disk with annular tear with extensive contrast dissection into the outer third of the annulus fibrosus (grade 4).

Discography is controversial, and there is no consensus about the usefulness of the procedure in the evaluation of low back pain. Proponents believe the test can identify symptomatic disk, or "pain generators," thereby serving as a screening tool to identify those patients who may benefit from minimally invasive intradiscal procedures, spinal fusion, or disk arthroplasty. Skeptics believe the test has too many false positives to be reliable.

Early investigators reported a very low rate of false positives, and it is generally accepted that asymptomatic, psychologically healthy individuals with normal disk morphology have a very low rate of painful disk injections. However, recent work by Caragee has identified a number of situations in which individuals without back pain have a high rate of false-positive disk injections. These include degenerative disk disease, previous disk surgery, chronic pain elsewhere in the body, somatization disorder, compensation issues, and extraspinal sources of pain, e.g., iliac crest donor-site pain.

The best usage of the test appears to be in defining the extent of a fusion among patients who already meet accepted criteria for a fusion procedure. An example of this is the patient with severe stenosis and spondylolisthesis at L4–L5, who is being considered for decompression and fusion. If adjacent segment disk degeneration is seen at L5–S1,

discography can be performed at that level. A positive discogram would suggest that the L5–S1 level should be included in the fusion, while a negative discogram would suggest that the adjacent level does not need to be included, and that surgery could be limited to the L4–L5 level. Even this seemingly well accepted use of discography has been challenged by recent work, showing that status of adjacent levels by provocative discography did not affect outcome following spinal fusion.

The weakest indication for discography is in the evaluation of the psychologically unstable patient in search of an anatomic diagnosis of a chronic pain state.

It should be emphasized that discography is not a test at the level of a gold standard in evaluating low back pain, and that test results should be interpreted with caution.

Bone density measurement

Bone mineral density (BMD) should be measured in all patients with vertebral compression fractures and in other individuals at increased risk for osteoporosis. Bone density testing can be used to establish a diagnosis of osteoporosis, to estimate future fracture risk, and to follow the response to treatment.

Dual-energy X-ray absorptiometry (DXA) is the most widely used test for measuring BMD. DXA can measure bone density in the lumbar spine and hip, two sites which are subject to the most clinically significant fractures. The DXA test report includes a measure of BMD in grams per square centimeter, a calculated T-score, and a calculated Z-score. The T-score represents the number of standard deviations (SD) a bone density is above or below the mean peak bone mass of the general population. T-scores are used to define the presence of osteoporosis. For example, a T-score between +1.0 and −1.0 is normal; a T-score between −1.0 and −2.5 indicates osteopenia (low bone mass); and a T-score below −2.5 indicates osteoporosis.

Selective nerve root block

Selective nerve root block (SNRB), done with fluoroscopic or CT guidance, involves localized injection of anesthetic agents and sometimes steroids, over a spinal nerve root. Although the procedure may provide long-term therapeutic benefit, the major role of SNRB is to serve as a diagnostic test to confirm whether a specific nerve root is symptomatic, when this is not clear on clinical grounds.

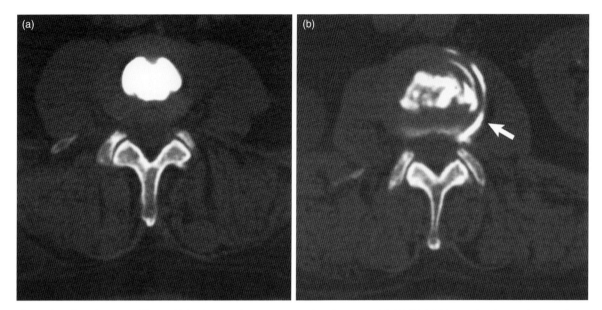

Figure 8.8. Post discogram CT scan. (a) Axial image depicting a normal nucleogram at L2–L3. (b) Axial image showing grade 4 annular tear at L3–L4, with extension of contrast into the outer annulus on the left (arrow).

Two responses should be assessed during the procedure: pain response to needle placement and pain response after anesthetic injection. If the patient's radicular pain is reproduced during needle placement and abolished with anesthetic injection, this is good confirmation of the symptomatic nerve root. Results must be interpreted with some degree of caution, as there is some risk of false-positive response due to spillover of anesthetic agents to adjacent levels.

Further reading

1. Carragee EJ, Alamin TF. Discography: a review. *Spine J* 2001; **1**:364–372.

2. Fenton DS, Czervionke LF (eds). *Image-Guided Spine Intervention*. PA: Saunders, 2003.

3. Public Health Advisory. *Update on Magnetic Resonance Imaging (MRI) Contrast Agents Containing Gadolinium and Nephrogenic Fibrosing Dermopathy*. Rockville, MD: United States Food and Drug Administration, December 22, 2006.

4. Shellock FG. *Reference Manual for Magnetic Resonance Safety, Implants and Devices*. Los Angeles, CA: Biomedical Research Publishing Company, 2007.

5. Weinstein JN, Rydevik BL, Sonntag VKH (eds). *Essentials of the Spine*. New York: Raven Press, 1995.

6. Willems PC, Elmans L, Anderson PG, van der Schaaf DB, de Kleuver M. Provocative discography and lumbar fusion: is preoperative assessment of adjacent discs useful? *Spine* 2007; **32**: 1094–1099.

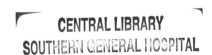

Disorders of the cervical spine: pre-operative assessment and surgical management

Clinical assessment and surgical evaluation

A wide range of disease processes affect the cervical spine. The differential diagnosis is shown in Table 9.1. Some of these disorders may require surgical management. Currently, the majority of surgical procedures performed on the cervical spine are done for disk herniations and cervical spondylosis; however, surgery may also be required for trauma, neoplasm, infection, inflammatory processes, vascular lesions, and congenital anomalies.

The importance of the clinical assessment and neurologic examination cannot be overemphasized. While the decision of what operation to perform (how to operate) is guided by imaging studies, the decision of whether and when to operate is largely made on clinical grounds. Establishing an accurate diagnosis is, therefore, of paramount importance.

Most patients with pain in the neck, or elsewhere in the spinal column, do not have a serious underlying illness and can be evaluated in an elective fashion; however, a small number of patients require more urgent evaluation. Symptoms which should prompt urgent or emergent evaluation are often referred to as "red flag" symptoms and include history of significant trauma, serious underlying medical illness, especially cancer or infection, weight loss, fever, and progressive neurologic deficit.

Neurologic examination should include an assessment of gait, motor and sensory function, and deep tendon reflexes. The head and neck should be examined for evidence of spinal deformity or head tilt, and for reproduction of neurologic symptoms with changes in position. The clinician should particularly search for a Spurling sign or Lhermitte sign. Spurling sign refers to the production of radicular pain when the patient extends the neck and looks over the shoulder on the symptomatic side. The presence of a Spurling sign usually indicates the presence of nerve root compression.

A Lhermitte sign refers to an electric shock sensation produced in the torso or extremities with changes in position of the head and neck, in particular cervical flexion. When present, a Lhermitte sign indicates the presence of a cervical cord lesion, which may be compressive (e.g., intramedullary cord tumor) or noncompressive (e.g., multiple sclerosis).

Motor loss from cervical nerve root compression may or may not be apparent to the patient, depending on the nerve root involved and the severity of the deficit. For example, C8 radiculopathy produces hand weakness, which is often detected very early by the patient, especially if the dominant hand is affected. In contrast, a patient with C7 radiculopathy may be unaware of profound triceps weakness, as there is less dependence on the triceps muscle in normal life activities.

C5 and C6 root lesions are intermediate in their impact on activities of daily living. A C5 radiculopathy, producing deltoid and external rotator weakness, can limit the patient's ability to lift objects overhead. Severe C6 motor loss can be bothersome as impaired biceps function may prevent the patient from feeding themselves, brushing their teeth, and shaving.

Diagnostic pitfalls

The following is a list of scenarios from the author's spine surgery practice, in which the correct diagnosis has been missed or delayed. In some cases, the patient has been referred for potentially inappropriate surgery, while in others, appropriate surgical referral has been delayed. The problem often results from an over-reliance on spine imaging studies, coupled with an inadequate clinical assessment of the patient.

1. Carpal tunnel syndrome vs. cervical spondylotic myelopathy. The patient with numb hands usually has carpal tunnel syndrome, not cervical myelopathy. Yet, patients with this symptom sometimes undergo magnetic resonance imaging (MRI) of the cervical spine and referral to a neurosurgeon for decompressive surgery on the

Table 9.1. Differential diagnosis of pain in the neck, shoulder, and arm, with or without neurologic involvement

1. Discogenic or degenerative disease

    A. Herniated intervertebral disk

    B. Degenerative cervical spondylosis with canal stenosis

    C. Synovial cyst of facet joint

2. Trauma

3. Tumor

    A. Primary intradural tumor of spinal cord or adjacent nerve roots

    B. Tumor of vertebral column or epidural space (or both)

      – Metastatic tumor

      – Plasmacytoma or multiple myeloma

      – Primary bone tumor (e.g., chordoma)

4. Infection

    A. Intervertebral discitis or osteomyelitis

    B. Epidural abscess

    C. Herpes zoster or other viral radiculopathy

5. Vascular lesion

    A. Neoplastic vascular lesion (e.g., cavernous malformation)

    B. Arteriovenous fistula

    C. Arteriovenous malformation

6. Inflammatory arthropathy (e.g., rheumatoid arthritis)

7. Syringomyelia

8. Brachial plexus lesion

9. Peripheral nerve lesion (e.g., carpal tunnel syndrome)

10. Shoulder disorder (e.g., rotator cuff tear)

11. Thoracic outlet syndrome

12. Noncompressive disorders of the spinal cord and peripheral nerves

    A. Motor neuron disease

    B. Primary lateral sclerosis

    C. Guillain–Barré syndrome

    D. Peripheral neuropathy

13. Metabolic bone disease

    A. Osteoporosis

14. Congenital bony anomalies (e.g., Klippel–Feil syndrome)

cervical spine. The diagnosis of carpal tunnel syndrome should be relatively straightforward on clinical grounds and can be confirmed with electromyography (EMG). Imaging of the cervical spine is not indicated and often just leads to confusion regarding the correct diagnosis and management.

> *Clinical pearl: Numb hands usually indicate carpal tunnel syndrome, not cervical cord compression.*

2. Amyotrophic lateral sclerosis (ALS) vs. cervical spondylotic myelopathy. ALS may produce findings similar to a compressive myelopathy. One distinguishing feature is that ALS often produces brain stem signs and prominent fasciculations in the tongue and other muscles. Also, patients with ALS generally do not have any sensory findings, in contrast to compressive myelopathy. EMG is an important diagnostic tool. In most cases, the diagnosis of ALS can be reliably established on clinical and neurophysiologic grounds. That said, distinguishing between ALS and cervical cord compression is sometimes difficult, even for an experienced neuromuscular specialist. As a result, an occasional patient who undergoes cervical decompression for cervical spondylosis later proves to have ALS.

> *Clinical pearl: If the patient with cervical myelopathy has no sensory findings but does have bulbar signs and prominent fasciculations, think ALS.*

3. Shoulder disorder vs. cervical radiculopathy. The patient with a shoulder disorder (tendonitis, subacromial bursitis, or rotator cuff tear) has localized tenderness over the greater tuberosity of the humerus, decreased range of motion, and shoulder pain with internal and external rotation and abduction. In contrast, the patient with cervical radiculopathy characteristically has pain beneath the scapula, aggravated by turning the head to the affected side (Spurling maneuver). The diagnostic impression can be confirmed with plain film radiography of the shoulder. EMG may be useful in excluding radiculopathy. Again, imaging of the cervical spine is generally not necessary and may simply serve to obscure and delay the correct diagnosis.

> *Clinical pearl: Anterior shoulder pain precipitated by internal and external rotation and abduction of the arm usually indicates a primary disorder of the shoulder, not cervical radiculopathy.*

4. Brachial plexus lesion vs. cervical radiculopathy. The diagnosis of brachial plexopathy should be considered in the patient with significant arm pain and weakness, with unremarkable imaging of the

cervical spine. In these cases, MRI of the brachial plexus should be performed to look for tumor, which may be benign or malignant (Figure 9.1). EMG may also be helpful in defining the location and severity of a plexus lesion.

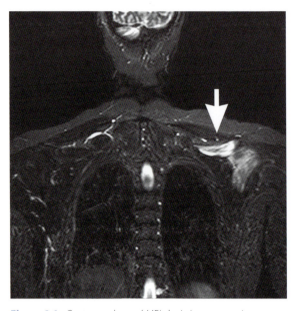

Figure 9.1. Contrast-enhanced MRI depicting metastatic tumor of left brachial plexus (arrow).

> *Clinical pearl: If the patient has significant arm pain and weakness, with unremarkable imaging of the cervical spine, look at the brachial plexus.*

5. False localizing level. A sensory level does not always correspond to the level of the cord lesion. A 47-year-old man presented with a myelopathy with a T4 sensory level. MRI of the thoracic spine was completely normal (Figure 9.2a). After a delay of several months, MRI of the cervical spine was obtained, and the study showed a large central disk herniation at C5–C6, with cord compression and signal change in the cord, consistent with myelomalacia (Figure 9.2b). The patient underwent anterior cervical decompression and fusion with allograft bone and plate. Neurologic recovery was compromised due to the delay in diagnosis.

> *Clinical pearl: A sensory level may be several segments downstream from the cord lesion.*

6. Odontoid fracture of the elderly. Older individuals often have advanced cervical spondylosis, which makes it difficult to discern fractures with plain film radiography, especially in the upper cervical region. An 80-year-old man presented to the

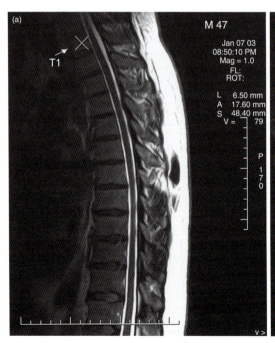
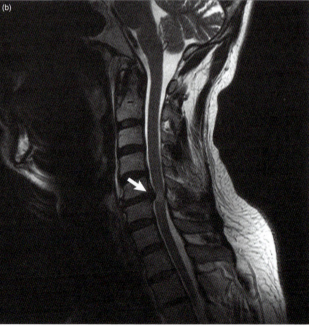

Figure 9.2. (a) Normal sagittal, T_2-weighted thoracic spine MRI in a patient with T4 sensory level myelopathy. (b) Cervical spine MRI in the same patient depicting a large midline disk herniation at C5–C6 with cord compression and myelomalacia (arrow).

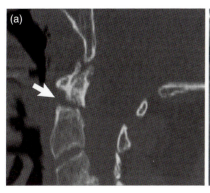
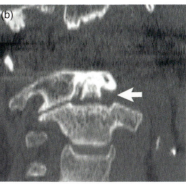

Figure 9.3. (a) Sagittal and (b) coronal CT scan of the cervical spine depicting an unstable, posteriorly displaced Type II odontoid fracture (arrow), which was not identified on plain radiographs.

emergency department with neck pain after a fall at home. Plain film radiography was negative. A CT scan of the cervical spine showed a Type II odontoid fracture (Figure 9.3), which required surgery. In most centers, CT scanning has become the procedure of choice for evaluating the patient with cervical spine trauma.

> *Clinical pearl: Plain film radiography can miss cervical spine fractures, especially in the elderly. CT is more sensitive and is the diagnostic procedure of choice in the evaluation of acute cervical spine trauma.*

Surgical indications and approaches

The clinical indications for surgery on the cervical spine include myelopathy, radiculopathy, and instability. Neck pain by itself is rarely an indication for surgery. Most operations are done for degenerative or discogenic processes, however a wide range of disorders may potentially require surgery.

Cervical spine procedures utilize anterior, posterior, or combined anterior–posterior approaches. In general, anterior approaches are used for lesions in the anterior spinal column. Posterior approaches are appropriate for lesions posterior to the cord and for virtually all intradural pathology. Combined techniques, so-called circumferential or 360° approaches, are used when there are compressive lesions both anterior and posterior to the cord and when extensive realignment and stabilization are required. When a 360° approach is used, the anterior and posterior portions may be done on the same day (single-stage) or on separate days (staged), depending on the clinical circumstances.

If significant deformity correction is required, the patient will almost always require an anterior or combined anterior–posterior approach. It is very difficult to achieve significant spinal realignment using just a posterior approach.

Complex fixed deformities may even require a posterior–anterior–posterior or 540° operation. In these situations, the spine is initially approached posteriorly with multiple facetectomies to release the posterior elements, followed by anterior decompression, deformity correction, and placement of instrumentation. In the final stage, the posterior incision is reopened for placement of lateral mass instrumentation.

Anterior techniques include discectomy, corpectomy, fusion with various bone grafting materials, and instrumentation. The most common anterior cervical operation is anterior cervical discectomy with bone graft and plate. The procedure may be performed at a single level or multiple levels, depending on clinical and radiographic findings. The steps of the procedure are outlined in Figure 9.4.

Posterior techniques include foraminotomy, discectomy, decompressive laminectomy, laminoplasty, fusion with various bone grafting materials, and instrumentation. One of the more common posterior operations is lateral mass fixation, which is used to prevent or treat kyphotic deformities of the cervical spine. Lateral mass fixation is often combined with laminectomy to decompress the neural elements. The steps involved in lateral mass fixation plus laminectomy are outlined in Figure 9.5.

Bone graft considerations

Current options for bone grafting include autograft, allograft, and synthetic implants. Autograft refers to bone transplanted from elsewhere in the patient's body, typically the iliac crest. Allograft, or homograft, refers to bone transplanted from another human. Allograft is usually harvested from a cadaver and maintained in a bone bank until it is needed. The

147

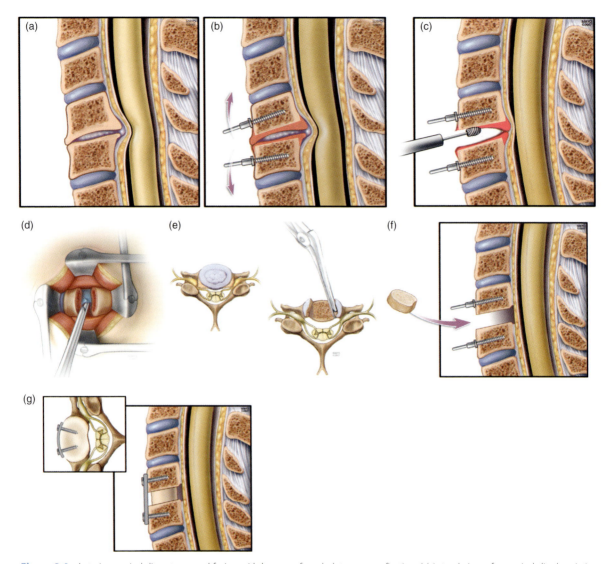

Figure 9.4. Anterior cervical discectomy and fusion with bone graft and plate – screw fixation. (a) Lateral view of a cervical disc herniation (disk–osteophyte complex) causing spinal cord compression. (b) Distraction posts in the adjacent vertebral bodies, preparing for distraction to open up the interspace. Note posts have been placed in divergent positions, to promote cervical lordosis after distraction is applied. (c) Removal of disk material and osteophytes with high-speed drill. (d) Removal of posterior longitudinal ligament. (e) Axial view depicting osteophyte removal with the Kerrison punch. This may also be accomplished with the drill or a variety of curettes and pituitary rongeurs. (f) Insertion of bone graft. (g) Final appearance of construct after placement of plate and screws. Note decompression of the spinal cord and restoration of cervical lordosis. Figure reproduced with permission from Mayo Foundation for Medical Education and Research.

relative merits of grafting materials have been widely debated. The key issues in this discussion include clinical efficacy, graft harvest morbidity, safety, cost, and availability.

The long-term goal of bone grafting is graft incorporation without creating any new spinal deformity. In this regard, autograft has significant advantages over allograft. Autograft contains bone morphogenetic proteins (BMPs), which are important in osteoinduction and in the production of osteoblasts. In contrast,

BMPs are limited in fresh-frozen allografts and absent in freeze-dried allografts.

The structure of the graft also plays a role in its incorporation. Cancellous bone provides a three-dimensional scaffold, which is a more favorable environment for osteoconduction than cortical bone. Cancellous allograft and autograft have been shown to have a faster rate of incorporation than cortical allograft.

The short-term goal of bone grafting is to maintain height of the interspace until the graft is

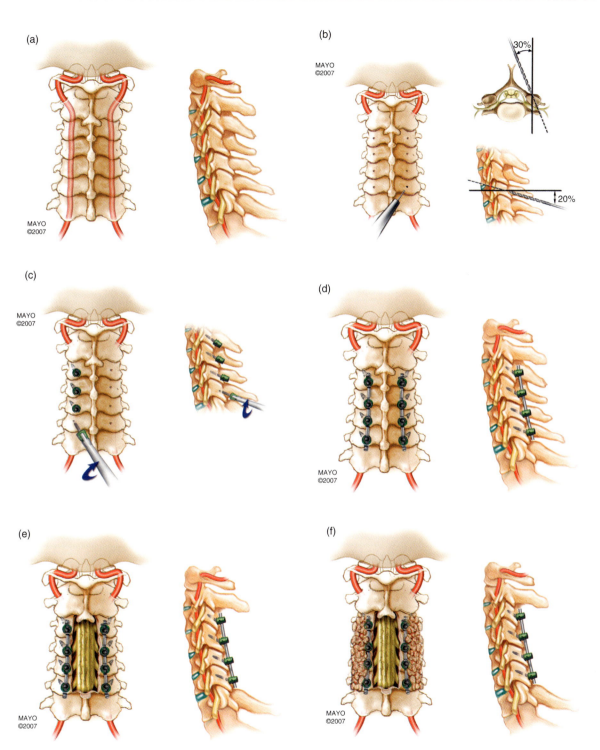

Figure 9.5. Posterior cervical fusion with lateral mass fixation, plus laminectomy. (a) Anteroposterior and lateral exposure of the cervical spine depicting relation of vertebral artery and nerve roots to bony landmarks. (b) Anteroposterior view depicting starting points for lateral mass screws, with drilling of one "starter" hole. Axial and lateral views depicting trajectories used for drilling the lateral masses. (c) Placement of lateral mass screws. (d) Completion of lateral mass screw–rod construct, C3–C6. (e) Completion of laminectomy. Note that laminectomy is generally done after placement of lateral mass instrumentation in order to avoid injuring the spinal cord by dropping instruments or implants on the exposure dura during placement of fixation devices. (f) Final appearance of the surgical site after placement of bone grafting materials. Care should be taken to keep all graft material lateral to the rod and away from the exposed dura. Figure reproduced with permission from Mayo Foundation for Medical Education and Research.

incorporated. This is important because significant disk space collapse may lead to kyphotic deformity and other morbidity. Variable degrees of loss of disk height are noted with either autograft or allograft, ranging from 20% to 50%.

Anterior cervical discectomy and fusion procedures date back to the 1950s. The first procedures were performed using the patient's own iliac crest bone (autograft). The graft harvest involves a separate incision over the iliac crest, and removal of an appropriately sized graft using an oscillating saw and/or osteotome. An alternative graft harvest site is the middle third of the fibula. Extensive clinical experience has shown iliac crest autograft to be an excellent graft material. Compared with allograft, iliac crest autograft is associated with higher fusion rates for one- and two-level anterior cervical fusions.

The main drawback to the use of iliac crest autograft is donor-site morbidity. Acute complications include wound hematoma, infection, iliac fracture, and meralgia parasthetica from injury to the lateral femoral cutaneous nerve. Donor-site pain is a significant issue for many patients and is often under-recognized by the surgical team. Acute pain at the donor site may be severe, and one-third of patients report some degree of pain one year after surgery.

These concerns led surgeons to employ allograft bone, in an effort to avoid donor-site complications associated with harvesting bone from the iliac crest or fibula. The use of allograft bone eliminates donor-site morbidity and decreases the operative time. Allograft fusion is a very important option when iliac crest bone is either not available due to previous harvesting, or cannot be used because of poor bone quality. Another advantage of allograft is that it can be more precisely machined than autograft specimens that are shaped in the operating room. In many cases, this allows for a better fit of allograft bone within the interspace.

The main drawback to allograft bone, relative to autograft, is that the fusion process has proven to be slower, with a higher rate of nonunion. This is especially true when two or more levels are fused. These concerns were addressed with the development of anterior plating systems which have made the use of allograft more appealing. The fusion rates seen in one- and two-level anterior cervical discectomy and fusion procedures, performed with allograft and plate, now approach those seen with iliac crest autograft.

There has been some concern regarding the safety of allograft relative to the risk of transmission of human immunodeficiency virus (HIV), hepatitis B, hepatitis C, and other viruses. There have been two reported cases of HIV transmission with fresh-frozen allografts, and both occurred early in the evolution of the HIV epidemic before routine screening techniques were used. There have been no reported cases of viral transmission with the techniques of donor screening and allograft preparation that are currently in use.

A comprehensive cost analysis comparing autograft and allograft is not available. Allograft bone represents an added expense, relative to autograft. However, this apparent saving associated with using autograft bone is offset by the cost of extra time in the operating room required to harvest and prepare the autograft, and by costs incurred when treating donor-site complications.

At the present time, most surgeons use allograft supplemented with plate-screw fixation when performing anterior cervical discectomy and fusion procedures.

Smokers represent a special circumstance. Smoking has a detrimental effect on the arthrodesis rate after anterior cervical fusion, and this effect is more pronounced with allograft than autograft. Therefore, autograft bone is often a better choice in smokers undergoing anterior cervical fusion. Iliac crest autograft should also be considered in other patients with risk factors for pseudarthrosis, including end-stage renal disease and fusions spanning three or more levels.

The major new technology in this area is synthetic interbody devices, which may be either nonabsorbable or absorbable. An example of a nonabsorbable device is the poly-ether-ether-ketone (PEEK) spacer; and an example of an absorbable device is the Macro-Pore spacer (Medtronic, Sofamor Danek, Memphis, TN). The advantages of synthetic devices are that they: can be made in unlimited quantities, do not carry a risk of disease transmission, are not associated with donor-site morbidity, and can be machined to perfectly fit the interspace. The major drawback to synthetic devices is their cost, especially when combined with BMP.

In preliminary studies using a PEEK spacer filled with BMP, investigators have achieved a 100% fusion rate regardless of the number of levels fused or the patient's smoking history. However, these encouraging results must be balanced by the recent observation that BMP has also been shown to be associated with local swelling and swallowing difficulties when used in the ventral cervical spine. In addition, use of BMP in the cervical spine is considered an off-label indication.

Provided the difficulties with BMP can be resolved, the use of synthetic interbody devices may permit "bone-free" cervical arthrodesis in the near future. Absorbable implants are discussed in more detail in Chapter 13.

Surgical complications

The spine surgeon must be well aware of potential complications associated with an operative procedure; however, it is also important for the neurologist to have a working knowledge of this topic, as patients often inquire about potential complications prior to surgical referral. The neurologist may also be asked to evaluate patients who have experienced these events after the surgical procedure.

Acute surgical complications include spinal cord or nerve root injury, vertebral artery injury, cerebrospinal fluid (CSF) leak, infection, graft/plate movement, esophageal injury, and airway compromise. The most ominous complications are quadriplegia and respiratory arrest due to airway compromise.

Neurologic deterioration

Neurologic complications may occur at the spinal cord or nerve root level. Quadriplegia may be acute, due to intra-operative cord injury, or delayed, due to post-operative extradural hematoma, bone graft migration into the spinal canal, or loss of alignment.

Any patient who awakens from a surgical procedure with a new neurologic deficit or develops a new deficit in the post-operative period must be investigated promptly. The decision to re-operate is largely made on clinical grounds; however, imaging studies may assist the surgeon in deciding what needs to be done when the patient is returned to surgery. Plain radiographs should be obtained to check for malalignment and problems with positioning of bone grafts and instrumentation, for example a screw projecting into the spinal canal. MRI can identify post-operative hematomas and fluid collections causing cord compression. In the case of deterioration after laminectomy, MRI is particularly helpful in identifying hematomas dissecting beneath laminae that were not removed at the initial procedure. In the case of deterioration after anterior cervical procedures, MRI can identify hematomas that have dissected beneath the vertebral body above or below the original

surgical site. Without this information obtained from the MRI, the surgeon might simply re-explore the surgical site and miss the compressive hematoma at re-operation.

In situations where the patient develops a new radicular pain or weakness after lateral mass fusion, a CT scan should be performed to look for evidence of nerve root or foraminal penetration by a misdirected screw. In these cases, the screw should be re-directed or removed. The surgeon should also avoid placing screws that are too long. On a lateral radiograph, the screw should not extend ventrally past the posterior margin of the vertebral body.

Often, the CT scan does not reveal any evidence of foraminal penetration by screws or instruments. In these cases, the radicular deficit is attributed to "lag screw effect." This complication occurs when there is a gap between the lateral mass and the rod or plate. Tightening of the lateral mass screw can cause the lateral mass to shift dorsally against the rod or plate, resulting in deformation of the neural foramen, with stretching or compression of the nerve root.

This complication can be minimized, although not completely avoided, by carefully contouring the plate or rod to approximate the alignment of the spine to the greatest extent possible. This will minimize any potential lag effect, with the concomitant shifting and deformation of the neural foramen during final tightening of a lateral mass screw.

Post-operative radiculopathy can affect any of the cervical nerve roots; however, the C5 root is particularly vulnerable. The reasons for this are unclear, but possibly relate to increased traction and tethering of the C5 root in the neural foramen, which could be exacerbated by the lag screw effect and also by posterior migration of the cord if laminectomy is performed.

The C8 root is also vulnerable in lateral mass fusion procedures, as the C7–T1 lateral mass is quite shallow, putting the C8 root at greater risk during screw placement.

Vascular injury

The vertebral artery may be injured during anterior or posterior cervical procedures.

Two risk factors for this complication during anterior procedures are an anomalous vertebral artery and failure of the surgeon to remain oriented to the midline. Prior to the procedure, the surgeon should carefully review pre-operative imaging studies, in order to verify the position of the vertebral artery at the intended level of surgery, as this vessel occasionally takes an anomalous course toward the midline. During the procedure, the surgeon must constantly stay oriented to the midline of the spine, in order to avoid dissecting or drilling too far laterally and damaging the vertebral artery.

The vertebral artery is also at risk during posterior procedures, in particular those in the upper cervical region. Lateral soft tissue dissection between the occiput and C1, and screw placement at C1 and C2 can result in injury to the vertebral artery. In the subaxial spine, the vertebral artery lies immediately ventral to the nerve root, and can be injured if the surgeon explores too far ventrally in search of an extruded disk fragment behind the nerve root.

Tumor cases are also problematic, as the tumor may encase or significantly displace the vertebral artery well away from its normal position. In these cases, magnetic resonance angiography (MRA) or CT angiography should be considered to more precisely define the location of the vertebral artery. In selected cases, a pre-operative balloon occlusion test may be helpful, to determine whether the affected vertebral artery can be safely sacrificed during the tumor resection.

If the vertebral artery is injured, ligation must usually be performed. Because the vessel is quite deep and is fixed by the transverse foramina, direct repair is difficult, but can sometimes be accomplished. Endovascular techniques may also be helpful in managing this complication.

The carotid artery can be injured during anterior cervical procedures. As this vessel is much more accessible than the vertebral artery, direct repair is often feasible.

Cerebrospinal fluid leak

Dural openings and cerebrospinal fluid (CSF) leakage can be seen with operations on the anterior or posterior cervical spine. Risks are increased with revision surgery. The risk of CSF leakage is markedly increased in anterior procedures on patients with ossification of the posterior longitudinal ligament (OPLL).

In some cases, a CSF leak is apparent during the surgical procedure, while in others it does not manifest until the post-operative period. Signs of a post-operative leak include postural headache, bulging of the surgical wound, or frank drainage of CSF through the incision. A CT or MRI may confirm a CSF collection at the surgical site, but imaging findings are often nonspecific and may not be able to distinguish between CSF and seroma fluid. In equivocal cases, a fluid collection can be aspirated percutaneously and analyzed for beta-2 transferrin, a protein that is found in CSF but not in other body fluids.

Once a leak is identified, direct repair should be attempted. Because of exposure limitations, it is often impossible to carry out direct repair of leaks occurring during anterior procedures. The dural opening should be covered with a small piece of Gelfoam or muscle. This is often adequate to seal the leak, as there is very little dead space in which CSF can accumulate following the procedure. With posterior procedures, the dura can be more widely exposed, thereby facilitating direct repair.

A variety of tissue sealants may be used to reinforce a dural repair. A short course of lumbar CSF drainage may also be beneficial.

Lumboperitoneal shunting may also be useful in refractory cases. This procedure should be used judiciously, as patients with lumboperitoneal shunts are at risk for overdrainage of CSF with subsequent development of subdural hematoma or acquired Chiari malformation. It is often advisable to remove or ligate the shunt 6–8 weeks post-operatively to prevent these complications.

Airway and swallowing complications

A potentially serious complication of operations on the anterior cervical spine is airway compromise, which may be caused by a hematoma or edema at the surgical site. Even a small hematoma may compress the airway and cause respiratory arrest.

Extensive anterior operations represent a particular risk for post-operative airway compromise. Specific risk factors that have been identified include: prolonged operative time (>10 hours), extensive blood loss (transfusion >4 units), high approach to the C2 level, multi-level approaches, asthma, and obesity. It is often best to keep such patients intubated overnight following surgery and arrange for careful extubation the next day under the direct supervision of an anesthesiologist or critical care specialist.

Hoarseness and dysphagia may occur after anterior operations on the cervical spine. These complications are usually mild and temporary, but are occasionally prolonged and quite bothersome, especially for individuals who engage in singing and public speaking. Initially, it had been thought that hoarseness was

---

more common with right-sided approaches due to greater vulnerability of the recurrent laryngeal nerve on that side; however, more recent data have shown that the incidence of hoarseness is equivalent between right-sided and left-sided approaches.

There are several potential causes of post-operative dysphagia, including injury to the nerves involved in swallowing, prevertebral swelling, direct esophageal injury during the procedure (either tearing of the esophagus or pressure from retractors), compression of the esophagus from a cervical plate or screw, and adhesion formation around the plate.

Patients should be observed carefully for signs of aspiration following operations on the anterior cervical spine. In high-risk patients, oxygen saturation should be monitored on an intermittent (spot check) or continuous basis. Swallowing function should be assessed and verified to be satisfactory before permitting oral intake. A speech pathologist can perform a formal swallowing evaluation if necessary. For patients that "fail" their post-operative swallowing study, nutrition should be maintained via a nasal or percutaneous gastrostomy (PEG) feeding tube until swallowing normalizes. Among patients undergoing extensive anterior cervical procedures, a feeding tube may be necessary in the early post-operative period in 15%–20% of cases. In almost all cases, swallowing function recovers and the feeding tube can be removed within 3 months of surgery.

Esophageal injury

The esophagus can be injured during operations on the anterior cervical and upper thoracic spine. If an esophageal tear is identified during the procedure, repair should be performed immediately. Often, the injury is not recognized at the time of surgery. Post-operative signs of esophageal injury include excessive neck pain, difficult or painful swallowing, subcutaneous emphysema of the neck and upper chest, and signs of infection, including fever and tachycardia. The diagnostic test of choice is an esophagogram with water-soluble contrast material. If a tear is identified, immediate re-operation and repair should be carried out. If a tear is not identified, management is less straightforward. Depending on clinical circumstances, the patient may be re-explored or may be managed with observation and placement of a nasogastric tube.

Esophageal injury is a serious complication. Left untreated, it can result in esophageal strictures, fistula formation, mediastinitis, and death.

Finally, it should be noted that esophageal injury may rarely occur as a complication of endotracheal intubation. Therefore, any patient who is currently intubated or has a history of recent endotracheal intubation, or who demonstrates any of the signs noted above, should be promptly investigated for possible esophageal injury.

Complications related to positioning

Peripheral nerve or plexus injury related to positioning may occur, especially during lengthy operations. Patients must be carefully positioned prior to surgery with meticulous padding of all pressure points in order to avoid these complications.

Wrong level surgery

Wrong level/wrong side/wrong patient surgery mishaps are occasionally seen and have been the subject of much recent attention. At many hospitals, pre-operative "time-outs," surgical site labeling and verification, and other measures have been instituted in an effort to avoid this type of problem. An example of wrong level surgery is shown in Figure 10.3.

Infection

Post-operative infection may occur after procedures at any level of the spinal column. Risk factors include diabetes, smoking, prolonged operations, repeat operations, and placement of instrumentation or other foreign bodies. A posterior cervical wound infection is shown in Figure 9.6.

The traditional approach to surgical wound infections was debridement and removal of all foreign bodies, including spinal instrumentation. The wound was packed open and allowed to heal secondarily with wet-to-dry dressing changes. Although these treatments eventually resolve the infection, there are several drawbacks to this strategy. First, it often takes several weeks or months for the wound to heal. Second, the process of wet-to-dry dressing changes requires daily nursing visits for the duration of the treatment and can be quite painful to the patient. And third, another operation is ultimately required to replace the explanted spinal instrumentation.

Improvements in antibiotic therapy in the early twenty-first century and a better understanding of spinal infections have made it possible to preserve spinal instrumentation in the vast majority of surgical wound infections.

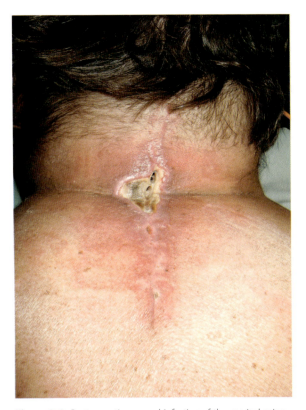

Figure 9.6. Post-operative wound infection of the cervical spine.

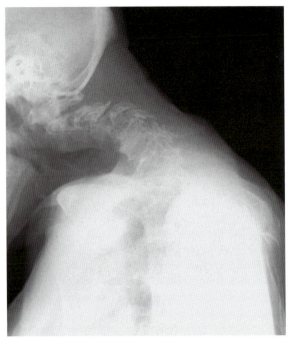

Figure 9.7. Lateral radiograph showing post-laminectomy kyphosis (swan neck deformity).

Management now includes surgical debridement and immediate re-closure of the wound over drains, with preservation of instrumentation. The patient typically receives 4–6 weeks of intravenous antibiotics tailored to the organism(s) cultured from the wound. In high-risk patients, this may be followed by a course of oral suppressive therapy.

For wounds that fail to heal with these measures, continuous wound suctioning with a Wound VAC (vacuum assisted closure) device may help. Similar to wet-to-dry dressing changes, Wound VAC therapy allows the wound to heal secondarily. The Wound VAC is lower maintenance and requires less nursing care and causes less discomfort than wet-to-dry dressing changes. In refractory cases, the involvement of a plastic surgeon may be necessary for rotation of muscle flaps to promote wound healing.

Late complications

Delayed surgical complications include progressive kyphosis (swan neck deformity) and other types of instability. Kyphotic deformities are usually seen after decompressive laminectomy, but may also occur after

anterior procedures. Post-operative deformity may represent a complication of surgery, inadequate correction of a pre-existing deformity, natural history, or some combination of these. Figure 9.7 depicts an example of swan neck deformity, which occurred after decompressive laminectomy.

Selected surgical disorders of the cervical spine

Cervical disk herniation with radiculopathy and/or myelopathy

Acute cervical disk herniation is usually seen in middle-aged persons, but may also affect the elderly. This problem is rarely seen in children and is uncommon in young adults. The patient usually presents with radicular pain and variable degrees of neck pain. Pain beneath the ipsilateral scapula is often a prominent finding. Typical physical examination findings include a positive Spurling maneuver and radicular weakness, which may range from mild to profound. More severe degrees of weakness should prompt more rapid evaluation and treatment. When present, long tract signs and other evidence of myelopathy should also prompt urgent evaluation. EMG and SNRB may be useful in confirming the clinical impression, and

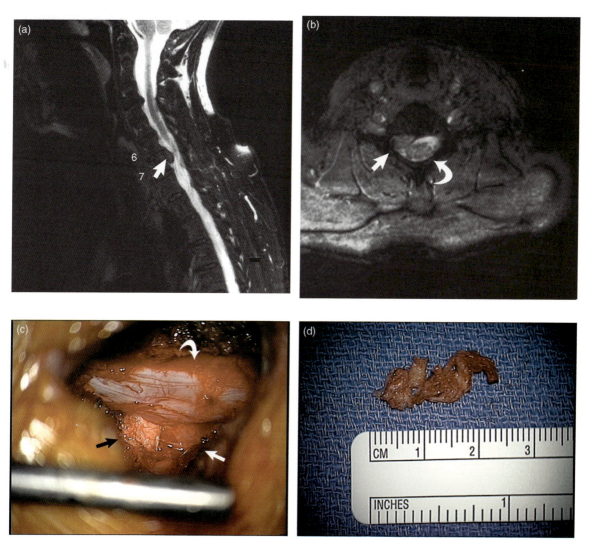

Figure 9.8. (a) Sagittal T$_2$-weighted MRI, with fat saturation, depicting a large cervical disk extrusion at C6–C7, right, with spinal cord compression and caudal migration of disk material (arrow). (b) Axial T$_2$-weighted MRI, depicting the disk extrusion (straight arrow), with compression and rotation of the spinal cord (curved arrow). (c) Intra-operative photomicrograph showing the extruded disk (black arrow) in the axilla of the nerve root (straight white arrow), lateral and ventral to the common dural sac (curved white arrow). Patient orientation: head to the right, feet to the left. (d) Photograph of the extruded disk fragment after removal.

may also be useful in pinpointing the symptomatic level if two or more levels are positive on imaging studies. MRI is the imaging procedure of choice. Surgery should be considered for intractable radiculopathy or myelopathy. A lateral soft disk herniation may be treated with either an anterior or a posterior approach, while a midline soft disk herniation or any hard disk (osteophyte) is generally best approached anteriorly.

Figures 9.8a and 9.8b depict a cervical spine MRI showing a lateral soft disk extrusion at C6–C7, right, with inferior migration of disk material. The finding of a lateral soft disk extrusion made the patient a good candidate for a posterior operation. The disk fragment was removed via a posterior approach. Figure 9.8c depicts a photomicrograph of the surgical site, showing the relationship between the disk fragment and the exiting nerve root and common dural sac. Figure 9.8d depicts the surgical specimen after removal. A fusion is usually not performed with a posterior discectomy. A hard collar is not required post-operatively, although patients sometimes use a soft collar for a few days as a comfort measure.

Figure 9.9a depicts the typical MRI findings of a midline cervical disk herniation at C5–C6. Since the

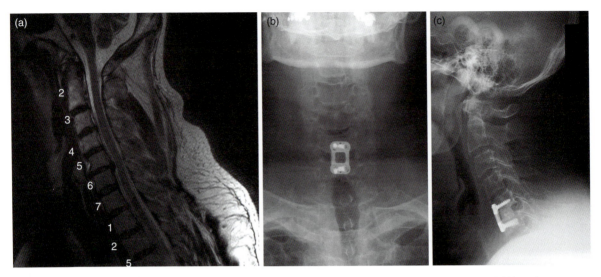

Figure 9.9. (a) Sagittal T$_2$-weighted cervical spine MRI depicting a disk herniation at C5–C6. (b) Anteroposterior and (c) lateral post-operative lateral radiograph depicting the expected appearance of the bone graft and plate–screw construct at C5–C6.

herniation was in the midline, an anterior approach was used. The patient underwent anterior cervical discectomy with allograft and plate. Figures 9.9b and 9.9c depict the post-operative plain film radiographs. Following this procedure, patients generally wear a hard cervical collar for 4–8 weeks, based on surgeon preference.

Surgery for a single-level disk herniation with radiculopathy is one of the most successful spine operations, with excellent results obtained in 85%–90% of cases, using either an anterior or a posterior approach.

Serious complications are uncommon. In a large series of more than 1000 patients undergoing first-time anterior cervical discectomy and fusion, the mortality rate was 0.1% and the overall morbidity was 19.3%, with most complications being mild and temporary. The following complications were observed: spinal cord injury 0.2%, esophageal perforation 0.3%, Horner syndrome 0.1%, wound infection 0.1%, instrumentation back-out 0.1%, and post-operative hematoma 5.6%, with surgical evacuation of the hematoma being required in 2.4%. The most common complications related to swallowing and voice quality. The incidence of post-operative dysphagia and symptomatic recurrent laryngeal nerve palsy were 9.5% and 3.1% respectively. These symptoms resolved within 3 months of surgery.

Recurrent disk herniation at a previously operated level is uncommon. This is especially true with anterior cervical discectomy and fusion, which involves a complete discectomy and generous removal of posterior osteophytes.

At the same time, it is now recognized that, with long-term follow-up over 5–10 years, patients undergoing cervical disk procedures are at risk for development of disk degeneration and osteophytes elsewhere in the spine, often at a level immediately adjacent to the previously operated level. This process has come to be known as "adjacent segment disease."

It is important to distinguish between radiographic and clinically significant adjacent segment disease. In many cases, patients just have radiographic evidence of progressive spondylosis without any clinical symptoms. However, in others, the degenerative process progresses to the point of causing symptomatic nerve root or spinal cord compression requiring re-operation.

The cause of adjacent segment disease has not been fully clarified. Some have postulated that a single-level fusion in the mid-cervical region produces significant alterations in spinal biomechanics, resulting in more stress on other spinal segments, leading to an increased rate of symptomatic degeneration at adjacent levels. Others have suggested that adjacent segment disease simply represents the natural history of cervical spondylosis. Indeed, it is well known that cervical spondylosis does progress slowly over time, whether surgical intervention is performed or not.

The incidence of adjacent segment disease following anterior cervical discectomy and fusion has been studied extensively, and several studies have shown that symptomatic adjacent segment disease develops at an annual rate of about 3%. Corresponding data for nonfusion, or motion-sparing, procedures are less extensive; however, a recent report showed an incidence of 0.7% for posterior cervical foraminotomy.

Based on these data, it appears that the fusion itself accelerates the process of adjacent segment disease, and that a motion-sparing operation is associated with a lower rate of adjacent segment degeneration. This has been the primary justification for the development of new motion-sparing procedures, specifically the disk arthroplasty, which is discussed in more detail in Chapter 13.

At the same time, it remains possible that the development of adjacent segment disease is more dependent on the natural history of cervical spondylosis and on the characteristics of the individual patient undergoing surgery than the procedure itself. It is premature to conclude that an anterior cervical fusion causes more adjacent segment disease than a motion-sparing procedure, either posterior foraminotomy or disk arthroplasty. Prospective studies will be needed to answer this important clinical issue.

Cervical spondylotic myelopathy

Cervical canal stenosis with myelopathy is generally a disease of the elderly, but can be seen in middle-aged persons, especially those harboring congenital spinal stenosis. The patient usually presents with upper and lower extremity symptoms, associated with variable degrees of neck pain. In the early stages, strength may be normal or almost normal. Fine motor skills in the hands are often affected. There may be subtle gait instability. In more advanced forms, there is marked weakness and spasticity of the upper and lower extremities. As the gait deteriorates, a cane or other ambulation aid may be required. If the patient has primarily gait instability, with minimal involvement of the upper extremities, normal pressure hydrocephalus is in the differential diagnosis. In these situations, the presence of upgoing toes and other long tract signs suggests the diagnosis of cervical myelopathy. MRI is the imaging procedure of choice.

Other conditions which may present in a similar manner and must be excluded through appropriate investigations include demyelinating disease, motor neuron disease, peripheral neuropathy, polyradiculitis (Guillain–Barré syndrome), syringomyelia, rheumatoid arthritis, post-polio syndrome, and pernicious anemia with vitamin B_{12} deficiency. Double crush syndrome, which refers to simultaneous compression of nerve root and peripheral nerve, must also be considered. The usual scenario is the patient with upper extremity symptoms who has evidence of both cervical myeloradiculopathy and carpal tunnel syndrome.

Rating scales

Several rating scales have been developed for quantifying the severity of cervical spondylotic myelopathy. Two of the most widely used scales are the Nurick disability scale and the modified Japanese Orthopaedic Association (mJOA) functional score.

With the Nurick scale, a patient is assigned a grade from 0 to 5, based on the degree of gait impairment. A patient with symptoms or signs of nerve root involvement, but no evidence of spinal cord dysfunction, would be a Nurick grade 0. At the other end of the spectrum, a patient with severe myelopathy, who is confined to chair or bed, would be a grade 5. The Nurick scale is shown in Table 9.2.

The mJOA score provides a more comprehensive assessment of lower extremity function and also provides an assessment of upper extremity motor function, sensation, and urinary symptoms. Scores range from 0 (complete absence of cord function) to 18 (normal cord function). This rating scale has been shown to have high interobserver and intraobserver reliability. The mJOA scale is shown in Table 9.3.

Natural history and approaches to treatment

The natural history of cervical spondylosis is variable, and some patients may experience long periods of

Table 9.2. Nurick disability score (for grading cervical myelopathy)

Grade	Signs and symptoms
0	Signs or symptoms of root involvement but no evidence of spinal cord disease
1	Signs of spinal cord disease but no difficulty walking
2	Slight difficulty in walking that prevented full-time employment
3	Difficulty in walking that prevented full-time employment or the ability to do all housework, but that was not so severe as to require someone else's help to walk
4	Able to walk only with someone else's help or with the aid of a frame
5	Chair-bound or bedridden

Source: Data from Nurick S. The natural history and results of surgical treatment of the spinal cord disorder associated with cervical spondylosis. *Brain* **95**:101–108, 1972. With permission from Oxford University Press.

Table 9.3. Modified Japanese Orthopaedic Association functional score (for grading cervical myelopathy)

		Score
I.	Motor dysfunction score of the upper extremities	
	Inability to move hands	0
	Inability to eat with a spoon but able to move hands	1
	Inability to button shirt but able to eat with a spoon	2
	Able to button shirt with great difficulty	3
	Able to button shirt with slight difficulty	4
	No dysfunction	5
II.	Motor dysfunction score of the lower extremities	
	Complete loss of motor and sensory function	0
	Sensory preservation without ability to move legs	1
	Able to move legs but unable to walk	2
	Able to walk on flat floor with a walking aid (i.e., cane or crutch)	3
	Able to walk up and/or down stairs without hand rail	4
	Moderate to significant lack of stability but able to walk up and/or down stairs without hand rail	5
	Mild lack of stability but able to walk unaided with smooth reciprocation	6
	No dysfunction	7
III.	Sensation	
	Complete loss of hand sensation	0
	Severe sensory loss or pain	1
	Mild sensory loss	2
	No sensory loss	3
IV.	Sphincter dysfunction score	
	Inability to micturate voluntarily	0
	Marked difficulty with micturition	1
	Mild to moderate difficulty with micturition	2
	Normal micturition	3

Source: From Benzel EC, Lancon J, Kesterson L, Hadden T: Cervical laminectomy and dentate ligament section for cervical spondylotic myelopathy. *J Spinal Disord* **4**:286–295, 1991. Reproduced with permission.

relatively stable symptomatology. For patients who present primarily with neck pain and have no evidence of myelopathy, a course of observation is appropriate, even if imaging studies show significant stenosis.

Conservative treatment, consisting of immobilization with a cervical collar, bed rest, and NSAIDs, may provide relief of acute symptoms, but has not been shown to be a long-term solution. Furthermore, chronic use of a cervical collar is not recommended, as this may lead to deconditioning of the cervical paraspinous musculature and weakening of the supporting structure of the cervical spine, further degrading spinal stability.

Once the examination shows clear-cut evidence of a myelopathy, surgery is usually required. There is no single operation that can be uniformly applied to all patients with this diagnosis. The surgical approach must be tailored to the clinical and imaging findings in each case.

The traditional surgical approach has been a decompressive laminectomy over the stenotic segments. This continues to be an appropriate operation for patients with multi-level stenosis and preserved lordosis. It should be emphasized, however, that patients who have lost lordosis are at risk for a postoperative kyphotic deformity and should be approached differently. These individuals should be considered for lateral mass fusion, in addition to laminectomy, in order to prevent post-operative sagittal plane deformities (swan neck deformity). Figure 9.10a depicts an MRI showing multi-level cervical stenosis and loss of lordosis, managed with laminectomy and lateral mass fusion. His 5-year postoperative lateral radiograph shows the expected appearance of the rod–screw construct, C2–T1, with maintenance of alignment (Figure 9.10b).

Anterior approaches may be useful for ventral compression involving one or two interspaces, while circumferential approaches are used for combined ventral–dorsal compression and for kyphotic deformities. Any patient with a significant sagittal plane deformity requires an anterior or circumferential approach. In these situations, a purely posterior operation will not provide adequate deformity correction.

Another surgical option used in some centers is cervical laminoplasty. Multiple variations in surgical technique have been described, but all are similar in that they expand the spinal canal by removing the ligamentum flavum and repositioning the laminae posteriorly.

The rationale for repositioning, rather than removing, the laminae is to prevent post-laminectomy membrane formation and to preserve spinal stability and cervical range of motion. Figure 9.11 depicts the radiographs of a patient treated in this manner.

Although there is substantial experience with laminoplasty, predominantly in Japan, the literature does not indicate any particular advantage of the technique. Neurologic outcomes and post-operative stability appear similar after laminectomy and laminoplasty. The role for laminoplasty is more established in

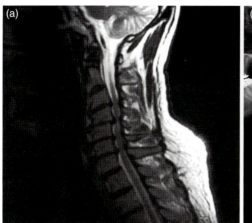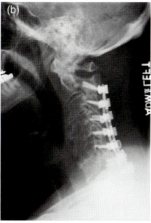

Figure 9.10. (a) Sagittal T$_2$-weighted cervical spine MRI depicting severe cervical canal stenosis with loss of lordosis. (b) Post-operative lateral radiograph depicting the expected appearance of the rod–screw construct at C2–T1.

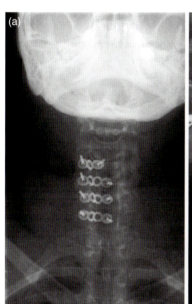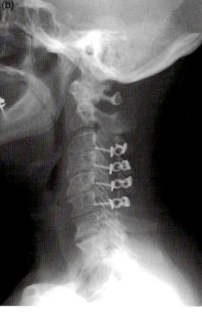

Figure 9.11. (a) Anteroposterior and (b) lateral post-operative radiographs depicting cervical laminoplasty.

children with spinal cord tumors. In these cases, preserving the laminae may prevent late deformity.

Regardless of the particular surgical technique used, surgical outcomes in patients with cervical spondylotic myelopathy are less favorable than in patients with radiculopathy and single-level disk herniation. Signal change in the cord, indicative of myelomalacia, usually does not resolve after surgical decompression, and is a predictor of poor or incomplete neurologic recovery. Sometimes a realistic goal of surgical intervention is simply to stabilize neurologic function and prevent future deterioration.

Cervical stenosis with deformity

In its more advanced forms, cervical spondylosis is associated with kyphosis and other deformities. In these cases, surgery often involves an attempt at restoring proper sagittal alignment, in addition to decompressing the spinal cord and stabilizing the spinal column.

Figure 9.12a depicts the sagittal MRI of a 60-year-old woman with rheumatoid arthritis, who developed subaxial stenosis with cord compression and a swan neck deformity. She underwent combined, single-stage,

159

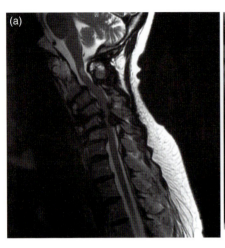
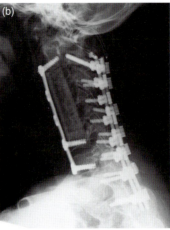

Figure 9.12. (a) Sagittal T$_2$-weighted cervical spine MRI depicting severe multi-level stenosis with kyphotic deformity. (b) Three-year post-operative lateral radiograph demonstrating circumferential reconstruction with improved sagittal alignment.

anterior–posterior decompression and fusion with instrumentation. Her 3-year post-operative lateral radiograph is shown in Figure 9.12b. Note the improved sagittal alignment, with partial correction of the swan neck deformity.

Ossification of the posterior longitudinal ligament (OPLL)

Seen most commonly in Japan, OPLL is a variant of cervical spondylosis, which is associated with abnormal bony overgrowth in the posterior longitudinal ligament. More advanced cases may cause compression of the spinal cord. OPLL is generally seen in middle-aged and older adults and is uncommon under the age of 30. OPLL is generally thought to be a part of the spectrum of age-related degenerative spine disease; however, unlike degenerative cervical spondylosis, these patients also have abnormal bone formation in the posterior longitudinal ligament, the pathogenesis of which is not fully understood. In addition, the OPLL mass is intimately involved with the ventral dura, resulting in a high incidence of CSF leakage and potential risk for spinal cord or nerve root injury during resection of the abnormal tissue.

The diagnosis is established with plain radiographs, CT, or MRI. The abnormal ossification may be confined to a single interspace or vertebral body, or may extend in a continuous or interrupted fashion over multiple spinal segments.

The primary indication for surgery is progressive myelopathy. The radiographic finding of OPLL, in the absence of myelopathy, does not mandate surgical intervention.

Both anterior and posterior operations have been used, and there are advantages and disadvantages to each.

The benefit of the anterior approach is that it provides direct access to the pathology, situated ventral to the spinal cord. The major drawback to the anterior approach is the high risk of dural injury and CSF leakage.

The benefit of the posterior approach is that it permits decompression and stabilization of the spine, while minimizing the risk of dural injury. The drawback of the posterior approach is that it provides only indirect decompression, with the OPLL mass remaining in place.

Similar to cervical spondylosis, there is no gold-standard operation that can be recommended for all patients with OPLL. One- or two-level OPLL can often be treated with anterior decompression and stabilization, while it may be preferable to treat multi-level disease posteriorly. Patients with extensive disease and kyphotic deformity may require circumferential operations. Beyond these general guidelines, the surgical approach must be individualized, based on the clinical and imaging findings in each case.

Trauma

Acute fracture and ligamentous injury may occur at any level of the spinal column. A spectrum of neurologic findings may be present, ranging from completely normal neurologic status to complete, high cervical quadriplegia. If a fracture is identified at one level, the clinician should evaluate the entire cervical spine carefully for other fractures at contiguous or noncontiguous levels.

Occipitocervical injury

Occipitocervical dislocation is an uncommon injury, which is usually fatal. The injury is grossly unstable, and survivors generally require occipitocervical fusion to stabilize the spine.

C1 fracture

The C1 (atlas) fracture, also known as Jefferson fracture, usually does not cause a neurologic deficit, because of the relatively large diameter of the spinal canal at that level and because of the tendency of fracture fragments to remain nondisplaced or displace outward, as opposed to displacing inward to impinge on the spinal cord. Much like a pretzel, the C1 ring usually fractures in two or more locations. A concurrent fracture of C2 may also be present, and imaging studies must be carefully scrutinized for this possibility. An isolated C1 fracture can usually be managed with bracing, and rarely requires surgical intervention. A combination C1–C2 fracture may be quite unstable and require surgical stabilization. Management of the combined C1–C2 fracture is usually dictated by the severity of the injury at C2.

C2 fracture

A variety of fractures can occur at C2, including odontoid fractures, Hangman's fracture (traumatic spondylolisthesis of the axis), and miscellaneous fractures involving the lamina and spinous process.

There are three types of odontoid fractures. Type I fractures involve the tip of the odontoid, above the transverse ligament. These fractures are so rare that there are insufficient outcomes data upon which to make definite recommendations for bracing or surgery. Treatment must be individualized, based on an overall assessment of fracture stability and other injuries.

Type II fractures involve the base of the odontoid. Despite extensive study, there are no clear-cut data regarding which fractures will heal with bracing alone and which fractures should be treated surgically. Patients with nondisplaced and minimally displaced fractures should be considered for a trial of immobilization in a Halo vest or cervicothoracic orthosis. The usual period of immobilization is 10–12 weeks.

Surgical stabilization should be considered for patients with an odontoid displacement of >6 mm at the time of diagnosis, failure to maintain alignment in a Halo vest, and nonunion of the fracture despite immobilization. A posteriorly dislocated odontoid fracture is particularly unstable, and early surgery

should be considered in these cases, regardless of the extent of displacement.

The standard surgical approach for an odontoid fracture is posterior fusion at C1–C2, using instrumentation and iliac crest bone graft. The traditional approach has been to use sublaminar wiring at C1 and C2 to maintain alignment and lock the bone graft in place. Recently, techniques of screw fixation have been developed, which involve screw placement in the lateral mass of C1 and pars interarticularis or lamina of C2.

Screw fixation provides more secure fixation, and is particularly useful when sublaminar wiring is precluded by previous laminectomy or damaged posterior elements. The benefits of screw fixation must be balanced against the increased risk of complications, particularly vertebral artery injury, which can occur with placement of screws at C1 or C2. Screw placement is particularly challenging at C1, and, in some cases, the lateral mass is too small to accept a screw. In these cases, the surgeon must be prepared to shift to an alternative strategy, such as posterior wiring or extension of the fusion to the occiput.

Type III odontoid fractures extend down into the body of C2. These fractures are more stable and can generally be managed with bracing. As compared with Type II fractures, Type III fractures have a larger area of cancellous bone on each side of the fracture, which promotes better healing.

Odontoid fractures are commonly seen in elderly individuals. One of the dilemmas associated with managing odontoid fractures in the elderly is that this patient group is the most likely to fail external immobilization and, at the same time, the least able to tolerate surgery. An external bone growth stimulator may be helpful in promoting fracture healing in patients in whom surgery represents an unacceptable risk.

The Hangman's fracture (traumatic spondylolisthesis of the axis) is a bilateral fracture through the pars interarticularis of C2. There may be an associated anterior subluxation of C2 on C3. Spinal cord injury is rare. In most cases, the injury is stable and can be managed with immobilization alone.

Miscellaneous fractures of C2 include those involving the spinous process, lamina, facets, lateral mass, or vertebral body. Most can be managed with immobilization.

Subaxial (C3–C7) injuries

Subaxial injuries include fractures of the vertebral body, facet, lateral mass, lamina, spinous process,

Table 9.4. Criteria for clinical instability of the cervical spine

Item	Points
Anterior elements destroyed or unable to function	2
Posterior elements destroyed or unable to function	2
Positive stretch test	2
Spinal cord injury	2
Nerve root injury	1
Abnormal disk narrowing	1
Developmentally narrow spinal canal	1
Dangerous loading anticipated	1
Neutral position radiographs	
Sagittal plane translation >3.5 mm or 20%	2
Relative sagittal plane angulation >11°	2
OR	
Flexion–extension radiographs	
Sagittal plane translation >3.5 mm or 20%	2
Sagittal plane angulation >20°	2
Unstable if total ≥5 points	

Source: Adapted from White AA III, Panjabi MM. The problem of clinical instability in the human spine: a systematic approach. In *Clinical Biomechanics of the Spine*, Second Edition. Philadelphia: Lippincott, 1990, pp. 277–378. With permission from Lippincott.

and ligamentous injury with perched or locked facets. These various injuries can occur in isolation or in combination. Injury stability should be assessed using the guidelines shown in Table 9.4, as discussed in the section "Stability of the cervical spine" later in this chapter. Patients scoring ≥5 points are considered to have unstable injuries and should be considered for surgical intervention.

Facet subluxation is the result of a severe flexion injury, and can be unilateral or bilateral. If complete subluxation has occurred, the facets are said to be locked. If the facet capsule has been partially disrupted, and the facets start to override but do not lock, the injury is known as perched facets.

Unilateral or bilateral locked facets are often associated with spinal cord or nerve root injury, with the risk being greater in patients with bilateral subluxation. Surgical intervention is usually required. An alternative strategy is to attempt reduction of the locked facets using traction. This is often unsuccessful. Even if the subluxation can be corrected using closed reduction, the injured facets are still unstable, and surgical stabilization will often be needed.

Figure 9.13a depicts the lateral radiograph of a man with a fracture-dislocation at C4–C5 with bilateral locked facets, following a motor vehicle accident. The CT scan is depicted in Figure 9.13b. Neurologic examination showed an incomplete spinal cord injury. He underwent surgery to decompress the spinal cord, and realign and stabilize the spinal column. Figure 9.13C depicts the post-operative lateral radiograph following circumferential reconstruction.

Cervical spine trauma is covered in more detail in the sections "Stability of the cervical spine" and "Spinal cord injury" later in this chapter.

Intradural tumor

Intradural tumors may be extramedullary or intramedullary. The most common intradural extramedullary tumors are meningioma and schwannoma. The most common intradural intramedullary tumors are astrocytoma and ependymoma. Patients typically present with axial pain and slowly progressive cervical myelopathy. MRI is the imaging procedure of choice. Contrast-enhanced scans should be obtained if neoplasm is suspected.

Observation may be appropriate for the occasional patient with minimal clinical findings or indeterminate findings on MRI; however, surgery is the recommended treatment in almost all symptomatic patients. The goal of surgery is to remove the tumor to the greatest extent possible, while preserving neurologic function and spinal stability.

Extramedullary tumors situated lateral or posterior to the spinal cord are more amenable to resection, while lesions ventral to the cord may present a significant surgical challenge. Figure 9.14 depicts a left-sided C2-level schwannoma with intradural and extradural components. The spinal cord was displaced posteriorly and to the right. The tumor was completely resected without any neurologic complications.

Surgical judgment concerning resectability of intramedullary tumors is particularly challenging. As a general rule, ependymomas have a better plane between tumor and cord, and are, therefore, more amenable to complete surgical resection. In contrast, astrocytomas often lack a well-defined plane and appear to merge into normal cord parenchyma. In these cases, complete removal is impossible without causing an unacceptable degree of neurologic morbidity, and the procedure may have to be limited to a biopsy.

Figure 9.15 depicts the sagittal MRI of an enhancing, intramedullary tumor at the cervicothoracic

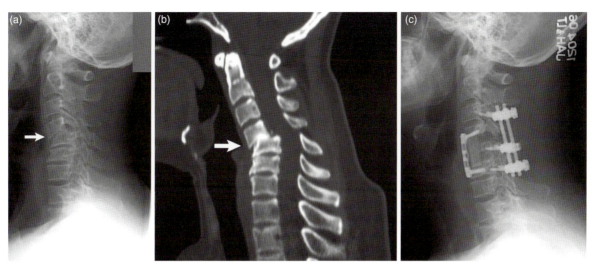

Figure 9.13. (a) Lateral radiograph of the cervical spine depicting fracture-dislocation at C4–C5 (arrow) with bilateral locked facets. (b) Sagittal CT scan confirming fracture-dislocation C4–C5. (c) Post-operative lateral radiograph depicting circumferential reconstruction with correction of deformity.

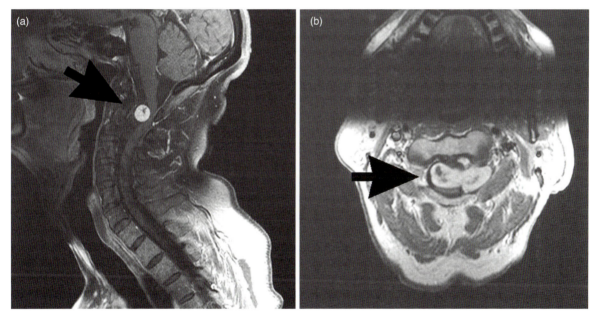

Figure 9.14. (a) Sagittal and (b) axial, T_1-weighted, contrast-enhanced cervical spine MRI depicting a left-sided C2-level schwannoma with intradural and extradural components. Note displacement of the spinal cord posteriorly and to the right (arrow).

junction, with associated syrinx extending from the craniocervical junction down to T10. The tumor, which proved to be an ependymoma, was completely resected, and the syrinx resolved.

Figure 9.16 depicts the MRI of a patient with an intramedullary cord lesion at the C5–C6 level. Excisional biopsy revealed a B-cell lymphoma.

Vascular lesions may also occur in the cervical region. Figure 9.17 depicts an intramedullary mass in the right side of the cord at the C1 level. The increased signal intensity within the lesion indicates acute or subacute hemorrhage. The dark ring at the periphery of the lesion (decreased signal intensity) indicates hemosiderin from chronic hemorrhage. These findings are consistent with a cavernous malformation (cavernoma). The management of vascular lesions of the cord is discussed in more detail in Chapter 10.

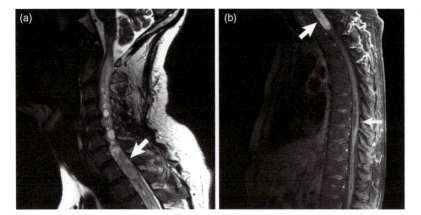

Figure 9.15. (a) Sagittal T$_2$-weighted cervical spine MRI depicting an ependymoma at the cervicothoracic junction, with associated syrinx occupying the entire cervical cord. Note the tumor, expanding the cord (arrow), and irregular syrinx extending rostrally. (b) Sagittal T$_1$-weighted, contrast-enhanced thoracic spine MRI, depicting the tumor (large arrow) and caudal extent of the syrinx (small arrow).

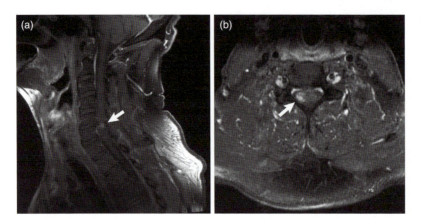

Figure 9.16. (a) Sagittal and (b) axial T$_1$-weighted cervical spine MRI with contrast enhancement, depicting an intramedullary mass lesion in the right side of the cord at the C5–C6 level (arrow). Excisional biopsy confirmed a B-cell lymphoma.

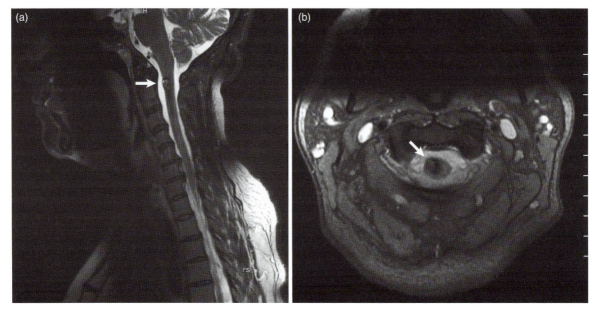

Figure 9.17. (a) Sagittal and (b) axial T$_2$-weighted cervical spine MRI depicting an intramedullary mass lesion in the right side of the cord at the C1 level. The increased signal intensity within the lesion and the ring of decreased signal intensity at the periphery are consistent with cavernous malformation with subacute and chronic hemorrhage.

(a)   (b)

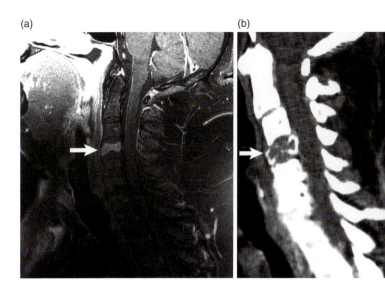

Figure 9.18. (a) Sagittal T$_1$-weighted cervical spine MRI with contrast enhancement depicting an enhancing lesion of the C4 vertebral body (arrow). (b) Sagittal CT scan depicting destruction of the C4 vertebral body (arrow). Findings are consistent with metastatic renal cell carcinoma.

Spinal metastatic disease

Metastatic tumors may occur at any level of the spinal column. Although somewhat more common in the thoracic and lumbar regions, metastatic tumors may also occur in the cervical spine. Figure 9.18 depicts the appearance of a C4 metastasis in a patient with known renal cell carcinoma. Surgery should be considered for patients with severe or progressive neurologic deficit, axial pain due to spinal deformity, failure of radiotherapy, or known radio-resistant tumor. Surgery may also be indicated for the occasional patient with a destructive lesion, without a known primary malignancy, in whom the diagnosis is in question. Any surgical strategy must be considered in the context of the patient's overall prognosis and extent of tumor burden elsewhere in the body. Metastatic disease is discussed in more detail in Chapter 10.

Syringomyelia

Syringomyelia refers to cystic cavitation of the spinal cord. The term hydromyelia is often used synonymously with syringomyelia; however, this is not technically correct. Hydromyelia refers to a cavity lined with ependymal cells, which represents simple dilatation of the central canal. The term syringomyelia is reserved for cases with extension into the cord parenchyma. In many cases, there is some overlap between the two disease processes, and the cystic process involves both the central canal and cord parenchyma. In these cases, the generic term hydrosyringomyelia, which encompasses both entities, is appropriate.

Hydromyelia is often associated with abnormalities of the foramen magnum, the most common

example of which is the Chiari malformation. Syringomyelia is often idiopathic, but may be associated with trauma or neoplasms, such as astrocytoma, ependymoma, or hemangioblastoma. Syringomyelia may extend through the entire extent of the cord from the foramen magnum to the conus medullaris. Rostral extension into the brain stem may also occur and is termed syringobulbia.

Patients with syringomyelia usually describe neck pain and have evidence of a cervical myelopathy on neurologic examination. The classic finding is a dissociated ("cape") sensory loss, which refers to loss of pain and temperature sensation, with preserved touch and joint position sense. The natural history is quite variable, although most patients progress slowly over years.

Magnetic resonance imaging is the imaging procedure of choice, as it nicely defines the syrinx in sagittal and axial planes. A contrast-enhanced study should be obtained to exclude neoplasm.

Computed tomography/myelography is less reliable in the diagnosis of syringomyelia. Delayed CT scans are required to look for diffusion of contrast media into the cyst. This technique is less sensitive than MRI. Myelography by itself is quite unreliable and should not be used as a stand-alone imaging modality for this diagnosis.

Treatment options include surgery and observation with serial imaging studies. A patient with minimal symptoms and idiopathic syringomyelia (nonenhancing cyst) may be safely followed until symptoms become more pronounced.

If the clinical picture warrants surgery, the procedure of choice is a syringo-subarachnoid shunt,

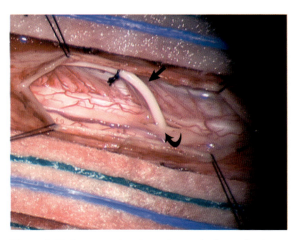

Figure 9.19. Intra-operative photomicrograph of a small syrinx (curved arrow) treated with a syringo-subarachnoid shunt (straight arrow).

which involves placement of a small drainage tube, with the proximal end in the cyst and the distal end in the spinal subarachnoid space. Figure 9.19 depicts an intra-operative photomicrograph of a small syrinx with drainage tube in place.

Surgery is recommended for a syrinx with an associated enhancing nodule or mass, which is almost always a tumor. The syrinx often resolves after removal of the tumor.

Management of hydromyelia due to Chiari malformation should start with decompression of the Chiari malformation. Once CSF flow dynamics at the foramen magnum are normalized, the hydromyelic cavity often resolves. The hydromyelic cavity should not be shunted initially as this is often unnecessary, and may even precipitate neurologic worsening by causing further tonsillar descent.

Rheumatoid disease of the cervical spine
Rheumatoid arthritis is a chronic systemic inflammatory disorder, which causes synovial proliferation, leading to destruction of joints and ligaments. There is a female preponderance and a peak onset in the fourth and fifth decades of life. The disease most commonly affects the joints of the hands and feet, followed by involvement of the cervical spine. The diagnosis is established by history, distribution of joint involvement, and a positive rheumatoid factor. The natural history is variable, but the clinical course tends to be chronic and progressive.

Rheumatoid arthritis generally affects the cervical spine in one of three ways: atlantoaxial instability, basilar invagination, or subaxial subluxation.

Neck pain in a rheumatoid patient warrants careful evaluation. Detailed neurologic examination should be performed, looking for evidence of cervical myelopathy. Neurologic examination in these patients is often particularly challenging due to rheumatoid deformities of peripheral joints. For example, it can be very difficult to ascertain whether apparent hand weakness is the result of spinal cord compression or rheumatoid deformities of the hands. Somatosensory evoked potentials may be helpful in this assessment.

Dynamic radiographs should be obtained to evaluate for instability, in particular at C1–C2. MRI should be obtained to evaluate for neural compression.

Indications for surgical intervention are similar to those used for other disorders of the cervical spine, and include myelopathy, radiculopathy, instability, and deformity. Atlantoaxial instability is generally managed with a posterior C1–C2 fusion or occipitocervical fusion. A trial of cervical traction may be appropriate to optimize alignment prior to surgery. Subaxial subluxation may be treated with anterior, posterior, or combined approaches, based on the level and extent of the disease.

Basilar invagination is associated with ventral migration of C1 and upward displacement of the odontoid through the foramen magnum, leading to progressive compression of the brain stem and upper cervical cord. A period of inline cervical traction is often helpful to attempt to reduce the odontoid out of the foramen magnum. Reducible cases can be managed with posterior occipitocervical fusion, with C1 laminectomy being added, if necessary, for dorsal compression.

Patients with fixed, nonreducible abnormalities require a circumferential approach, including transoral resection of the odontoid, followed by posterior occipitocervical fusion, with upper cervical laminectomy as needed.

Transoral odontoidectomy is associated with significant morbidity. Through resection of the odontoid and associated ligaments, the procedure often causes C1–C2 instability, even when performed in nonrheumatoid patients with stable spines at baseline. Thus, posterior stabilization is often required. Most procedures are performed for extradural lesions. If the dura is opened, it is extremely difficult to obtain a watertight dural closure, resulting in an increased risk of meningitis. Soft tissues in the posterior pharynx heal slowly, and there is often prolonged difficulty with swallowing and phonation.

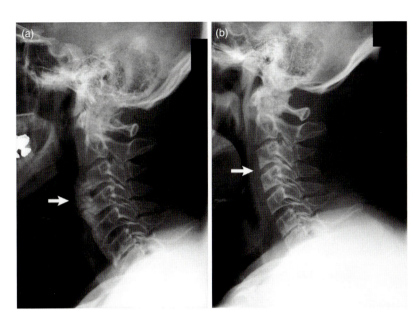

Figure 9.20. (a) Lateral radiograph of the cervical spine depicting large anterior osteophytes at C3–C6, most severe at C3 and C4 (arrow). (b) Post-operative radiograph depicting complete removal of osteophytes (arrow).

Dysphagia secondary to anterior cervical osteophytes

Large osteophytes projecting off the anterior cervical spine represent an uncommon cause of dysphagia. It is not uncommon to see anterior cervical osteophytes develop with advancing age. These are usually of no clinical consequence; however, very large osteophytes may occasionally cause dysphagia. Before considering surgical removal, other causes of dysphagia should be excluded, and a careful swallowing study should be performed to confirm that the osteophytes are indeed the source of the patient's swallowing difficulties. A typical case is depicted in Figure 9.20a, which shows large anterior osteophytes at C3–C6, maximal at C3 and C4. Anterior osteophytectomy was performed with excellent resolution of the patient's dysphagia symptoms. Figure 9.20b depicts the post-operative radiograph showing complete removal of the osteophytes.

C1–C2 facet arthropathy

An often overlooked cause of neck pain is C1–C2 facet arthropathy, which may be amenable to an arthrodesis procedure. These patients typically present with severe localized pain at the craniocervical junction, which lateralizes to the side of the abnormal facet joint. Pain is consistently reproduced by cervical extension and by looking over the shoulder on the affected side. High-resolution CT with coronal cuts often identifies the problem better than MRI. If the pain is abolished with a diagnostic injection of the

facet joint, C1–C2 fusion often provides excellent long-term pain relief. Figure 9.21 depicts the CT scan of a patient with severe, focal, left-sided upper cervical pain. Note the severe arthritic changes in the left C1–C2 facet joint, as compared with the asymptomatic right side. Posterior C1–C2 fusion provided complete relief of pain.

Fusion may also be beneficial in selected patients with subaxial facet arthropathy, who experience a favorable response to diagnostic facet injection.

Cervical epidural hematoma

Spinal epidural and subdural hematomas have previously been thought to be uncommon, but are being seen with increasing frequency, as a result of increased usage of warfarin and other anticoagulants in the elderly. The clinical history is usually one of severe neck pain followed by rapidly progressive myelopathy. Symptoms often arise spontaneously, with no history of significant antecedent trauma or unaccustomed physical activity. Management includes urgent reversal of anticoagulation and hematoma evacuation via laminectomy. Figure 9.22 depicts an MRI showing a cervical epidural hematoma at C3–C5, on the left. The patient had been on warfarin for atrial fibrillation. Emergency laminectomy was performed to evacuate the hematoma.

Thoracic outlet syndrome

Although not a spinal disorder, thoracic outlet syndrome should be considered in the differential

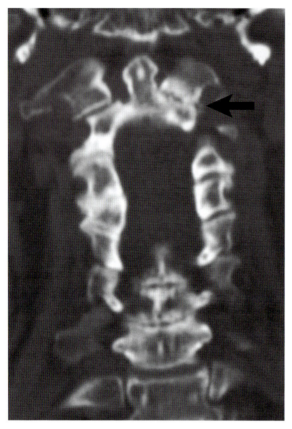

Figure 9.21. Coronal CT scan depicting severe degenerative change in the left C1–C2 facet joint (arrow), as compared with the normal right side.

diagnosis of the patient with unexplained pain in the neck, shoulder, and arm. Thoracic outlet syndrome is a controversial entity, which is often overdiagnosed and overtreated. Patients with a variety of nonspecific neck and upper extremity symptoms have been diagnosed with thoracic outlet syndrome and subjected to ill-advised surgical procedures. True thoracic outlet syndrome is quite uncommon, but does exist. Vascular and neurologic forms have been described.

Thoracic outlet syndrome is a diagnosis of exclusion. No single finding or combination of findings is diagnostic. This diagnosis should be considered in the differential diagnosis of the patient with shoulder and arm symptoms. More common disorders, including cervical disk herniation and spondylosis, median or ulnar nerve compression, brachial plexitis, and Pancoast tumor must be excluded.

The thoracic outlet is located at the apex of the lung, bordered by the first rib below and the clavicle above. The subclavian artery and vein and brachial plexus pass through this small opening. If the thoracic outlet is compromised, the potential exists for vascular and/or neurologic symptoms to occur. Thoracic outlet syndrome has been subdivided into vascular and neurologic forms. The more common of the two forms, vascular thoracic outlet syndrome, is further subdivided into two subgroups: arterial, with compression of the subclavian artery, resulting in upper extremity pallor and ischemia, and venous, with compression of the subclavian vein, resulting in upper extremity swelling and edema.

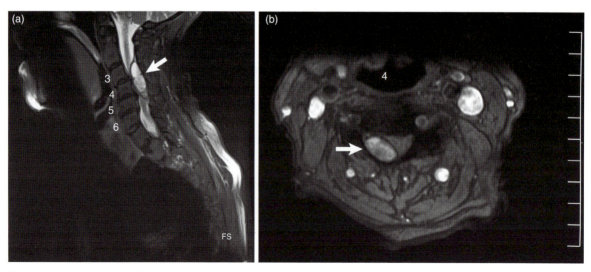

168

Figure 9.22. (a) Sagittal and (b) axial T$_2$-weighted cervical spine MRI depicting an epidural hematoma in the right posterior aspect of the spinal canal, extending from C3 to C5, causing severe spinal cord compression.

Physical examination findings are notoriously unreliable. The most common examination maneuver for the vascular component of this syndrome is the Adson test, in which the radial pulse is assessed while the patient sits with the arms dependent, takes and holds a full breath, extends the neck, and turns the head to the side. Alternative techniques involve assessment of the radial pulse during shoulder hyperabduction and during shoulder bracing in an exaggerated military position. With any of these procedures, obliteration of the radial pulse on the affected side, with preservation on the nonaffected side, constitutes a positive test.

It is generally agreed that all of these maneuvers have poor sensitivity and specificity. Positive results are thought to be somewhat useful if the maneuver reproduces the patient's symptoms, in addition to abolishing the radial pulse.

If suspected on clinical grounds, arterial or venous vascular thoracic outlet syndrome must be confirmed with arteriography. If vascular compression is identified, transaxillary resection of the first rib may be of benefit.

True neurologic thoracic outlet syndrome is a rare condition, primarily seen in adult women, and is usually unilateral, resulting from an anomalous cervical rib or constricting fibrous bands causing compression of the C8 and T1 roots or lower trunk of the brachial plexus.

Neurologic manifestations typically include C8 and T1 radiculopathy or a lower trunk plexopathy. In more advanced forms, wasting of the intrinsic hand muscles may be noted. These findings should be confirmed with EMG studies.

Imaging studies may show rudimentary or fully formed cervical ribs; however, this finding must be interpreted cautiously since an estimated 1% of the population has cervical ribs, and most of these individuals are asymptomatic.

Treatment of neurologic thoracic outlet syndrome should be conservative whenever possible. If the main symptoms are shoulder pain and paresthesias, a program of shoulder strengthening exercises, local heat, and analgesics should be pursued.

Surgery should only be considered for severe pain and unequivocal neurologic compromise. The usual approach is resection of the anomalous rib and/or fibrous bands through a supraclavicular approach. Posterior subscapular approaches have also been described. Sectioning of the scalenus muscles has largely been abandoned.

Whether it is done for vascular or neurologic thoracic outlet syndrome, surgery is associated with a significant risk of further damage to the brachial plexus, and should therefore be done only by surgeons experienced in the technique.

Thoracic outlet syndrome is difficult to diagnose and even more difficult to treat successfully. Of the two forms, vascular thoracic outlet syndrome is somewhat more common and somewhat easier to diagnose with objective angiographic criteria. First rib resection may be beneficial. Neurologic thoracic outlet syndrome is less common; this diagnosis should be made only after carefully excluding other causes of neural compression. Treatment should be conservative whenever possible, with surgery being an option in highly selected cases.

Clinical issues
Stability of the cervical spine

Spinal stability is an important concept, which has been studied extensively from clinical and biomechanical standpoints. At a basic level, stability of the cervical spine implies that there is no significant deformity or neural compression, and that neither of these will develop during physiological loading. Stated differently, a stable cervical spine provides adequate structural support for the head and neck and protection of the spinal cord and nerve roots during normal life activities. The cervical spine may be rendered unstable by a variety of disease processes including trauma, tumor, infection, rheumatoid arthritis, and degenerative spondylosis. Although it is not possible to predict with certainty whether a particular patient's cervical spine is stable, guidelines have been developed to assist the clinician in making this determination.

Stability of the upper cervical spine is difficult to quantify as a result of the unique anatomy and wide range of motion in this region. Potentially unstable situations include Type II odontoid fracture, ligamentous injury at C1–C2, producing a translation of >4 mm on dynamic radiographs, destruction of the odontoid by tumor, and iatrogenic instability, for example following transoral odontoid resection. A posteriorly displaced Type II odontoid fracture is particularly unstable.

In contrast, stability of the mid and lower cervical spine has been somewhat easier to categorize. White and Panjabi have published specific guidelines for the assessment of the stability of the mid and lower cervical spine (Table 9.4). Points are assigned for damage to the anterior or posterior spinal elements, injury to the spinal cord or nerve roots, developmental narrowing of the spinal canal, anticipation of dangerous loading (e.g., heavy laborers, participants in contact sports, and motorcyclists), and deformities demonstrated on neutral or dynamic radiographs. In equivocal cases, a stretch test is performed by applying incremental traction, starting with 4.5 kg (10 lbs) and increasing in 4.5-kg (10-lb) increments every 5 min, up to 33% body weight (30 kg or 65 lbs max). Lateral radiographs and neurologic examination are assessed after each increase in traction weight. The test is considered positive if radiographs show a separation of >1.7 mm or change in spinal alignment of >7.5°, or if there is a change in neurologic findings. The stretch test is contraindicated in the presence of obvious instability.

A score of 5 points or more indicates an unstable spine. For example, a patient with a burst fracture of C5 with cord compression (2 points), spinal cord injury (2 points), and kyphotic deformity of 20° (2 points) would have a total of 6 points and be considered unstable.

Although helpful, this protocol does have several drawbacks. First, the score cannot be interpreted rigidly, as it is possible for a patient scoring less than 5 points to have an unstable spine and a patient scoring more than 5 points to have only minimal symptoms. Second, the protocol is somewhat outdated in that it relies on criteria based on plain radiographs, rather than more sophisticated spinal imaging tests, such as CT and MRI, which are increasingly used in the evaluation of the cervical spine. Third, some of the listed maneuvers are contraindicated in certain patients; and, of necessity, application of the protocol varies from one patient to the next. For example, the patient with a grossly unstable spine should not undergo a stretch test or flexion–extension radiographs. Therefore, this stability protocol should be used and interpreted cautiously.

A stability checklist represents only one component of the evaluation of the patient with a potentially unstable cervical spine and is no substitute for careful repeated neurologic and radiographic assessment of the patient.

Clearing the cervical spine

Cervical spine clearance after trauma is a major clinical and public health issue. More than one million patients are treated for blunt trauma and potential cervical spine injuries each year in emergency departments in U.S. hospitals each year. Because of concerns about missing potentially catastrophic injuries, cervical spine radiographs have been obtained liberally in this patient population. More than 98% of these studies are negative, and the incidence of acute spinal injury is only 1%. Although not an expensive service, cervical spine radiographs add significantly to healthcare costs due to high volumes of usage.

Concerns about maintaining patient safety, while at the same time addressing practice efficiency and costs, have led to the development of guidelines for the imaging requirements in patients who have sustained cervical spine trauma. These guidelines continue to evolve.

It should be emphasized that clearance of the cervical spine is based on a combination of clinical and imaging findings.

Current recommendations are that low-risk patients can be cleared without any imaging studies. Patients in this category must meet the following five criteria: no midline cervical tenderness, no focal neurologic deficit, normal alertness, no intoxication, and no painful, distracting injury.

Patients who do not meet these criteria should be maintained in a hard cervical collar until the cervical spine can be cleared.

For patients with intermediate and high risk of cervical spine injury, helical CT scanning has replaced plain film radiography as the imaging modality of choice. CT has a sensitivity of 96% in the detection of cervical spine fracture, compared with 64% for plain radiography. The superior sensitivity of CT is even more beneficial in the elderly, in whom advanced degenerative changes may mask findings of acute trauma on plain radiographs. Another benefit of CT is that the examination can be performed faster and with less patient manipulation than plain radiographs. Because most trauma patients undergo a CT head scan immediately upon arrival, adding a scan of the cervical spine to the initial imaging study is straightforward, and expedites decisions about cervical spine clearance and subsequent management. The CT scan of a patient who sustained a fracture-dislocation at C5–C6 is depicted in Figure 9.23.

The major area of controversy in cervical spine clearance continues to be the management of the patient who is unconscious from severe head or multisystem trauma. At some centers, cervical spine precautions are discontinued if the CT scan is negative. The

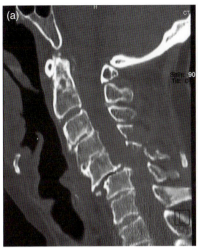 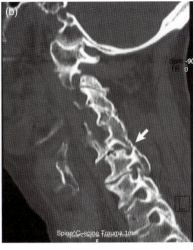

Figure 9.23. (a) Mid-sagittal cervical spine CT scan depicting a fracture-dislocation at C5–C6. (b) Paramedian sagittal cuts depicting a facet fracture at C5–C6 (arrow).

limitation of this strategy is that CT scanning can miss the infrequent, occult, unstable ligamentous injury.

At the other end of the spectrum, some investigators believe that cervical spine clearance is a process which requires the participation of an awake, co-operative patient, and that it is impossible to clear the cervical spine of an obtunded patient, regardless of what imaging studies are performed. This viewpoint requires leaving the hard collar in place until the patient regains consciousness and can be assessed clinically. There are two drawbacks of this strategy: first, prolonged use of an immobilizing collar complicates nursing care and basic hygiene, and may result in skin breakdown; and second, the severely head-injured patient may remain unconscious for a prolonged period of time, or may never regain consciousness at all.

An intermediate strategy is to obtain further imaging with MRI, upright lateral radiographs, or lateral flexion–extension radiographs. MRI is useful in selected cases. MRI can demonstrate compression, edema, or hemorrhage of the cord; traumatic disk herniations; and ligamentous injuries. Major disadvantages of this technique include prolonged scanning times and difficulty in imaging patients on advanced life support. These factors may preclude MRI in the unstable, multiple trauma patient. In addition, some centers do not have MRI capability.

Lateral flexion–extension, or dynamic, radiographs performed with physician supervision may also play a role in excluding ligamentous instability; however, it is often difficult to obtain a technically satisfactory study in the trauma setting.

Optimal dynamic radiographs require an awake, co-operative patient, with a slender neck, who is able to assume a sitting or standing position for the imaging study. Even under these ideal circumstances, it is sometimes difficult to visualize the lower cervical spine and cervicothoracic junction.

When dealing with an unconscious trauma patient who must be imaged in the recumbent position obtaining technically adequate lateral radiographs is even more challenging. In these situations, the study is often technically inadequate, and fails to visualize the area of greatest concern, the lower cervical spine and cervicothoracic junction.

Cervical spine clearance continues to be challenging in this patient population. The author's preference is to evaluate the patient with MRI whenever possible to assist with the clearance process. However, until validated protocols are developed, there will continue to be variability in how these patients are managed.

Spinal cord injury

Spinal cord injury (SCI) is most commonly seen in young men, age 18–30, but may occur in all ages from infancy to advanced age. There are approximately 10 000 cases of SCI in the USA each year. It is estimated that 10% of these occur during athletic events.

Patients with acute spinal trauma report pain at the site of injury. The unconscious patient should be considered to have a cervical spine injury until proven otherwise with appropriate imaging studies. General physical examination may reveal bruising, tenderness, and muscle spasm at the site of injury. A detailed neurologic examination should include motor testing, sensory testing (light touch, pinprick, joint position sense) of the entire body including the perianal region, deep tendon reflexes, rectal tone, and bulbo-cavernosus reflex.

The neurologic assessment can reveal a wide spectrum of findings from a totally normal examination to a complete spinal cord transection. It is important to distinguish between complete and incomplete SCI. Patients with complete cord injuries rarely improve, while patients with incomplete cord injuries may experience substantial neurologic recovery. A syndrome of SCI without radiographic abnormality (SCIWORA) has been described in children.

Incomplete SCI syndromes can occur and should be carefully documented. The central cord syndrome is characterized by weakness that is more profound in the upper extremities than the lower extremities. Brown–Sequard syndrome is a unilateral SCI, often caused by penetrating trauma. These patients have loss of motor function and joint position sense ipsilateral to the injury, and loss of pain and temperature sensation contralateral to the injury.

The physician should be aware that patients with acute spinal injury may have other severe injuries, including head injury, which require rapid diagnosis and treatment. The clinical assessment must be supplemented with appropriate radiographic studies.

The basic principles of management of acute spinal injury include immobilization, airway management, and cardiovascular resuscitation. Pharmacologic treatment is indicated for acute SCI. For patients seen within 3 hours of injury, high-dose methylprednisolone is administered intravenously, with an initial bolus of 30 mg per kilogram, followed by a continuous infusion of 5.4 mg per kilogram for 23 hours. For patients seen between 3 and 8 hours following injury, the methylprednisolone infusion is continued for 48 hours. For patients seen more than 8 hours following injury, methylprednisolone should not be given. This high-dose "steroid protocol" has been considered to be the standard of care; however, the clinical trials underlying this treatment have come under renewed scrutiny. As a result, some authorities now consider high-dose steroids for SCI to be a treatment option, rather than a standard.

Patients with acute, unstable fractures of the cervical spine should be placed in traction to immobilize the spine. Some spinal injuries can be managed non-operatively with bracing, while others require surgery to decompress neural elements and to realign and stabilize the spinal column. An active rehabilitation program is needed for patients with SCI. The acute management of the injury should be carried out as

expeditiously as possible, so that the patient can be mobilized and get into rehabilitation as soon as possible. This is especially important in the elderly. Rapid mobilization will help minimize the complications of bed rest, including deep venous thrombophlebitis, skin breakdown, and pneumonia.

Pain management in spinal cord injury

Most research on SCI has focused on a "cure" for the injury, while relatively less attention has been directed at symptom management. One of the major problems faced by individuals with SCI is chronic pain. There have been very few studies on pain associated with SCI; however, clinical experience indicates that it is a common and bothersome problem, which is often refractory to treatment. Pain associated with SCI often has a major impact on quality of life, interfering with sleep and other normal life activities.

Chronic pain in SCI is difficult to treat because it has different causes. Neuropathic pain below the level of injury, often referred to as below-level pain, is generally a central pain related to the spinal cord trauma, and is present in approximately one-third of patients 5 years following SCI. Neuropathic pain within two vertebral segments above or below the injury, known as at-level pain, may have both a peripheral component, related to nerve root injury, and a central component, of spinal cord or supraspinal origin. At-level pain is seen in approximately 40% of patients 5 years following SCI. Above-level neuropathic pain also occurs. The type of pain is often the result of compressive mononeuropathies associated with repetitive motion in the use of wheelchairs and other assistive devices.

Visceral nociceptive pain presents as abdominal discomfort, not necessarily related to bowel, bladder, or kidney dysfunction. Unfortunately, visceral pain often continues to evolve following the injury. One study showed an incidence of visceral pain of 10% 5 years following injury, increasing to 22% at 10 years, and 32% at 15 years. In addition, visceral pain is often described as severe or excruciating.

A third type of pain seen in SCI is musculoskeletal pain arising from vertebral column deformities, muscle spasms, and overuse of the upper extremities. This type of pain also progresses with time. Musculoskeletal pain may not be noted in the immediate post-injury phase, but is present in more than 50% of patients 5 years following injury.

It is not unusual for a patient with SCI to have multiple types of pain at the same time; for example, above-level musculoskeletal pain, at-level neuropathic pain due to nerve root injury, below-level neuropathic due to cord injury, and visceral pain. Given the heterogeneity of pain mechanisms seen in SCI, it is not surprising that it has been difficult to devise effective treatment.

A variety of analgesic medications have been used for SCI-related pain, including acetaminophen, NSAIDs, opioids, anticonvulsants, and antidepressants. None has shown a consistent benefit in clinical studies, and more than two-thirds of SCI patients report that medications provide little or no relief for their pain symptoms. At the same time, there is significant variation from patient to patient, likely due to the fact that pain mechanisms are so varied. This means that there is a subset of SCI patients who experience significant benefit from anticonvulsants, while another subgroup benefits from antidepressants, and so on.

Medication side-effects may be greatly magnified in the patient with SCI and must be taken into account when selecting an analgesic regimen. For example, tricyclic antidepressants are commonly used to treat neuropathic pain, but may cause constipation and urinary retention. Tricyclics may be well tolerated if bowel function is relatively normal, but may cause an unacceptable degree of constipation in a patient with neurogenic bowel.

Further complicating matters is that pain in SCI often changes and gets worse with time, thus requiring ongoing adjustments in the analgesic regimen. The optimal analgesic regimen is therefore highly variable, and must be tailored to each individual patient.

Physical therapy, massage, and cognitive restructuring techniques, such as hypnosis, may also be of benefit for SCI patients with chronic pain.

Facet blocks and other spinal injections, often used for treatment of common discogenic and degenerative back problems, have been underutilized in patients with SCI. Clinical studies have shown that intra-articular spinal injections can be as effective in providing pain relief in patients with SCI as in the general population of patients with back pain. Spinal injection therapy should therefore be considered as a treatment option for selected SCI patients with chronic pain.

Chronic pain is SCI has multiple causes and is often difficult to treat. The optimal approach would include an individualized analgesic regimen coupled with physical medicine, pain psychology approaches, and spinal injections.

Steady progress has been made in the management of SCI, and mortality has been significantly reduced. Despite these improvements, traumatic SCI remains a devastating condition that impacts on every aspect of the victim's life.

Cervical orthoses

Spinal orthoses are sometimes needed for the non-operative management of spinal injuries and for immobilization following surgical procedures. These devices are designed to restrict motion of the spinal column in order to facilitate healing after injury or surgery. In addition to providing the necessary degree of immobilization, a cervical orthosis must be comfortable and adaptable to a wide range of body sizes and shapes. Currently available cervical orthoses are made of lightweight, MRI-compatible materials, and are vastly superior to previous devices. Numerous cervical orthoses, in a wide range of sizes, are now available. Custom-made orthoses can be fabricated for individuals with unique clinical requirements and for those with unusual body shapes and sizes.

There are no well-defined protocols for selecting an orthosis. The plethora of available devices, coupled with the absence of well-defined guidelines for their use, sometimes makes it difficult for the clinician to select the most appropriate cervical orthosis. In choosing an orthosis, the clinician must consider a number of factors, including the patient's diagnosis and expected degree of instability, size and body habitus, age, smoking status, bone quality, and anticipated degree of compliance with wearing the device.

The support provided by these devices varies considerably. Among currently used devices, the Halo vest provides the highest degree of immobilization, followed by the broad category of cervicothoracic orthoses (CTO), and rigid collars in that order.

Halo vest

In previous years, the Minerva plaster jacket was frequently used for patients requiring rigid immobilization. This device was extremely heavy, made hygiene and skin care very difficult, and did not provide optimal immobilization. Starting in the 1960s, the Minerva plaster jacket was gradually replaced by the Halo vest, which consists of a metal ring attached to the skull and connected to a vest by means of four upright supports. Initially made of plaster, the vest is now made of lightweight plastic. The ring and fixation

173

Despite extensive efforts, no gold standard technique for iliac crest reconstruction has emerged. The procedure is not widely used at the present time.

Fixed versus dynamic cervical plates

Anterior cervical fusion procedures were originally done with bone grafting alone, without supplemental internal fixation. Fusion failure proved to be a significant problem, with pseudarthrosis rates as high as 24% being reported. Anterior cervical plating systems were introduced to enhance fusion rates.

Compared with the noninstrumented technique, plating results in better fusion rates, which approach 100% in single-level procedures. Although plating represents a definite technical advance, plate-related failures, including graft or plate fracture, extrusion, and pseudarthrosis, continue to occur. This is especially problematic with longer constructs.

There is some evidence that the problem lies in the design of the plate. The first systems consisted of "fixed" plates, which provide immediate rigid fixation, but do not allow for any plate shortening as the graft undergoes the expected degree of resorption. A fixed plate assumes more of the weight-bearing load as the graft resorbs, thereby shielding the graft from compression. This is significant because structural bone grafts heal faster in compression. The end result is an increased likelihood of pseudarthrosis.

In an effort to overcome the limitation of fixed plates, various "dynamic" plating systems have been developed. These systems are designed to allow vertical migration over time. As the graft resorbs, the plate shortens. Theoretically, this process allows for maintenance of load sharing between the plate and the graft, with fusion being more likely to occur because the graft remains under compressive force.

Although fixed plates may play a role in the development of pseudarthrosis following anterior cervical fusion procedures, there are likely other contributing factors. For example, overly aggressive curetting of the endplates may increase the risk of the graft telescoping into the vertebral body. The choice of graft material may also be a factor. Fibular grafts have a smaller circumference and a smaller "footprint" on the vertebral endplate, which may also increase the risk of graft subsidence. Iliac crest autograft or allograft has a larger circumference and a larger footprint on the vertebral endplate, which may decrease the risk of graft subsidence. Thus, surgical technique and choice

of graft material may have as much impact on the rate of pseudarthrosis as the design of the plate.

There is no consensus on the benefits of dynamic plating. Most surgeons believe there is little benefit from using a dynamic plate with a single-level anterior cervical discectomy and fusion. There is more enthusiasm for the use of these devices on longer reconstructions.

Variable-angle screws represent another option for creating a dynamic anterior cervical fusion construct. A common strategy is to place standard fixed-angle screws at the lower end of the construct and variable-angle screws at the other levels. The variable-angle screws allow for a modest degree of graft resorption and subsidence, while still keeping the graft under compression.

Emerging technology and new surgical procedures

The most widely publicized recent development in cervical spine surgery is the disk arthroplasty, or artificial disk. The first device to enter routine clinical practice in the USA was the Prestige ST Cervical Disc System (Medtronic Sofamor Danek), which gained FDA approval in 2007. Several other disk arthroplasty systems are under development or in clinical trials. Another area of current investigation is synthetic and biological materials to facilitate the process of spinal fusion and eliminate the need to harvest autogenous bone for grafting. Further details on these topics are found in Chapter 13.

Conclusions

Acute neck pain is a very common symptom, which usually does not require sophisticated imaging studies or extensive evaluation. Most patients experience symptom resolution without active treatment. A few patients have neck pain in the context of major trauma, systemic illness, such as cancer or infection, or progressive neurologic deficit. For these individuals, a fairly extensive differential diagnosis must be considered and prompt investigation carried out.

The most common indications for surgery on the cervical spine include intractable radiculopathy or myelopathy due to cervical disk herniation or spondylosis. Neck pain by itself is rarely an indication for surgical intervention. Prophylactic surgery for nonsymptomatic spondylosis is rarely indicated. Surgical approaches may be anterior, posterior, or combined.

Surgery for a single-level cervical disk herniation is associated with excellent clinical outcomes, using either anterior or posterior approaches. Surgical outcomes in cervical spondylotic myelopathy are less predictable. Often, a reasonable goal is to simply stabilize the patient's current neurologic function and prevent further deterioration.

Spinal cord injury is predominantly a disease of young men, but may occur at any age. Steady progress has been made in the management of spinal cord injury; however, this remains a devastating, life-altering illness.

Emerging technology in the treatment of the cervical spine includes the artificial disk and biological materials to enhance spinal fusion.

Further reading

1. Benzel EC, Lancon J, Kesterson L, Hadden T. Cervical laminectomy and dentate ligament section for cervical spondylotic myelopathy. *J Spinal Disord* 1991; **4**:286–295.

2. Clark CR (ed) *The Cervical Spine*, Fourth Edition. Philadelphia: Lippincott Williams & Wilkins, 2005.

3. Deutsch H, Haid R, Rodts G, Mummaneni PV. The decision-making process: allograft versus autograft. *Neurosurgery* 2007; **60**:S98–102.

4. Fenton DS, Czervionke LF (eds). *Image-Guided Spine Intervention*. Philadelphia: Saunders, 2003.

5. Foster JB. Pain in SCI: elusive causes and management challenges. *Appl Neurol* 2006; **2**:10–16.

6. Fountas KN, Kapsalaki EZ, Nikolakakos LG, et al. Anterior cervical discectomy and fusion associated complications. *Spine* 2007; **32**:2310–2317.

7. Grogan EL, Morris JA, Dittrus RS, et al. Cervical spine evaluation in urban trauma centers: lowering institutional costs and complications through helical CT scan. *J Am Coll Surg* 2005; **200**:160–165.

8. Heller JG, Silcox DH, Sutterlin CE. Complications of posterior cervical plating. *Spine* 1995; **20**:2442–2448.

9. McLaughlin MR, Haid RW, Rodts GE (eds). *Atlas of Cervical Spine Surgery*. Philadelphia: Saunders, 2005.

10. Nurick S. The natural history and results of surgical treatment of the spinal cord disorder associated with cervical spondylosis. *Brain* 1972; **95**:101–108.

11. Popp JA (ed). *The Primary Care of Neurological Disorders*. Rolling Meadows, IL: American Association of Neurological Surgeons, 1998.

12. Ratliff JK, Cooper PR. Cervical laminoplasty: a critical review. *J Neurosurg (Spine 3)* 2003; **98**:230–238.

13. Resnick DK (ed). Special issue on cervical myelopathy. *Spine J* 2006; **6**:175S–317S.

14. Ropper AH, Brown RH (eds). *Adams and Victor's Principles of Neurology*, Eighth Edition. New York: McGraw-Hill, 2005.

15. Schultz KD, McLaughlin MR, Haid RW, Comey CH, Rodts GE, Alexander J. Single-stage anterior-posterior decompression and stabilization for complex cervical spine disorders. *J Neurosurg (Spine 2)* 2000; **93**: 214–221.

16. Stiell IG, Wells GA, Vandemheen KL. The Canadian C-spine rule for radiography in alert and stable trauma patients. *JAMA* 2001; **286**:1841–1848.

17. Vaccaro AR, Betz RR, Zeidman SM (eds). *Principles and Practice of Spine Surgery*. Philadelphia: Mosby, 2003.

18. White AA III, Panjabi MM. The problem of clinical instability in the human spine: a systematic approach. In: *Clinical Biomechanics of the Spine*, Second Edition, eds. White AA III, Panjabi MM. Philadelphia: JB Lippincott, 1990. pp. 277–378.

19. Winn HR (ed). *Youman's Neurological Surgery*, Fifth Edition. Philadelphia: Saunders, 2004.

Disorders of the thoracic spine: pre-operative assessment and surgical management

Clinical assessment and surgical evaluation

The disorders seen in the thoracic spine are similar to those seen in other regions of the spine, although there are a few notable differences.

Compression fractures due to osteoporosis and osteolytic tumor are among the most common surgical disease processes in the thoracic region. Acute traumatic fractures also occur in the thoracic spine, but are less common than fractures in the cervical and lumbar regions because of the relative stiffness of the thoracic spinal column due to support from the rib cage and chest wall. When acute fractures do occur, they are usually seen at the cervicothoracic junction or thoracolumbar junction, rather than in the mid-thoracic region.

Disk herniations and degenerative stenosis are much less common in the thoracic spinal column than in the cervical and lumbar regions, again as a result of buttressing provided by the ribs and chest wall.

In addition to diseases within the spinal column itself, the possibility of referred pain from extraspinal structures, such as a dissecting aneurysm of the thoracic aorta, must be considered. The differential diagnosis of thoracic spine disorders is shown in Table 10.1.

Diagnostic pitfalls
Thoracic lesion masquerading as lumbar spinal stenosis

The patient with a thoracic cord lesion usually presents with lower extremity symptoms and may undergo lumbar magnetic resonance imaging (MRI) as the initial diagnostic modality. If lumbar canal stenosis is identified, a lumbar decompressive laminectomy is often performed. Lumbar decompressive surgery does not help and may further obscure the situation, as subsequent investigations are directed at potential complications of the lumbar procedure, rather than looking elsewhere for the diagnosis.

A careful clinical assessment should help avoid this situation. The patient with symptomatic lumbar spinal stenosis usually has gradually progressive lower extremity symptoms with minimal or no bladder dysfunction, and would not be expected to have evidence of a myelopathy on neurologic examination. In contrast, the patient with a thoracic cord lesion usually has neurologic deficits that tend to be more severe and rapidly progressive, with long tract signs.

Intradural tumor and spinal dural arteriovenous fistula are two thoracic cord lesions that are sometimes misdiagnosed initially as lumbar spinal stenosis.

> *Clinical pearl: If the patient with lower extremity symptoms, with presumed lumbar canal stenosis, has long tract signs, significant, rapidly progressive lower extremity weakness, or significant loss of sphincter control, look at the thoracic cord.*
>
> *Clinical pearl: Any patient who has progressive neurologic deterioration after lumbar decompressive laminectomy should have an investigation of the thoracic cord.*

Inflammatory lesion versus intramedullary tumor

Thoracic cord lesions with indeterminate or nonspecific findings on MRI often present a clinical challenge. Both clinical and imaging factors must be considered in determining whether to follow the lesion or to operate for excision or biopsy. A clinical course that is rapidly progressive or waxing and waning, coupled with MRI findings of a weakly enhancing or nonenhancing lesion without cord enlargement, suggests an inflammatory process. A clinical course that is slowly progressive and MRI findings of a uniformly enhancing lesion with cord enlargement suggest neoplasm. This is discussed in more detail later in this chapter in the section "Spinal cord biopsy."

Table 10.1. Differential diagnosis of lesions of the thoracic spine, with or without neurologic involvement

1. Discogenic or degenerative disease

   A. Herniated intervertebral disk

   B. Degenerative cervical spondylosis with canal stenosis

   C. Synovial cyst of facet joint

2. Trauma

   A. Acute traumatic fracture or fracture-dislocation

   B. Osteoporotic vertebral compression fracture

3. Tumor

   A. Primary intradural tumor of spinal cord or adjacent nerve roots

   B. Tumor of vertebral column or epidural space (or both)

   – Metastatic tumor

   – Plasmacytoma or multiple myeloma

   – Primary bone tumor (e.g., chordoma)

4. Infection

   A. Intervertebral discitis or osteomyelitis

   B. Epidural abscess

   C. Herpes zoster or other viral radiculopathy

5. Vascular lesion

   A. Neoplastic vascular lesion (e.g., cavernous malformation)

   B. Arteriovenous fistula

   C. Arteriovenous malformation

6. Inflammatory arthropathy (e.g., ankylosing spondylitis)

7. Syringomyelia

Clinical pearl: Before performing a biopsy of a spinal cord lesion, make sure the patient does not have an inflammatory process, such as multiple sclerosis.

Upper thoracic fracture

Plain radiographs are less sensitive than computed tomography (CT) scanning for the detection of acute fractures of the thoracic spine. This is a particular concern in the upper thoracic spine and cervicothoracic junction. Swimmer views and oblique views may be attempted; however, even with these additional views, the soft tissues of the upper torso may prevent adequate visualization of the spinal column. Figure 10.1 depicts the CT scan of a T3 compression fracture that was missed on plain radiographs.

Clinical pearl: If an acute thoracic spine fracture is suspected, CT scanning is the imaging procedure of choice.

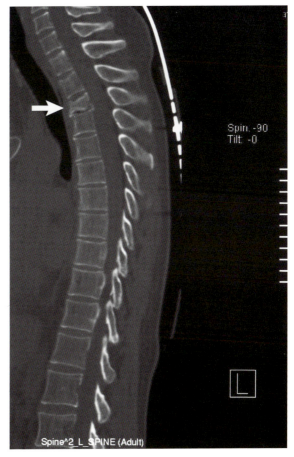

Figure 10.1. Sagittal CT scan depicting an acute traumatic T3 compression fracture, which was missed on plain radiographs (arrow).

Surgical indications and approaches

The surgical approach is determined by the nature, location, and extent of the pathology, in the context of the overall general medical condition of the patient.

Lesions ventral to the spinal cord generally require an anterior approach, while lesions posterior to the cord and intradural lesions are usually treated with a posterior or posterolateral approach. Circumferential or 360° approaches are used for compressive lesions situated both anterior and posterior to the cord and when extensive realignment and stabilization are needed. The anterior and posterior portions may be done on the same day or on separate days, depending on the clinical situation.

Anterior operations on the mid and lower thoracic spine are performed through a lateral thoracotomy approach. Anterior operations on the upper thoracic spine may require a trans-sternal approach,

179

as it is often not possible to reach the upper thoracic vertebrae from the side via a thoracotomy. In patients with long, slender necks, the T1 level can sometimes be reached successfully via a supraclavicular incision, similar to the approach used in anterior cervical operations.

Posterior operations include direct posterior approaches and posterolateral approaches.

Surgical complications

Spinal cord injury

The most dreaded complication of surgery on the thoracic spine is post-operative paraplegia from spinal cord injury, which may be either immediate or delayed. Immediate paraplegia may result from cord damage during removal of intramedullary or extramedullary tumors or disk herniations, inadvertent placement of instrumentation into the spinal canal, or excessive deformity correction. The thoracic cord is especially vulnerable to ischemic injury due to its limited blood supply.

Intra-operative somatosensory evoked potential monitoring is now widely used during operations on the thoracic spine. Although this monitoring does not detect changes in motor function, it has made these operations safer. Motor evoked potential monitoring is available in some centers but is technically more difficult to perform. This technique is not widely used.

The most common cause of delayed paraplegia is post-operative hematoma. In cases where deformity correction has been performed, an overly aggressive correction may cause acute paraplegia, and loss of correction post-operatively may precipitate a progressive myelopathy.

Any patient with a new neurologic deficit should be promptly investigated with MRI or CT/myelography to look for hematoma or other treatable cause. When spinal instrumentation is used, the potential exists for implants to be placed in suboptimal positions. Screws are particularly difficult to place in the upper thoracic region due to small pedicle size, and also in the previously operated spine, where scar tissue and deformity may obscure normal anatomic landmarks. Figure 10.2 depicts a right T1 pedicle screw medially directed into the spinal canal. The advent of sophisticated image guidance systems has lowered the risk of this complication.

Cerebrospinal leak

As with any spine surgery, dural openings with associated cerebrospinal fluid (CSF) leak may be

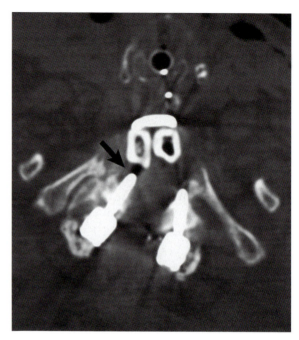

Figure 10.2. Axial CT scan depicting malposition of a right T1 pedicle screw, medially directed into the spinal canal (arrow).

encountered. These may be a consequence of the underlying problem, such as trauma or calcified transdural disk herniation, or a consequence of the surgical approach. In most cases, the leak can be repaired during the operation, utilizing primary closure, sometimes reinforced with a dural patch and/or a variety of biologic tissue sealants. An external lumbar drain is sometimes utilized post-operatively to assist with the repair. If these measures are not successful, re-operation to repair the leak may be needed.

Infection

Infection can occur after operations at any region of the spine. Risk factors include diabetes, smoking, prolonged operations, repeat operations, and placement of spinal instrumentation. Spinal infection is usually not apparent immediately following the operation. The patient typically presents 1–4 weeks post-operatively. The usual clinical manifestation is a draining surgical wound, without fever or signs of systemic infection. The white blood cell count is often normal, while the erythrocyte sedimentation rate (ESR) and C-reactive protein (CRP) are usually elevated. Surgical debridement and several weeks of intravenous antibiotics are usually required. Instrumentation can usually be preserved.

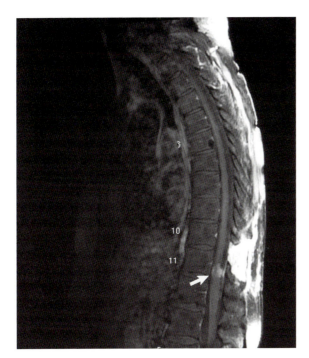

Figure 10.3. Wrong level surgery. Sagittal T_1-weighted MRI with contrast enhancement, depicting an intradural meningioma at T11 (arrow) and post-surgical changes of a surgical approach at T10, the level above the lesion.

Wrong level surgery

Localizing the correct anatomic level is a critical component of any spine procedure. This is accomplished through careful review of pre-operative and intra-operative imaging studies, and inspection of anatomic landmarks. During the procedure, the level is confirmed with fluoroscopy or anteroposterior and lateral radiographs. This process involves placing a clamp or other radiopaque marker on an exposed vertebra, taking a radiograph or fluoroscopic image, and counting up from the sacrum or down from C1 to positively identify the exposed spinal segment.

Localizing the correct level with intra-operative fluoroscopy or radiographs is generally straightforward, but may be difficult when the spinal column is not well visualized, for example in patients with obesity or osteoporosis. Localization may also be problematic in patients with an atypical number of vertebrae, e.g., four or six lumbar type vertebrae, or a transitional segment, e.g., "lumbarized S1 segment."

Lesions in the mid and upper thoracic region may also be difficult to localize in the operating room because of a lack of distinct anatomic landmarks and suboptimal imaging. For lesions in the thoracic spine where intra-operative confirmation of the correct

level is anticipated to be difficult, it is sometimes helpful to take the patient to the radiology suite prior to surgery, localize the lesion fluoroscopically, and place a mark on the skin overlying the lesion.

Wrong level surgery may occur at any level of the spinal column. Figure 10.3 depicts the thoracic spine MRI of a patient with an intradural meningioma at T11, who had a negative exploration at T10. In this case, the surgical approach was one level too high.

Selected surgical disorders of the thoracic spine

Vertebral compression fracture

Vertebral compression fracture (VCF) is a very common disorder, which develops in patients with osteoporosis and osteolytic tumor. These fractures cause significant morbidity and pain. There are 700 000 new cases of VCF each year in the United States. By way of comparison, there are approximately 5000, 10 000, and 30 000 new cases of motor neuron disease, multiple sclerosis, and subarachnoid hemorrhage, respectively. This gives some perspective on the magnitude of the problem of VCF, as compared with other common neurologic disorders.

Osteoporosis is a systemic skeletal disease, associated with progressive loss of bone density and bone quality. Patients with osteoporosis are vulnerable to VCF, which often occurs after minimal or no trauma. VCF is known to occur in post-menopausal women and elderly persons of both genders. Other risk factors include cigarette smoking, excessive alcohol intake, sedentary lifestyle, spinal radiation therapy, chronic corticosteroid therapy, and end-stage liver or kidney disease. Organ transplant recipients are at particularly high risk for osteoporotic VCF because of their underlying disease process and because they require long-term treatment with steroids and other immunosuppressive drugs.

Osteoporosis of the elderly is known as primary osteoporosis, while osteoporosis associated with steroid therapy, end-stage liver disease, premature menopause, or other metabolic disorders is referred to as secondary osteoporosis. Patients with secondary osteoporosis often develop bony disease at an earlier age and have more advanced disease at the time of diagnosis than patients with primary osteoporosis.

Patient evaluation

Any patient with acute, severe back pain should undergo appropriate imaging studies, looking for

VCF and to assess the age of any fractures that are identified. This latter issue is important because patients with acute VCF are often candidates for vertebral augmentation, while chronic VCF may not be amenable to treatment.

Plain film radiography, radionuclide bone scanning, CT scanning, and MRI can play a role in the diagnosis of VCF. Plain radiographs and CT scanning are useful in establishing the presence of a VCF, but do not indicate whether the fracture is acute or chronic. A bone scan provides information about fracture age, with an acute fracture showing radionuclide uptake and a chronic fracture not showing uptake. The most useful study is MRI, which is able to identify VCF and also provide information about fracture age. The sagittal T_1- and T_2-weighted images with fat saturation are particularly sensitive for the diagnosis of acute VCF.

Some patients with acute VCF are not able to tolerate a full MR examination because of severe pain, but may be able to complete a limited examination. In these cases, it is helpful to start with sagittal T_1- and T_2-weighted (fat saturation) sequences, as it may be possible to establish a diagnosis and plan treatment based on these sequences, even if a full examination cannot be completed. Another option for the patient in severe pain is to obtain the MRI under general anesthesia. If acute VCF is suspected based on other imaging studies, it may be desirable to plan to proceed directly to vertebral augmentation immediately following completion of the MRI under the same anesthetic. This strategy avoids a second intubation and a second general anesthetic.

Unfortunately, there are situations in which MRI is absolutely contraindicated, often due to the presence of a metallic foreign body. The usual situation in this patient population is a cardiac pacemaker. In these cases, the radiographic diagnosis of VCF must be confirmed with some combination of plain radiographs, radionuclide bone scanning, and CT scanning.

Osteoporotic VCF is most commonly seen at the thoracolumbar junction, but may occur at any level from the sacrum to the mid-thoracic region. Fractures above the T6 level are uncommon and usually represent osteolytic tumor, rather than a benign fracture from osteoporosis.

If a VCF is identified, a bone density study should be performed, and the patient should be considered for systemic therapy for osteoporosis, in addition to local therapy with vertebral augmentation.

Conventional treatment

Historically, treatment options for VCF have been limited and ineffective. Conservative management has included narcotic analgesics, bracing, and periods of bedrest. This treatment regimen is often not effective and has its own complications. Narcotic pain medications frequently cause constipation and confusion or hallucinations in the elderly. Braces are often uncomfortable and poorly tolerated. Bedrest aggravates osteoporosis, and increases the risk of additional complications of immobility in the elderly; including decubitus skin ulceration, pneumonia, deep venous thrombosis, and pulmonary embolism.

At the other end of the therapeutic spectrum, major reconstructive surgery is occasionally performed, but these procedures are poorly tolerated by this frail patient population, and there is a high risk of medical complications and implant failure. As a result, conservative treatment (or no treatment at all) has been the usual approach for the vast majority of patients with VCF. Unfortunately, many of these patients have ongoing, severe pain, and have been unable to resume their usual physical activities.

Another patient group at risk for VCF are those with osteolytic tumors, including metastatic carcinoma and myeloma. Similar to VCF caused by osteoporosis of nonmalignant origin, VCF secondary to osteolytic metastasis or myeloma often responds poorly to conservative treatment, and major spinal surgery with instrumentation and bone grafting may not be appropriate due to limited life expectancy and poor medical condition.

It is now recognized that VCF is a common disorder that is sometimes overlooked and undertreated. These fractures cause significant morbidity, and conventional therapy is often of limited benefit. These factors have stimulated increasing interest in the prompt diagnosis of VCF and in new, percutaneous methods of fracture stabilization that relieve pain and allow early return to activity.

Percutaneous techniques of vertebral augmentation

The first percutaneous vertebral augmentation procedure was vertebroplasty, which was initially reported in 1987, as a technique for treating painful vertebral hemangiomas. Indications for treatment were subsequently expanded to include VCF due to osteoporosis and tumor. The procedure involves the injection of polymethylmethacrylate (PMMA) into a diseased vertebral body. The injectate is in very liquid form and is injected into the vertebral body under high pressure.

The procedure was later modified to include the use of an inflatable balloon tamp (balloon) to create a cavity within the vertebral body prior to PMMA deposition. This new technique came to be known as kyphoplasty. There are three balloon sizes currently available: 10, 15, and 20 mm. The choice of balloon size is based on the size of the vertebral body, with 10-mm balloons generally used in the mid-thoracic region, 15-mm balloons in the lower thoracic region, and 20-mm balloons in the lumbar region. After careful placement in the vertebral body, the balloons are slowly inflated under anteroposterior and lateral fluoroscopic guidance. The balloon inflation creates a cavity for PMMA deposition, and, in many cases, restores the height of the fractured vertebral body and improves sagittal alignment.

Patients with an allergy to iodine should be pre-treated with corticosteroids, as balloons occasionally burst during the filling process. Aside from the potential for allergic reaction to iodine, the bursting of a balloon usually has no clinical consequence.

When kyphoplasty is performed, the injectate has a firmer consistency, like toothpaste, and is injected under low pressure.

There are many similarities between vertebroplasty and kyphoplasty. Both can be performed in an operating theater or in a radiology special procedures suite, using general anesthesia or conscious sedation plus local anesthesia. Prophylactic antibiotics are administered intravenously or mixed in the PMMA prior to injection. Both procedures involve percutaneous, transpedicular placement of needles and other instruments into an affected vertebral body for the purpose of injecting PMMA. High-quality fluoroscopic imaging is needed in order to assure accurate instrument placement and PMMA deposition. It is generally more efficient to do vertebral augmentation with biplane fluoroscopy or with two portable units that can remain in a fixed position, although it is possible to do the procedure with a single fluoroscopic unit.

Bone biopsy is performed prior to PMMA injection. This should be done in all patients, even when the imaging suggests a benign VCF. Bone biopsy adds no risk to the procedure and will detect an occasional unsuspected tumor, often multiple myeloma.

Bilateral injection is usually performed, but a unilateral injection is sometimes feasible in the thoracic region if instrument placement can be achieved via a more lateral entry site (extrapedicular approach). PMMA volume ranges from 2 to 6 ml

per side. Any segment from the mid-thoracic level to the sacrum is potentially treatable with either technique.

Patients may ambulate immediately following the procedure, as their general condition permits. There is no need for post-procedure bracing, as the PMMA hardens almost immediately. Patients are generally maintained in the hospital overnight and discharged the day following the procedure; however, in some cases, the procedures may be performed on an out-patient basis. Both vertebroplasty and kyphoplasty are usually performed as a stand-alone procedure, but can be done in conjunction with an open procedure. For example, a patient with a VCF plus degenerative spinal stenosis might undergo vertebral augmentation and a decompressive laminectomy under the same anesthetic.

There is a trend toward early treatment of a VCF, rather than trying weeks of often-futile conservative treatment.

Although there are many similarities between these two procedures, there are some important differences as well.

The primary difference is that kyphoplasty involves creation of a cavity in the fractured vertebral body using an inflatable bone tamp (balloon). The cavity created during the course of the balloon inflation during a kyphoplasty procedure permits a low-pressure injection of relatively firm PMMA into the vertebral body, thereby lowering the risk of PMMA extravasation and embolus.

In contrast, there is no cavity creation with vertebroplasty, and a high-pressure injection of a more liquid injectate is required to fill the vertebral body, thereby increasing the risk of PMMA extravasation into the spinal canal or paraspinal soft tissues and embolus to the lungs and other distant sites.

Second, kyphoplasty has the potential to correct a kyphotic deformity and improve spinal biomechanics via inflation of the balloon tamp, which can reduce the fracture, restore vertebral body height, and improve local and global sagittal alignment. In one study, more than 5° of correction was achieved in thirty of fifty-two VCF (58%), with a mean improvement in global sagittal alignment of 14.2°. By comparison, vertebroplasty is basically an in situ fracture stabilization procedure and does not have the capacity to reduce a VCF and improve sagittal alignment.

The steps utilized in balloon kyphoplasty are outlined in Figure 10.4.

183

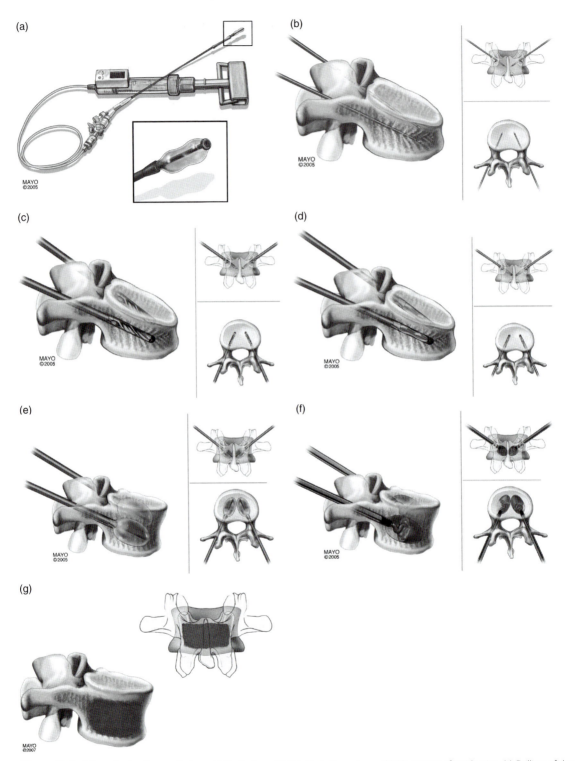

Figure 10.4. Balloon kyphoplasty technique. (a) Illustration of inflatable balloon tamp. (b) Placement of guide pins. (c) Drilling of the vertebral body to create a channel for the balloon. (d) Balloon placement. (e) Balloon inflation. Note restoration of height of the fractured vertebral body. (f) PMMA deposition into cavities created by balloons. (g) Final appearance of PMMA in the vertebral body. Figure reproduced with permission from Mayo Foundation for Medical Education and Research.

Treatment outcomes

Excellent outcomes have been achieved with both vertebroplasty and kyphoplasty. Several large studies have shown excellent and sustained pain relief and improved functional capacity with either technique. Kyphoplasty also improves the height of the affected vertebral body and improves kyphosis in more than 50% of cases. Results are better if treatment is carried out within 3 months of onset.

Vertebral augmentation has also been shown to be safe and effective in patients with VCF due to osteolytic tumor. Several investigators have obtained a mean improvement in the visual analog scale (VAS) pain score of 5 points after kyphoplasty treatment of a pathologic VCF. This degree of improvement is highly significant and is similar to the results obtained with typical osteoporotic VCF.

Vertebral augmentation can be combined with radiotherapy in osteolytic spinal tumors. When adjuvant radiotherapy is required, it can be administered immediately following the vertebral augmentation procedure. This represents an advantage over conventional reconstructive surgery, where radiotherapy would have to be delayed, sometimes for several weeks, in order to allow for wound healing.

Complications

Serious complications are uncommon. Potential complications include spinal cord or nerve root injury from PMMA leakage, infection, pulmonary embolus from PMMA, rib fractures from positioning, and medical complications related to anesthesia. Atrial fibrillation and other cardiac dysrhythmias are not infrequent in this elderly patient population. Cerebral embolism of PMMA with cerebral infarction has been reported after vertebroplasty in a patient with a right to left cardiac shunt.

Preliminary multicenter data on 603 fractures in 340 patients revealed a complication rate of 0.7% per fracture and 1.2% per patient. In this series, there were four serious complications related to instrument misplacement and PMMA injection into the spinal canal, including epidural hematoma and incomplete spinal cord injury. PMMA extravasation into the adjacent intervertebral disk or paraspinal soft tissues occurs in 10%–15% of cases, usually with no clinical consequences.

Neurologic complications may be seen with either vertebroplasty or kyphoplasty, and may occur acutely or in a delayed fashion. Neurologic symptoms presenting on a delayed basis are often heralded by recurrent back pain. Imaging studies in cases with acute deterioration typically show cord compression due to PMMA extrusion into the spinal canal. Subacute cases typically demonstrate fracture progression with retropulsion of bone fragments into the spinal canal. Open surgery to decompress the spinal cord is often required. Stabilization may also be needed.

Although neurologic deterioration is uncommon following vertebral augmentation, physicians performing these procedures should maintain a high index of suspicion and be prepared to respond in an emergent manner when a neurologic complication is identified.

New fracture development

Since osteoporosis is a systemic process, it is not surprising that patients are at risk for fracturing another vertebra following augmentation of an acute VCF. Approximately 10%–20% of patients with primary osteoporosis develop new VCF within 12 months of the index procedure, typically adjacent to the index level. Patients with secondary osteoporosis are at even higher risk.

An important clinical issue is whether treatment of the initial fracture predisposes to new fractures by altering spinal biomechanics. In one large study of balloon kyphoplasty, the incidence of new fractures was 11% among patients with primary osteoporosis, but 48% among patients with secondary osteoporosis.

An alternative explanation is that subsequent fractures simply represent the natural history of a systemic skeletal disease process. This viewpoint is supported by studies on the natural history of untreated VCF, showing a 20% incidence of new fractures following diagnosis of the index fracture.

Regardless of the mechanism, new VCF can often be successfully treated with additional augmentation procedures.

The risks of PMMA dislodgement and recurrent fracture of a treated level are low with either technique, but are probably slightly higher with vertebroplasty. In one study of vertebroplasty, there was a 2.5% incidence of further compression at the treated level. There are anecdotal reports of this event occurring following kyphoplasty as well, but the incidence is probably less than 1%.

Figure 10.5A depicts the sagittal CT scan of a patient with VCF at L1. Figure 10.5B depicts the pre-procedure lateral radiograph showing 50% loss of anterior vertebral body height. Figure 10.5C depicts the post-procedure lateral radiograph showing

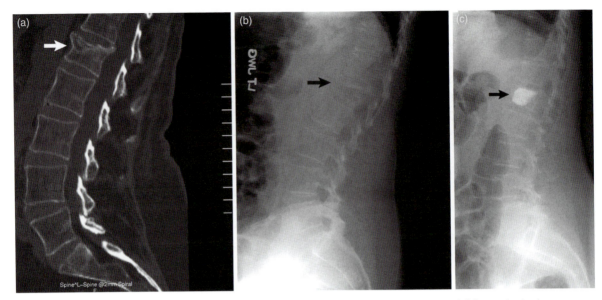

Figure 10.5. (a) Sagittal CT scan and (b) lateral radiograph depicting L1 VCF (arrow). (c) Lateral radiograph following kyphoplasty demonstrating excellent PMMA placement and near-complete height restoration of the L1 vertebral body (arrow).

PMMA deposition in the L1 vertebral body, with near-complete height restoration of the anterior vertebral body.

Vertebral augmentation cannot be performed if the vertebral body is too severely compressed (vertebra plana) or if there is significant compromise of the spinal canal.

Figure 10.6 depicts the CT scan of a patient with severe VCF at T3, T5, T7, and T8 with kyphotic deformity. Vertebra plana is seen at T5 and T7. Vertebral augmentation is not technically feasible because these two vertebral bodies are too severely compressed to permit introduction of instruments and PMMA.

Figure 10.7a depicts the sagittal T_2-weighted MRI of a patient with a severe osteoporotic VCF with retropulsion of bone into the spinal canal, causing severe spinal stenosis and cauda equina syndrome. This patient was not a candidate for simple vertebral augmentation. Reconstructive surgery was needed for decompression and stabilization. Figures 10.7b and 10.7c depict the post-operative radiographs.

Vertebral augmentation in the high thoracic region

Fractures above the mid thoracic region are uncommon and usually indicate osteolytic tumor, rather than a benign fracture from osteoporosis. The standard percutaneous kyphoplasty and vertebroplasty techniques, used for fractures between T6 and L5, have distinct limitations in the upper thoracic region.

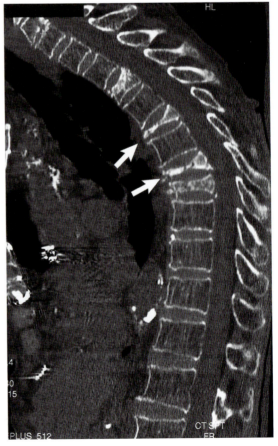

Figure 10.6. Thoracic spine CT scan depicting multiple VCF at T3, T5, T7, and T8. Note vertebra plana at T5 and T7 (arrows).

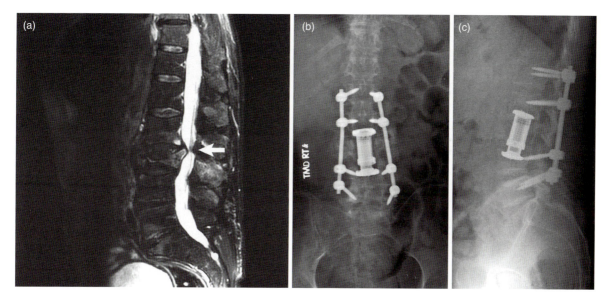

Figure 10.7. (a) Sagittal T$_2$-weighted lumbar MRI depicting a severe osteoporotic L3 VCF with retropulsion of bone into the spinal canal and severe canal stenosis (arrow). (b) Anteroposterior and (c) lateral post-operative radiographs, depicting circumferential decompression and stabilization.

The shoulders and soft tissues of the upper torso interfere with fluoroscopic imaging, especially in the lateral plane. Without high-quality imaging, there is a risk of placing instruments or PMMA in the spinal canal. The small size of the pedicle and vertebral body also contribute to the difficulty associated with high thoracic vertebral augmentation. The combination of technically difficult fluoroscopy and a small anatomic target make it difficult to carry out percutaneous vertebral augmentation in the upper thoracic region, especially at T1–T3. In these cases, it may be necessary to do the procedure open, and place instruments and PMMA using image guidance or direct visualization of anatomic landmarks, or a combination of the two. Image guidance may be helpful in assuring accurate placement of instruments and PMMA.

Since the vertebral body is quite small, the surgeon should use at most a 10-mm balloon. Often the vertebral body is too small to accept even a 10-mm balloon. In these cases, the procedure may be done without a balloon, using a vertebroplasty technique.

The vertebral bodies of the cervical spine are too small to be safely treated with percutaneous vertebral augmentation using techniques that are currently available.

PMMA augmentation of acute traumatic vertebral fractures

With VCF due to osteoporosis or tumor, the goals of treatment are fracture reduction and pain relief.

These patients often do not have a prolonged life expectancy, therefore fracture healing has not been a primary focus of treatment.

In contrast, patients with high-impact, traumatic vertebral fractures are often much younger at the time of injury. Since these patients may live for decades, treatment strategies have focused on fracture healing, as well as improving symptoms. As a result, acute traumatic vertebral fractures have generally been treated with bracing or reconstructive surgery. Vertebral augmentation has not been used in this patient population, as it has been felt that an inert material such as PMMA would interfere with bone healing.

Recently, however, vertebral augmentation on young patients with acute traumatic fractures has been reported. The procedure appears to be safe and effective in relieving pain, and, in many cases, obviates the need for reconstructive surgery. Although these preliminary results are encouraging, the long-term fate of PMMA injected into the spines of young individuals, who may survive for decades, is unknown. Further work will be needed to define the role of vertebral augmentation in acute traumatic VCF.

Future directions in vertebral augmentation

Technical refinements continue to be made in the instruments used to cannulate and prepare the vertebral body and inject the cement. Enhanced balloon technology may provide for better fracture reduction.

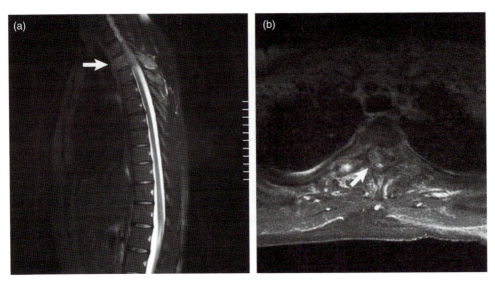

Figure 10.8. (a) Sagittal T$_2$-weighted MRI and (b) axial contrast enhanced, T$_1$-weighted thoracic MRI depicting metastatic leiomyosarcoma in the T3 vertebral body (arrow). Tumor extends into the epidural space and displaces the spinal cord to the left.

Preliminary work has been done with sophisticated computer-assisted image guidance systems to optimize instrument placement and cement delivery.

Alternatives to PMMA are being studied, as the long-term durability of PMMA in the spine is unknown, and may be a concern in young patients undergoing vertebral augmentation. This has stimulated interest in vertebral augmentation with biologic implants that will integrate into the spine. This is discussed in more detail in Chapter 13.

Indications for the procedure continue to expand. Kyphoplasty has recently been reported for treatment of VCF in organ transplant recipients and fibrous dysplasia of the spine, and for sacral insufficiency fractures.

The ultimate advance in the care of these patients involves the prevention of VCF through pharmacologic intervention.

Spinal metastatic disease

Metastatic tumors may occur at any level of the spinal column, and are more common in the thoracic spine, due to the fact that the thoracic spine is the largest region of the spinal column. The most common tumors are squamous cell carcinoma of the lung in men and carcinoma of the breast in women. Once a metastatic lesion is identified, it is essential to image the entire spine to evaluate for tumor at other levels.

The typical presenting symptom is localized spinal pain at the level of the lesion. If the tumor encroaches into the spinal canal or neural foramina, the patient may develop evidence of spinal cord or nerve root compression.

Metastatic tumors generally begin in the anterior portion of the spinal column, and then spread to the epidural space. The extent of disease is quite variable. The bony disease may be confined to a single level or may affect multiple levels. Likewise, epidural disease, if present, may occur at a single level or may span multiple levels.

Figure 10.8 depicts the MRI of a 30-year-old woman with metastatic leiomyosarcoma in the T3 vertebral body. Tumor extends into the epidural space and displaces the spinal cord to the left.

Less commonly, metastatic lesions affect only the posterior elements of the spinal column. Figure 10.9 depicts the MRI of a 48-year-old man with metastatic renal cell carcinoma. Tumor originates in the laminae of T8 and T9, and encroaches into the posterior epidural space. In this unusual case, there was no tumor in the anterior spinal column and ventral epidural space.

Intradural metastatic lesions are rare, and neurologic progression is often rapid. Carcinoma of the lung and other systemic tumors can metastasize to the spinal cord and subarachnoid space. Primary brain tumors, notably medulloblastoma, ependymoma, and glioblastoma, can also spread to the spinal cord and spinal subarachnoid space through a process known as drop metastasis.

The mainstays of treatment for spinal metastatic disease are radiotherapy and surgery. Management

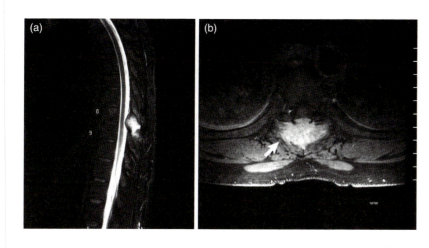

Figure 10.9. (a) Sagittal and (b) axial T$_2$-weighted thoracic MRI of a 48-year-old man with metastatic renal cell carcinoma. Tumor originates in the laminae of T8 and T9, and encroaches into the posterior epidural space (arrow).

strategies must take into account the type of tumor, location and extent of the spinal disease, extent of systemic tumor burden, the patient's age, neurologic and general medical status, and overall prognosis.

Aggressive treatment is often warranted for young patients with a single metastatic lesion and a favorable prognosis; while a more conservative approach may be more appropriate in elderly patients with extensive disease and limited life expectancy.

Spinal metastatic disease encompasses a heterogeneous group of patients, and it is not possible to outline a rigid protocol for selecting a surgical approach. Surgery should be considered for patients with severe or progressive neurologic deficit, axial pain due to spinal deformity, failure of radiotherapy, or known radio-resistant tumor. Biopsy may also be indicated for the occasional patient with a destructive lesion, without a known primary malignancy, in whom the diagnosis is in question and cannot be obtained by less invasive means.

The traditional operation has been posterior decompression via laminectomy. It is now recognized that, in many cases, laminectomy as a stand-alone procedure has limited effectiveness because, in most cases, the bulk of disease burden is ventral to the cord, and posterior decompression may predispose to kyphotic deformity. Nevertheless, laminectomy still has a role to play in patients with cord compression over multiple segments with preserved spinal alignment. Supplemental posterior instrumentation is often used to prevent post-operative deformity.

Anterior, transthoracic approaches are often appropriate for patients with a short segment of disease (one or two level), significant ventral cord compression, and kyphotic deformity. Circumferential, or

"360°," surgery may be needed for patients with significant ventral and dorsal compression and instability.

A significant recent development in the management of spinal metastatic disease has been the introduction of vertebral augmentation, using either vertebroplasty or balloon kyphoplasty, to treat painful compression fractures caused by metastatic tumor. This technique is primarily used for benign, osteoporotic compression fracture, but has been demonstrated to be safe and efficacious for malignant fractures as well. It should be considered in cases where there is little or no epidural tumor and no cord compression. Vertebral augmentation is a minimally invasive technique, which provides excellent pain relief, may obviate the need for major reconstructive surgery, and allows for immediate initiation of radiotherapy. This procedure is discussed in more detail in the previous section.

Intradural tumor

The clinical presentation, surgical management, and pathologic findings of thoracic intradural tumors are virtually identical to those of intradural tumors of the cervical spine. The reader is referred to Chapter 9 for discussion of these lesions.

Thoracic disk herniation

Although significantly less common than disk herniations in the cervical and lumbar regions, disk herniations are also seen in the thoracic spine. Symptoms usually include variable degrees of localized axial back pain, radicular pain from compression of the exiting nerve root, and myelopathic findings from cord compression. The diagnosis may be confirmed with MRI or CT/myelography.

189

remove a cavernous malformation has a similar impact on neurologic function as a hemorrhage from the malformation. However, these new post-operative deficits usually resolve with time, leaving the patient with stabilized or improved neurologic function.

Spinal dural arteriovenous fistula

One of the more common spinal vascular abnormalities is the dural arteriovenous fistula. These lesions produce symptoms by causing venous hypertension within the spinal cord, rather than by bleeding. Diagnosis is often delayed because symptoms may initially be mild and nonspecific, and because symptoms are sometimes mistakenly attributed to benign degenerative changes in the lumbar spine. These factors often result in delays in imaging the thoracic spine.

Although patients with dural arteriovenous fistula often present with minimal and nonspecific symptoms, they frequently have severe and progressive neurologic deficits later in their clinical course. In particular, the presence of severe bladder dysfunction should suggest that the patient may have a dural arteriovenous fistula, rather than the more common diagnosis of lumbar spinal stenosis.

Patients are sometimes subjected to misdirected decompressive operations on the lumbar spine, after which there is often some degree of neurologic deterioration. The mechanism for this worsening is thought to be exacerbation of venous hypertension in the spinal cord due to abdominal compression during the lumbar procedure.

The MRI usually shows intramedullary T_2 signal change and may reveal abnormal vessels on the dorsal aspect of the cord. MRA, including MR aortography, may be helpful in defining the general region of the fistula, however selective spinal angiography is needed to precisely define the location of the fistula. A schematic diagram of a dural arteriovenous fistula is depicted in Figure 10.12.

The original surgical approaches to these lesions involved removing the arterialized vein from the dorsal surface of the cord. It is now felt that removing the arterialized vein is not necessary and may add to the risk of the procedure. The current strategy is to obliterate the fistula by simply dividing the draining vein just distal to the fistula. The vein is left in place. In almost all cases, operative treatment results in improvement or stabilization of neurologic function.

These lesions have also been treated with endovascular techniques. This approach has some appeal because it is less invasive; however, it has been shown

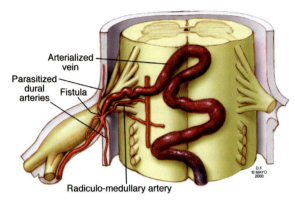

Figure 10.12. Schematic diagram of a dural arteriovenous fistula, which is fed by radicular arteries entering the spinal canal along with the nerve root. Note the prominent arterialized vein on the dorsal surface of the cord. From Atkinson JLD, Miller GM, Krauss WE, Marsh WR, Piepgras DG, Atkinson PP, et al. Clinical and radiographic features of dural arteriovenous fistula, a treatable cause of myelopathy. *Mayo Clin Proc* 2001; **76**:1120–1130. Used with permission of Mayo Foundation for Medical Education and Research.

to be less predictable in terms of fistula obliteration and neurologic recovery. Therefore, the primary treatment for dural arteriovenous fistula is surgical obliteration.

Arteriovenous malformation

True AVMs represent a diverse group of vascular lesions. Treatment options include surgical excision alone, surgery after embolization, and embolization alone. Because it represents definitive treatment, surgery is preferred for lesions that can be completely removed with minimal neurologic risk. Endovascular techniques should be considered in situations where there appears to be an unacceptable risk associated with surgery.

Spinal trauma
Acute fracture

Acute fractures occur most commonly at the thoracolumbar junction, followed by the cervicothoracic junction. These regions are vulnerable, because they represent zones of transition between the relatively immobile thoracic spine and the more flexible lumbar spine below and cervical spine above.

The usual mechanisms of injury are high-energy events, including motor vehicle accidents, falls, and blows to the back. Patients with acute thoracic fractures require a careful evaluation for evidence of multi-system trauma, as there is significant potential for visceral, extremity, and head injury.

The spine should be examined by log-rolling the patient. Note should be made of abrasions, lacerations, anatomic deformities, and any areas of muscle spasm and tenderness.

A careful neurologic examination should be performed. Patients with a spinal cord injury, either complete or incomplete, should receive the methylprednisolone spinal cord injury protocol. For patients seen within 3 hours of injury, methylprednisolone is administered intravenously, with an initial bolus of 30 mg per kilogram, followed by a continuous infusion of 5.4 mg per kilogram for 23 hours. For patients seen between 3 and 8 hours following injury, the methylprednisolone infusion is continued for 48 hours. For patients seen more than 8 hours following injury, methylprednisolone should not be given.

Until recently, this high-dose "steroid protocol" was considered to be the standard of care; however, the clinical trials underlying this treatment have come under renewed scrutiny. As a result, high-dose steroids for spinal cord injury are now considered by some authorities to be a treatment option, rather than a standard.

These injuries should be imaged with CT scanning, as significant fractures may be overlooked on plain radiographs. MRI should be performed if there is any neurologic deficit.

Common fracture patterns include the wedge compression fracture, burst fracture, Chance fracture (horizontal fracture through the posterior arch and pedicles, extending into the posterior aspect of the vertebral body), and fracture-dislocation.

The stability of thoracic fractures is often evaluated using the three-column model, which is discussed in Chapter 11. Injuries that are felt to be stable can be managed with external bracing, while unstable injuries may require surgical stabilization. The goal of treatment is to optimize fracture healing in order to facilitate early rehabilitation and prevent late spinal deformity.

Penetrating spinal trauma

The most common type of penetrating spinal injury is a gunshot wound to the spine resulting from assault with a handgun. In civilian gunshot wounds, the extent of injury is primarily caused by the bullet itself. In contrast, high-powered military weapons often cause more widespread damage from shock waves and cavitation.

These patients often have acute, life-threatening injuries to the chest or abdomen that require immediate attention and take priority over the spinal injury. Once the patient is stabilized, neurologic evaluation is needed.

Corticosteroids are not recommended for spinal cord injury associated with gunshot wounds, because these medications do not improve neurologic outcome and are associated with an increased risk of complications.

There is only a limited role for surgical intervention. Studies of patients with spinal cord injury in the setting of gunshot wound failed to show any neurologic recovery after treatment with laminectomy. It has also been shown that surgery increases the risk of spinal instability, CSF leakage, and infection. Furthermore, surgery does not diminish the incidence of late pain, as compared with patients managed nonsurgically. For these reasons, a conservative approach is generally recommended for patients with gunshot wounds to the spine.

At the same time, there are a few situations in which surgery may be beneficial. Potential indications for early surgery include:

1. Injury to the cauda equina (if neural compression by bullet or hematoma can be demonstrated)
2. Neurologic deterioration, suggestive of hematoma
3. Spinal instability (very uncommon sequela of isolated spinal gunshot wound)
4. CSF leak
5. Wound debridement to prevent infection (more important in military wounds or when bullet has traversed the gastrointestinal tract)

Potential indications for late surgery including:

1. Migrating bullet
2. Lead toxicity
3. Late instability

Figure 10.13 depicts the imaging studies of a 50-year-old woman, who sustained a spinal gunshot wound with a 45-caliber handgun. The entry wound was in the right lateral chest wall. Figure 10.13a and 10.13b depict plain thoracic radiographs showing the bullet in the right side of the spinal column at T5. Figure 10.13c depicts the axial CT scan, showing the bullet embedded in the lamina and transverse process at T5 on the right. There was no compromise of the spinal canal or neural foramen.

Chest tube drainage was required for injury to the right lung. The neurologic examination was normal. Surgery was not required. She was re-evaluated 3 years post-injury. There was no evidence of bullet

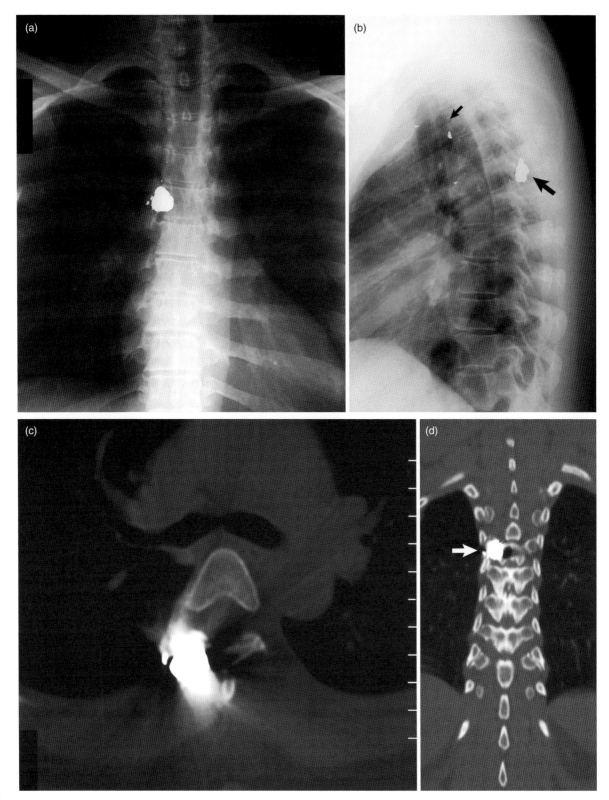

Figure 10.13. (a) Anteroposterior and (b) lateral radiograph depicting a 45-caliber bullet in the right side of the spinal column at T5. Lateral radiograph shows additional fragments (arrow). (c) Axial and (d) coronal CT scans depicting the bullet in the right T5 lamina and transverse process.

migration, spinal instability, or lead toxicity. The bullet was left in place.

Spinal deformity

Spinal deformities include scoliosis (coronal plane deformity or coronal plane imbalance) and kyphosis (sagittal plane deformity or sagittal plane imbalance). Patients may have scoliosis, kyphosis, or a combination of the two.

Spinal deformities are best assessed on standing, full-torso anteroposterior and lateral radiographs, which include the entire spinal column.

Scoliosis is defined through a process in which coronal plane balance is determined with a plumb line placed on the anteroposterior radiograph, extending caudally from the C7 vertebral body. If the line falls more than 25 mm from the mid-sacrum, coronal plane imbalance, or scoliosis, exists. Another definition of scoliosis is any coronal plane deformity measuring greater than $11°$.

Kyphosis is defined through a process in which sagittal balance is determined with a plumb line placed on the lateral radiograph, extending caudally from the C7 vertebral body. If this line falls in front of the sacrum, the patient is said to have positive sagittal balance or sagittal plane imbalance. If present, this finding is very significant because even small degrees of sagittal plane imbalance can produce significant back pain and disability.

Scoliosis is a common problem. It is estimated that there are 500 000 adults in the USA with curvatures exceeding $30°$. There are three major subgroups of scoliosis: congenital, idiopathic (juvenile), and degenerative.

Congenital scoliosis is characterized by the presence of vertebral anomalies, including hemivertebrae, failure of segmentation, and complete absence of one or more vertebral segments. Congenital scoliosis is often associated with neural tube defects and other congenital anomalies.

Idiopathic scoliosis is the most common spinal deformity and refers to spinal curvatures detected in otherwise healthy children and adolescents. In contrast to congenital scoliosis, these individuals have no neurologic or musculoskeletal disorder or other identifiable cause for the curvature. By definition, radiographic studies show no developmental vertebral abnormalities. The presenting symptoms are usually curvature progression and cosmetic deformity, rather than pain.

Degenerative scoliosis is seen in middle-aged and elderly individuals as a part of the degenerative cascade in the spine. In contrast to idiopathic scoliosis, patients with degenerative scoliosis often present with pain and neurologic abnormalities. Cosmetic issues tend to be less significant in the adult population.

Evaluation of the patient with spinal deformity should include a standard neurologic exam and should also include a search for examination findings that are specific for spinal deformity. The spine should be examined with the patient standing upright, bending forward at the waist, and prone. Note should be made of the relative heights of the iliac crest and shoulders, and the presence or absence of a rib hump. Positioning of the hips and knees should be evaluated while the patient is standing. Patients with sagittal plane imbalance must extend the hips and flex the knees in order to maintain an upright position.

Imaging assessment should include standing anteroposterior and lateral 36-in (92-cm) radiographs of the entire spinal column to identify the deformity and to measure the extent of coronal and sagittal plane imbalance. Lateral bending views are often helpful in assessing the flexibility of the deformity. Lateral flexion and extension views may also be helpful, especially for deformities in the lumbar region. MRI or CT/myelography is indicated for any patient with a neurologic deficit. Bone density should be measured; this is particularly important in patients being considered for surgical intervention. Discography is of limited importance in the initial evaluation of the deformity, but may play a role in surgical planning. In particular, discography may be useful in determining the caudal extent of a lumbar fusion. For example, when the clinical issue is whether to stop the fusion at L5 or extend it to the sacrum, a negative discogram at L5–S1 would support a decision to stop the fusion at L5, while a positive discogram at that level would suggest the fusion should include the sacrum.

Management of the patient with idiopathic scoliosis must take into account the natural history of the disorder without treatment, the impact of curvature progression, and the risks of treatment.

Data on the natural history of idiopathic scoliosis indicate that 68% of patients have progression after skeletal maturity. Thoracic, thoracolumbar, and lumbar curvatures greater than $50°$, progress at an annual rate of $1°$, $0.5°$, and $0.24°$ respectively. Thoracic curvatures less than $30°$ tend not to progress. Left untreated, severe curvature progression may have significant deleterious effects, including pain, impaired respiratory function, and socioeconomic limitations.

Treatment options include observation, non-operative management with bracing, and surgery. It is not possible to specify a precise algorithm for treatment, but the following general guidelines are useful. A curvature less than 30° can be followed, while those measuring greater than 50–60° should usually be considered for surgery. Intermediate curvatures measuring 30–50° may be considered for bracing or surgery depending on the skeletal maturity of the patient and rate of curve progression, if known.

The goal of surgery in idiopathic scoliosis is to prevent curvature progression and to restore normal coronal and sagittal plane balance to the greatest extent possible, while at the same time sparing as many motion segments as possible. When surgery is recommended, determination of the proximal and distal extent of the fusion should be based on whether the curvatures are major or minor. Whenever possible, the minor curve should be excluded from the fusion. The fusion should be planned and performed in a way that permits the proximal and distal vertebrae to be both neutral and stable post-operatively.

Most adults with acquired spinal deformity should have a trial of conservative management before considering surgical intervention. Physical therapy should be instituted in all cases, and diagnostic or therapeutic injections, including selective nerve root blocks, facet blocks, and epidural injections, may also be useful. Overweight patients should be placed on a weight reduction regimen. Although bracing may modify curvature progression in children and adolescents, this form of treatment is not effective in the adult with spinal deformity.

If surgery is contemplated, the patient must have an adequate level of fitness in order to withstand major reconstructive surgery and then be able to participate in a post-operative rehabilitation program. Pre-operative assessment should include a careful evaluation of cardiac and pulmonary function, as surgical procedures for spinal deformity are often quite prolonged and may involve extensive blood loss. In addition, these patients often have baseline impairment of pulmonary function due to the spinal deformity.

Correction of adult spinal deformities is among the most demanding of spine operations. While deformities in children and adolescents are usually flexible and often amenable to correction with a single anterior or posterior approach, adult deformities are often rigid and require a more complex operative strategy, including release procedures and circumferential approaches. The goal of surgery in the adult with degenerative spinal deformity is to normalize coronal and sagittal balance to the greatest extent possible, while at the same time, sparing as many motion segments as possible. The desired endpoint is to create a balanced spine, rather than absolute correction of the curvature. An additional goal is the creation of a solid fusion to prevent future deformity. Surgery in this patient population may also involve a laminectomy to treat neural compression from spinal stenosis. Pedicle subtraction osteotomy may be needed for correction of sagittal plane imbalance. Because of the complex procedures needed to treat rigid deformities and the presence of medical co-morbidities, complication rates are higher in adult deformity cases than those in children and adolescents.

Although symptoms may not be totally relieved, long-term surgical results are generally satisfactory. Comparative outcome studies of patients with scoliosis treated surgically and nonsurgically showed better relief of pain and fatigue in the surgical group.

Scheuermann kyphosis

Scheuermann kyphosis is the most common kyphotic deformity in the pediatric population. This disorder is more common in males and usually presents in adolescence, just prior to the onset of puberty.

The underlying cause is unknown, but appears to involve both genetic and environmental factors. Multiple genetic studies have shown a strong hereditary component.

Characteristic MRI findings included vertebral wedging, vertebral endplate irregularity, diminished anterior vertebral growth, and disk degeneration. Patients with Scheuermann kyphosis have more disk degeneration on MRI than normal individuals. Histopathologic studies have shown disorganized enchondral ossification, a reduction in collagen, and an increase in mucopolysaccharides in the endplate. It is not known whether these changes are cause of the disorder or the result of abnormal loading of the kyphotic spine.

Two distinct curve patterns have been described: thoracic and thoracolumbar. The thoracic pattern is more common and is associated with compensatory hyperlordosis of the cervical and lumbar spine. The thoracolumbar pattern is less common, but is thought to be more likely to progress in adulthood.

The reported incidence of Scheuermann kyphosis ranges from 1% to 8%. The true incidence is likely higher, as mild cases may be missed or attributed to poor posture.

The natural history is not well documented, and there are conflicting reports on the severity of pain, physical disability, and rate of curve progression. Neurologic complications are uncommon, but dural cysts and thoracic disk herniation have been described in small case series and case reports.

The most common reasons for seeking medical attention are pain and cosmetic issues related to the kyphotic deformity. Adolescents are often most concerned about the deformity. Adults are more likely to seek medical treatment because of pain; although pain is not a significant issue in all cases.

Treatment options include physical medicine, bracing, and surgery. Aggressive rehabilitation, with exercises and modalities, has been shown to provide modest symptomatic relief.

Bracing has been widely regarded as being effective in skeletally immature patients. Three separate studies have shown improvement in kyphosis, with some loss of correction after bracing is discontinued. These reports have significant limitations, in that all were retrospective and lacked a control group. Data available at the present time do not allow the physician to predict whether bracing will correct the deformity or prevent its progression. Well-designed prospective studies with control groups are needed to more accurately assess the role of bracing in these patients.

A variety of surgical procedures have been employed, including posterior instrumented fusion and combined anterior-posterior approaches. Both posterior only and combined anterior-posterior procedures have been shown to be effective in correcting the kyphotic deformity.

Serious complications are uncommon but have been reported. Major acute complications include permanent paraplegia, wound infection, hemothorax, and pneumothorax. Pulmonary function can be negatively impacted by anterior surgery. Delayed complications include development of junctional kyphosis at either end of the construct and pseudarthrosis.

The indications for surgery and the optimal surgical technique remain unclear. Critical appraisal of the role of surgery is hampered by the fact that most of the literature consists of retrospective clinical series with differing surgical indications and procedures. Relative to bracing, it appears that surgery provides better deformity correction at a cost of a small risk of potentially serious complications.

The lack of understanding of the natural history of Scheuermann kyphosis has made it difficult to assess the role of bracing and surgery in the management of these patients. Further information is needed on the rate of curve progression, particularly those between 70° and 90°, to guide clinicians in making evidence-based treatment recommendations.

Meningeal diverticulum with CSF leak: a cause of intracranial hypotension

Intracranial hypotension is a clinical syndrome of CSF hypovolemia, which results in positional headache and other neurologic symptoms. Causes of intracranial hypotension are classified as spontaneous (primary) and secondary (trauma and iatrogenic). The secondary cases are often easier to recognize, because the patient has a history of significant spinal trauma or recent therapeutic procedures, either injections or surgery, which have the potential to cause a CSF leak. The spontaneous cases are often more difficult to identify.

The most common cause of a spontaneous spinal CSF leak is a meningeal diverticulum. These lesions may occur at any level of the spinal column, but have a predilection for the lower cervical and upper thoracic spine. Mechanical stress and connective tissue disorders appear to be risk factors.

Because the predominant complaint is headache, the first imaging study is usually an MRI brain examination, which shows diffuse meningeal enhancement, brain sag, tonsillar descent, and sometimes subdural fluid collections. The presence of low-lying cerebellar tonsils may lead to the incorrect diagnosis of Chiari I malformation.

When the diagnosis of spinal CSF leak is suspected, imaging of the spine should be carried out. CT/myelography, MRI, and radionuclide cisternography may be performed. CT/myelography is the most reliable modality for identifying the precise site of a spinal CSF leak. At this time, MRI is less sensitive than CT/myelography; however, ongoing technical refinements may enable MRI to ultimately replace CT/myelography as the imaging test of choice for this problem. Radionuclide cisternography is useful to distinguish between cranial and spinal sources of the leak, and can define the general region of a spinal leak, but is rarely helpful in identifying the actual site of the leak.

Once identified, spinal leaks may initially be managed with short periods of bed rest, intravenous fluid, and pharmacologic therapy, including oral caffeine, theophylline, and steroids. These noninvasive measures are rarely successful, and more active treatment is generally required. The initial procedure is

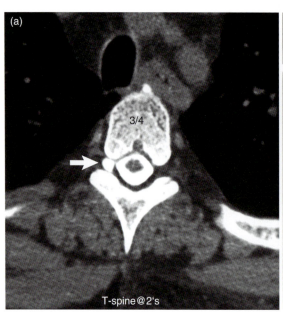 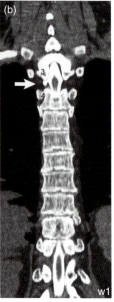

Figure 10.14. (a) Axial and (b) coronal CT/myelogram depicting a meningeal diverticulum at T3–T4, right (arrow).

usually an autologous epidural blood patch. Serial injections may be required. The injection site for the blood patch has not been standardized. Some investigators recommend a targeted blood patch at the site of the leak, while others have had success performing a "blinded" blood patch, with injection in the lumbar canal and allowing for rostral diffusion of blood in the epidural space. It is unclear whether precise identification of the leak increases the success rate of the blood patch procedure.

Surgical management is reserved for patients who fail multiple epidural blood patches. Surgical options include primary repair of the occult dural tear and packing of the epidural space. Short-term surgical results are excellent; however, clinical experience is limited, and long-term results are unknown.

Figure 10.14 depicts a meningeal diverticulum of the right T3 nerve root. The presenting symptom was low pressure headache. Symptoms were relieved after surgical repair of the diverticulum.

There is now increasing recognition that intracranial hypotension may occur as the result of meningeal diverticula and other spinal pathology. The majority of cases respond to epidural blood patches, with surgery being an option for refractory cases.

Clinical issues
Spinal cord biopsy
One of the most difficult decisions facing the neurologist or neurosurgeon is whether to recommend a spinal cord biopsy in a patient with an unexplained cord lesion. Clinicians are now confronted with this scenario with increasing frequency due to the widespread availability of high-resolution MRI, which is disclosing increasing numbers of spinal cord abnormalities. The primary diagnostic consideration usually lies between neoplastic and non-neoplastic conditions. MRI is sometimes unable to distinguish between the two, and, in these situations, a spinal cord biopsy may be needed.

Cord biopsy has a high rate of complications and often does not yield a specific diagnosis. However, there are occasional situations in which the information gained from a biopsy may be worth the risk, for example metastatic tumor and lymphoma.

The major concern is that a spinal cord biopsy carries significant risk of neurologic worsening and other complications. The overall complication rate of the procedure exceeds 20%.

Further complicating matters is the fact that the biopsy often does not yield a specific diagnosis. This is due in part to the fact that only small fragments of tissue are removed during the biopsy, which can make interpretation difficult, even for an experienced neuropathologist. It is not unusual for the biopsy to be abnormal, but not diagnostic. In these situations, the diagnosis remains uncertain, and it is impossible to make specific treatment recommendations.

Given the unfavorable risk/benefit ratio associated with biopsy, cord lesions should be diagnosed through less invasive means whenever possible.

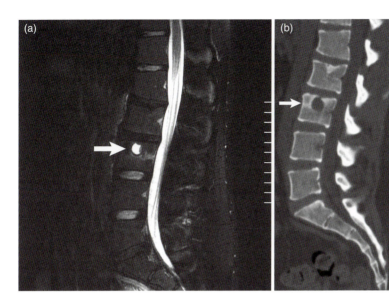

Figure 10.15. (a) Sagittal T$_2$-weighted MRI with fat saturation, and (b) sagittal CT scan, depicting a well-defined, rounded lesion in the L3 vertebral body (arrow).

The clinical findings are helpful. Severe, rapidly progressive neurologic deficits or a waxing and waning clinical course usually suggest an inflammatory process. Cord tumors are generally not associated with advanced neurologic deficits.

Demyelinating disease should be excluded with MRI of the brain and CSF examination. Granulomatous diseases, such as sarcoid and tuberculosis, should be excluded with a chest radiograph and appropriate systemic evaluations.

Magnetic resonance imaging characteristics of the lesion may be helpful in reaching a diagnosis. Lesions that do not expand the cord, that demonstrate only minimal, patchy enhancement, and that regress on follow-up imaging are more likely to be inflammatory than neoplastic.

Despite exhaustive work-up, the diagnosis of an intramedullary cord lesion occasionally remains elusive, and biopsy must be considered. It is impossible to recommend a precise algorithm for spinal cord biopsy. The clinical findings, especially the rate of neurologic decline, systemic evaluation, and MRI findings must all be considered. Overall, a conservative approach is recommended. If there is any doubt, it is often best to continue to follow the patient and repeat the MRI in 3–6 months, before deciding to biopsy.

If the decision is made to proceed with biopsy, the surgeon should be prepared to completely remove any surgically curable lesions, such as ependymoma or astrocytoma.

Management of the indeterminate bony lesion

Another clinical issue, which is vexing at times, is the management of a vertebral lesion that has indeterminate characteristics on imaging studies. The differential diagnosis usually includes tumor, infection, and benign degenerative changes. When confronted with this situation, the clinician must decide whether to recommend biopsy or a period of observation with follow-up imaging studies.

Although safer than a spinal cord biopsy, vertebral bone biopsy is not completely risk-free, and the risk/benefit ratio of the procedure must be carefully considered. On one hand, a conservative approach is often appropriate if the bony abnormality is asymptomatic or minimally symptomatic, and has a benign appearance on imaging studies. These patients can be followed with repeat imaging in 3–6 months.

On the other hand, if a lesion is causing significant pain and imaging findings are suggestive of cancer or infection, it is often best to proceed with biopsy.

Bony lesions in the lower thoracic and lumbar regions can be safely biopsied via percutaneous, CT-guided approaches. Lesions in the cervical and upper thoracic regions are less amenable to percutaneous biopsy due to the small size of the vertebrae and the close proximity of the spinal cord. In these cases, open biopsy is often needed.

Figure 10.15 depicts the lumbar MRI and CT scan of a 21-year-old man with low back pain. He was

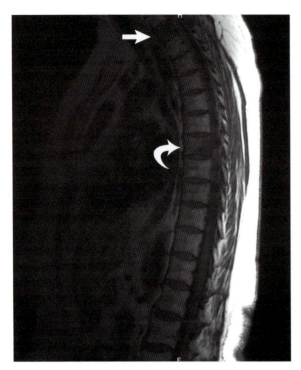

Figure 10.16. Sagittal T$_1$-weighted MRI depicting a destructive lesion in the T1 vertebral body (straight arrow) and a smaller lesion in the T7 vertebral body (curved arrow). Biopsy revealed metastatic carcinoma at both levels.

The imaging characteristics and location of the bony lesions and the patient's history of breast cancer all pointed toward a diagnosis of spinal metastatic tumor. Biopsy was performed and showed metastatic carcinoma at both levels.

The indeterminate spine lesion, in the setting of hepatic or renal failure, represents a special circumstance. These patients are often immunosuppressed and, therefore, have an increased incidence of fungal osteomyelitis and other opportunistic infections. Patients with chronic renal failure on long-term hemodialysis are at risk for dialysis spondyloarthropathy, which may progress to spinal instability, causing significant back pain and neurologic symptoms.

Patients being evaluated for organ transplantation, who are found to have indeterminate spine lesions during the pre-transplant evaluation, may require biopsy, in order to exclude infection or neoplasm prior to being listed for a transplant. In such cases, the need to proceed urgently with transplantation may mandate an immediate biopsy, rather than a period of observation and serial imaging, which would otherwise be an option.

otherwise healthy and had no "red flag" signs. The studies show a well-demarcated, rounded lesion in the L3 vertebral body. Although there was some surrounding edema, the lesion appeared benign, as there was no fracture, bony infiltration, or soft tissue mass in the epidural space or paraspinal region. Bone scan showed no uptake. The lesion was followed. A 6-month follow-up MRI demonstrated a stable appearance to the L3 lesion with reduction in the surrounding marrow edema. Biopsy was not performed. The lesion may have represented a large subchondral cyst. Although the precise nature of the abnormality was indeterminate without histologic confirmation, the stable appearance of the lesion on serial MRI studies strongly suggested the lesion was benign.

Figure 10.16 depicts the thoracic MRI of a 64-year-old woman with upper dorsal spine pain and a personal history of breast cancer. The study showed mixed sclerotic and lytic changes in the T1 and T7 vertebral bodies, with an epidural soft tissue mass at T1. These imaging findings were highly suggestive of malignancy rather than benign osteoporosis. Also, the location of the bony lesions in the upper thoracic region favored a malignant, rather than a benign, etiology.

Conclusions

The most common indications for surgery on the thoracic spine include trauma, tumor, infection, vascular lesions, deformity, and spondylosis. Although much less common than disk herniations in the cervical and lumbar regions, thoracic disk herniations do occur and often require surgical intervention. Thoracic spine lesions may be treated via anterior, posterior, and combined approaches. New technology includes minimally invasive thoracoscopic surgical techniques and computer-assisted image guidance to facilitate accurate placement of pedicle screws and other implants.

Further reading

1. Atkinson JLD, Miller GM, Krauss WE, et al. Clinical and radiographic features of dural arteriovenous fistula, a treatable cause of myelopathy. *Mayo Clin Proc* 2001; **76**:1120–1130.

2. Cohen AA, Zikel OM, Miller GM, Aksamit AJ, Scheithauer BW, Krauss WE. Spinal cord biopsy: a review of 38 cases. *Neurosurgery* 2003; **52**:806–816.

3. Fischer G, Brotchi J. *Intramedullary Spinal Cord Tumors.* New York, Thieme, 1996.

4. Fourney DR, Schomer DF, Nader R, et al. Percutaneous vertebroplasty and kyphoplasty for painful vertebral

body fractures in cancer patients. *J Neurosurg* 2003; **98** (Suppl 1):21–30.

5. Harrop JS, Prpa B, Reinhardt MK, Lieberman I. Primary and secondary osteoporosis: incidence of subsequent vertebral compression fractures after kyphoplasty. *Spine* 2004; **29**:2120–2125.

6. Heary RF. Evaluation and treatment of adult spinal deformity. *J Neurosurg Spine* 2004; **1**:9–18.

7. Hott JS, Feiz-Erfan I, Kenny K, Dickman CA. Surgical management of giant herniated thoracic discs: analysis of 20 cases. *J Neurosurg Spine* 2005; **3**:191–197.

8. Inamasu J, Guiot BH. Intracranial hypotension with spinal pathology. *Spine J* 2006; **6**:591–599.

9. Kim DH, Vaccaro AR. Osteoporotic compression fractures of the spine: current options and considerations for treatment. *Spine J* 2006; **6**:479–487.

10. Lee JY, Vaccaro AR, Schweitzer KM, et al. Assessment of injury to the thoracolumbar posterior ligamentous complex in the setting of normal-appearing plain radiography. *Spine J* 2007; **7**:422–427.

11. Lowe TG, Line BG. Evidence based medicine: analysis of Scheuermann kyphosis. *Spine* 2007; **32** (Suppl): S115–119.

12. Patel A, Vaccaro AR, Martyak GG, et al. Neurologic deficit following percutaneous vertebral stabilization. *Spine* 2007; **32**:1728–1734.

Chapter

11

Disorders of the lumbar spine: pre-operative assessment and surgical management

Clinical assessment and surgical evaluation

The differential diagnosis of disease processes affecting the lumbar spine is similar to that for other regions of the spine. A listing of the more common lumbar spine disorders is shown in Table 11.1. Most lumbar operations are currently done for degenerative and discogenic disorders; however, a number of other disease processes, including trauma, neoplasm, infection, inflammatory processes, vascular lesions, and congenital abnormalities, may also require surgical intervention.

Although low back pain is generally a benign and self-limited condition, a small number of patients have a serious underlying disease, and the clinician is again reminded to look for "red flag" symptoms, which should prompt urgent or emergent evaluation.

Neurologic examination should include an assessment of gait, tension signs (Lasègue sign or straight leg raising), motor and sensory function, and deep tendon reflexes. If cauda equina syndrome is suspected, rectal tone and perianal sensation should be assessed. Long tract signs, if present, should prompt investigation of higher levels, especially the thoracic cord.

The back should be carefully inspected for deformities, scars, and other cutaneous abnormalities. Hair patches (hypertrichosis) may indicate the presence of congenital anomalies, such as spinal dysraphism (Figure 11.1). Any patient confined to bed is at risk for skin breakdown, with the sacrum being a common site of involvement.

Diagnostic pitfalls

As with other regions of the spinal column, it is essential to make an accurate diagnosis before surgery or other treatment can be considered. Following is a list of diagnostic pitfalls in the lumbar spine, in which the patient may wind up in the surgeon's office with a lesion that is not surgical, and sometimes not even in the spine.

1. Pelvic/abdominal pathology. Diseases of the abdomen and pelvis may masquerade as spinal disorders. A classic example of this is abdominal aortic aneurysm presenting with low back pain (Figure 11.2).

> *Clinical pearl: When reviewing any spine imaging study, carefully scrutinize paraspinal and intra-abdominal structures for evidence of abdominal aortic aneurysm, retroperitoneal tumor, and other extraspinal lesions.*

2. Degenerative joint disease (DJD) of the hip. It can sometimes be difficult to distinguish between symptomatic DJD of the hip and lumbar spinal stenosis with neurogenic claudication. To a large extent, this is a clinical diagnosis, as imaging studies of the hip and spine are both likely to be abnormal. If the hip is symptomatic, the patient will typically have pain in the hip and groin, without distal radiating pain. Pertinent physical examination findings include tenderness of the hip joint and pain with flexion, abduction, and external rotation of the hip (FABER maneuver, aka Patrick test). In contrast, if the spine is symptomatic, the patient will usually have leg pain radiating below the knee and hip maneuvers will not be painful. Diagnostic injection of the hip is often useful in sorting out whether the hip is symptomatic.

> *Clinical pearl: If the pain is in the hip and groin, think hip disease. Check hip maneuvers and obtain a radiograph of the hip.*

3. Vascular claudication. Vascular and neurogenic claudication both cause radiating leg pain, which is precipitated by walking. To gain relief, the patient with neurogenic claudication must flex the lumbar spine by sitting, squatting, or bending forward at the waist. In contrast, the patient with vascular claudication does not have to flex the back, but only has to stop walking in order to

Table 11.1. Differential diagnosis of pain in the low back and leg, with or without neurologic involvement

1. Discogenic or degenerative disease

    A. Herniated intervertebral disk

    B. Lumbar spondylosis

    C. Synovial cyst of facet joint

    D. Degenerative disk disease

2. Trauma

3. Tumor

    A. Primary intradural tumor of spinal cord or adjacent nerve roots

    B. Tumor of vertebral column or epidural space (or both)

       – Metastatic tumor

       – Plasmacytoma or multiple myeloma

       – Primary bone tumor (e.g., chordoma)

4. Infection

    A. Intervertebral discitis or osteomyelitis

    B. Epidural abscess

    C. Herpes zoster or other viral radiculopathy

5. Vascular lesion

    A. Neoplastic vascular lesion (e.g., cavernous malformation)

    B. Arteriovenous fistula

    C. Arteriovenous malformation

6. Inflammatory arthropathy (e.g., ankylosing spondylitis)

7. Referred pain from abdominal or pelvic lesion

    A. Abdominal aortic aneurysm

    B. Gastric/pancreatic carcinoma

8. Noncompressive disorders of the spinal cord and peripheral nerves

    A. Motor neuron disease

    B. Guillain–Barré syndrome

    C. Peripheral neuropathy

9. Metabolic bone disease

    A. Osteoporosis

10. Congenital anomalies

    A. Myelodysplasia

experience pain relief. Also, the patient with vascular claudication has diminished pedal pulses on physical examination.

> Clinical pearl: Always check the pedal pulses in the patient who presents with claudication symptoms.

4. Viral radiculopathy. Herpes zoster (shingles) may affect lumbar nerve roots and cause radicular pain. Herpes zoster represents a cause of noncompressive radiculopathy.

> Clinical pearl: When evaluating a patient with radiculopathy, always look for the characteristic herpetic lesions that appear in the dermatome of the affected nerve root.

5. Intradural pathology. Cauda equina tumors and other intradural lesions can mimic lumbar disk herniations. Magnetic resonance imaging (MRI) or computed tomography (CT)/myelography must be performed in patients with radicular pain and neurologic deficits. As noted in Chapter 8, CT scanning without intrathecal contrast does not visualize the subarachnoid space, and is therefore not able to exclude intradural pathology. Figure 11.3 depicts the lumbar MRI of a patient with radicular pain who had a nerve sheath tumor of the upper cauda equina.

> Clinical pearl: When evaluating the patient with lumbar radiculopathy, always obtain an MRI or CT/myelography to exclude intradural pathology.

6. Thoracic lesion. Lower extremity symptoms are often attributed to the lumbar spine; however, the possibility of a thoracic cord lesion should always be considered. An occasional patient has undergone decompressive laminectomy for clinically insignificant lumbar stenosis, only to be found to have a thoracic cord lesion on subsequent evaluation. Look for a sensory level, hyperreflexia, and other signs of a cord lesion on neurologic examination. Figure 11.4 depicts a thoracic MRI showing a T4 meningioma, in a woman who was referred for neurosurgical evaluation of leg weakness, initially thought to be due to lumbar stenosis.

> Clinical pearl. If the patient with lower extremity symptoms has long tract signs, the lesion is probably in the thoracic region (or higher).

7. Sequestered disk herniation. The typical disk herniation remains in continuity with the disk space; however, sequestered fragments may migrate away from the disk space to lie behind the superior or inferior vertebral body. Axial MRI images that are taken only through the disk spaces may miss sequestered fragments. Figure 11.5a depicts a sagittal MRI "scanogram," indicating that axial cuts were only performed at the

203

(a) (b)

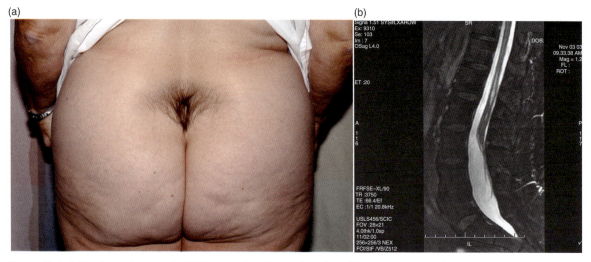

Figure 11.1. (a) Lumbosacral hair patch, highly suggestive of spinal dysraphism. (b) Sagittal T$_2$-weighted MRI showing tethered cord with low-lying conus medullaris.

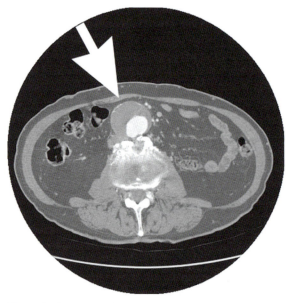

Figure 11.2. CT scan of the abdomen depicting an abdominal aortic aneurysm (arrow).

> Clinical pearl. Don't rely solely on axial MRI through the disk spaces. Be sure to obtain at least one sequence of axial images through the vertebral bodies.

8. Nonorganic pain syndromes. When evaluating a patient with spine pain, the clinician must always be alert to the possibility of a nonorganic pain state. Overly dramatic pain descriptions, nonanatomic pain drawings, exaggerated responses to physical examination maneuvers, and give way on muscle testing are all suggestive that the patient's symptoms may not have an organic basis. In 1980, Waddell defined a set of physical examination findings characteristic of these patients (see Table 4.4). If present, these signs do not establish a psychological diagnosis, but do suggest that the clinician should proceed cautiously, and perhaps recommend psychological assessment, before proceeding with surgery or other invasive procedures.

interspace level. Figure 11.5b depicts an axial MRI taken through the interspace, which was completely normal. Figure 11.5c depicts an axial MRI taken through the vertebral body, which shows an extruded disk fragment, which had migrated caudally (rostrally) away from the L3–L4 interspace. This finding is further confirmed on a sagittal MRI (Figure 11.5d).

Surgical indications and approaches

The clinical indications for surgery on the lumbar spine include radiculopathy, cauda equina syndrome, and instability. Mechanical or discogenic back pain is a controversial indication for surgery, discussed later in this chapter.

Most lumbar procedures are done through a posterior approach, including common operations done

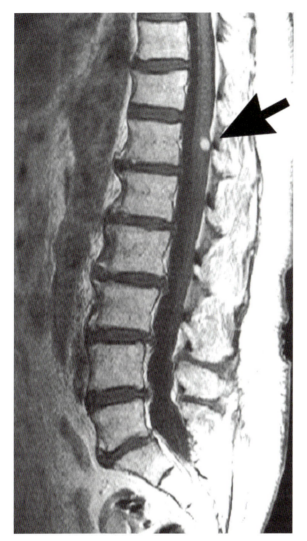

Figure 11.3. Sagittal T$_1$-weighted lumbar spine MRI, with contrast enhancement, depicting a small schwannoma of the upper cauda equina.

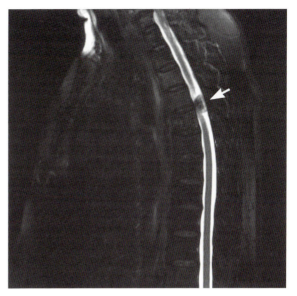

Figure 11.4. Sagittal T$_2$-weighted thoracic spine MRI with fat saturation, depicting a T4 intradural meningioma, in a woman initially thought to have a lumbar syndrome.

for disk herniation and spinal stenosis. Similar to other regions of the spine, virtually all lumbar intradural lesions are resected via a posterior approach.

Anterior approaches are utilized in selected cases, typically for fusion and disk arthroplasty. Circumferential or 360° approaches may be required in situations where the spine is extremely unstable or extensive deformity correction is required.

Surgical complications

Acute complications include neurologic injury (spinal nerve roots or cauda equina), CSF leak, and infection. Neurologic injury may occur during the operative procedure or following the procedure as a consequence of an epidural hematoma. A typical postoperative CSF leak and pseudomeningocele are depicted in Figure 11.6.

Vascular complications

An uncommon, but potentially life-threatening complication is great vessel injury, affecting the aorta, vena cava, or iliac vessels. Vascular injury is more common during anterior lumbar operations, but may occur during posterior procedures as well. Great vessel injury is immediately apparent during anterior lumbar procedures, as the vessels are directly exposed from the surgical approach. In contrast, great vessel injury may not be immediately apparent during posterior, laminectomy procedures. In some cases, the injury is heralded by a gush of arterial blood into the operative field; however, if bleeding is contained within the retroperitoneal space, it may not enter the surgical field. In these situations, intra-abdominal bleeding may not be detected for many hours or even days after the procedure.

Another uncommon, but potentially serious, vascular complication of anterior lumbar procedures is intra-arterial embolization from manipulation of the aorto-iliac vessels, resulting in distal embolization of atheromatous debris. Patients with aorto-iliac occlusive disease are at higher risk for this complication.

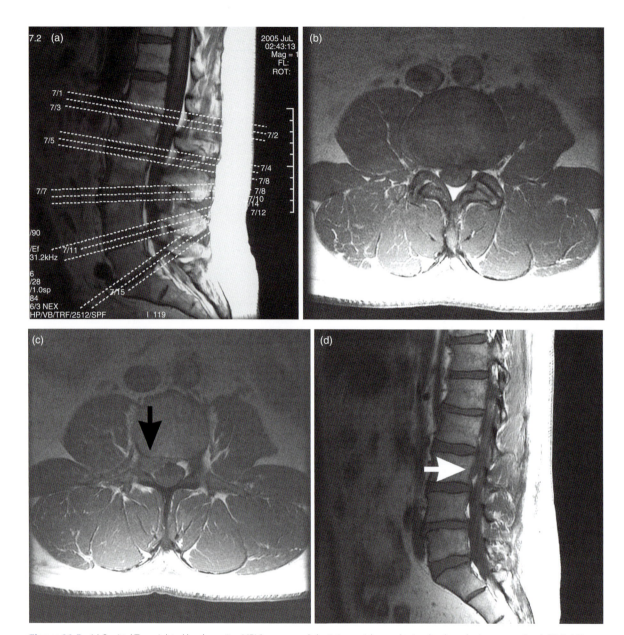

Figure 11.5. (a) Sagittal T_1-weighted lumbar spine MRI "scanogram" depicting axial cuts obtained only at the interspace level. (b) Axial image through the L3–L4 interspace is completely normal. (c) Axial image through the L4 vertebral body, depicting an extruded disk fragment, which had migrated caudally away from the interspace (arrow). (d) Sagittal image depicting disk fragment behind the L4 vertebral body (arrow).

As there is no intra-operative bleeding, the problem may not be immediately apparent. The patient usually reports leg pain in the early post-operative period. The diagnosis may be further delayed if the leg pain is attributed to nerve root irritation, and treated with a course of steroids or simply observed. The key to the diagnosis is the observation that the symptomatic leg is cool with diminished pulses. Prompt recognition of the problem and immediate consultation with a vascular surgeon or interventional radiologist are needed. Blood flow to the extremity must be promptly restored in order to avoid irreversible limb ischemia leading to amputation.

While leg pain following lumbar operations is most commonly caused by nerve root irritation, leg pain after anterior procedures may be ischemic in nature. Any patient with new leg pain following anterior lumbar surgery should be assumed to have

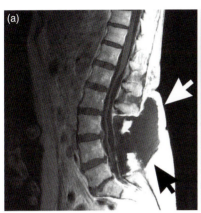 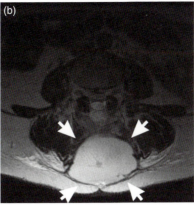

Figure 11.6. (a) Sagittal T_1-weighted and (b) axial T_2-weighted lumbar spine MRI depicting a CSF leak with a large, post-operative pseudomeningocele (arrows).

ischemic pain until proven otherwise and should be promptly investigated.

Blindness

Post-operative blindness is a rare but devastating complication, which may result from inadvertent pressure on the eyes or ischemic optic neuropathy. This event is associated with prolonged operations in the prone position with hypotension and significant blood loss. Post-operative blindness has been reported more often after operations on the lumbar and thoracic spine, but may occur after procedures at any level of the spine. This complication is not unique to spinal surgery and has been reported following prostate and vascular surgery. The American Society of Anesthesiologists has established a registry for tracking these cases in the USA.

The American Society of Anesthesiologist has recommended that high-risk patients be positioned so that their heads are level with or higher than the heart, and that the head and neck be maintained in a neutral position (without significant neck flexion, extension, lateral flexion or rotation), whenever possible. The recommendation was also made to consider the use of staged spine procedures in high-risk patients.

Although there are no published data to suggest there is a transfusion threshold that would eliminate the risk of post-operative vision loss related to anemia, some surgeons and anesthesiologists now recommend blood transfusion to maintain the hemoglobin >10 g/dl in high-risk patients, a more liberal transfusion policy than had been used previously.

Sexual dysfunction

Men undergoing anterior approaches to the lower lumbar spine and lumbosacral junction are at risk for retrograde ejaculation, as a result of damage to the presacral nerves.

Complications related to positioning

Peripheral nerve injury can occur with any operative position. These injuries are classified as either pressure palsies or traction palsies. Virtually any peripheral nerve can be affected. The prone position, which is commonly used for operations on the lumbar spine, is most commonly associated with compression injuries to the lateral femoral cutaneous, femoral, and ulnar nerves, and traction injury to the brachial plexus. Diabetes is an added risk factor, and extremes in body habitus, either marked obesity or emaciation, may also make peripheral nerves more vulnerable to peri-operative injury.

When the patient is positioned for surgery after induction of anesthesia, all pressure points should be carefully padded and awkward positioning of the extremities should be avoided. Efforts should be made to avoid excessive traction or pressure on the brachial plexus. These measures will decrease the incidence of peripheral nerve injuries, but cannot completely eliminate this complication.

When spine surgery is performed in the prone position, the head is often secured in a headrest with three or four sharp pins. If the skull is not intact, these pins can penetrate the dura, produce a CSF fistula, and potentially injure the brain. Injury to the middle meningeal artery may cause an epidural hematoma. In order to prevent this type of complication, the calvarium should be carefully inspected for evidence of previous craniotomies and other skull defects, prior to application of the headrest.

Laceration of the scalp, face, or eyes may occur if the head holder slips during the procedure.

Late complications

The most common late, or delayed, complication of lumbar discectomy is recurrent disk herniation. The most common late complications of spinal fusion are pseudarthrosis and loss of spinal alignment.

Additional risk factors

Surgical complication rates are increased in the setting of diabetes mellitus, chronic steroid therapy or other forms of immunosuppression, smoking, repeat operations, and spinal instrumentation.

Selected surgical disorders of the lumbar spine

Lumbar disk herniation

Similar to the cervical spine, symptomatic lumbar disk herniation is predominantly a disease of middle-aged adults. It is somewhat less common in the elderly and is an infrequent occurrence in children and teenagers.

The primary indication for surgical treatment of a lumbar disk herniation is intractable radicular pain, not back pain. Rarely, patients present with bladder and bowel dysfunction secondary to cauda equina syndrome. The diagnosis is confirmed with MRI or CT/myelography. Microdiscectomy remains the gold standard for surgical management. Surgery is elective for radiculopathy with little or no weakness, urgent for radiculopathy with severe weakness, and emergent for cauda equina syndrome.

Lumbar discectomy as a treatment for herniated lumbar intervertebral disks was first reported in the 1920s. After initial modifications, the procedure was basically unchanged until the operating microscope was introduced as a technical adjunct in 1978. This resulted in better illumination and magnification of the operative field. The operation came to be known as lumbar microdiscectomy or microsurgical discectomy, which is done through a smaller incision with less dissection than a standard discectomy. Microdiscectomy is generally regarded as a technical modification of standard discectomy, rather than a distinctly different procedure.

Currently the procedure is done through a small posterior incision, which is centered over the disk space. Most surgeons use some form of magnified vision, either loupes or an operating microscope. Variable amounts of laminar bone, ligamentum flavum, and medial facet are removed as needed to provide access to the disk herniation, which is then removed. The open surgical approach permits exploration for sequestered disk fragments and decompression of bony foraminal stenosis. In some centers, the procedure is now done through tube retractors of various sizes to limit dissection of paraspinal tissues. Patients are usually dismissed from the hospital within 24 hours of surgery and return to work within 2–6 weeks.

Extensive published data indicate that surgical results are generally excellent. Success rates as high as 95% have been reported in single surgeon series. Results obtained in routine clinical practice are not as robust, but are still excellent. In a prospective study of 219 patients undergoing lumbar discectomy, performed by multiple surgeons in community hospitals, with 1-year minimum follow-up, sciatica was improved in 81.3% of patients, and 86.5% of patients would choose surgery again. Operative complication rate was 6.0%, including dural tear – 2.2%, neural injury – 0.4%, and intra-operative bleeding (>500 ml) – 3.4%. The re-operation rate at 1-year follow-up was 6.5%. These data are important because they show the outcomes that can be expected in routine, contemporary, clinical practice.

Lumbar discectomy is generally well tolerated, and serious complications are uncommon. In one large, population-based study, the following complications were reported: mortality – 0.06%, major neurologic complications – 0.3%, deep infection – 0.3%, and major cardiovascular complications – 0.19%.

Although lumbar discectomy is not without risk, these data indicate that the risk of serious complication is extremely low in routine clinical practice.

SPORT study, Part I (lumbar disk herniation)

The SPORT study (Spine Patient Outcomes Research Trial) was a very large clinical trial, which analyzed outcomes in three common spinal disorders: lumbar disk herniation, degenerative lumbar spondylolisthesis, and lumbar spinal stenosis.

Part I, published in 2006, was a prospective study of patients with symptomatic lumbar disk herniation treated surgically and nonsurgically. There were two components to the study: a randomized clinical trial and an observational cohort.

In the randomized trial, patients with lumbar radiculopathy of more than 6 weeks' duration and imaging-confirmed disk herniation were randomized in a 1:1 ratio to surgery or nonoperative treatment. Anticipating that significant numbers of patients with symptomatic disk herniation would refuse randomization due to a strong desire to pursue a specific treatment strategy, the investigators included an observational cohort for patients who qualified for the study, but refused randomization.

Patients were followed for two years, and outcomes were assessed using well-established outcomes measures, including the SF-36, Oswestry Disability Index, and sciatic bothersomeness index.

Patients in the surgical arm underwent microdiscectomy at the symptomatic level. The procedure was well tolerated, with minimal complications. The most common complication was CSF leak (4%). Reoperation for a new disk herniation was required within one year of the index procedure in 4% of patients.

Patients in the nonoperative treatment arm received a variety of standard interventions including patient education, nonsteroidal anti-inflammatory medications, activity modification, physical therapy, and injections. Conservative treatment was also well tolerated. No patient developed a cauda equina syndrome or any other serious complication. This finding addresses the concern often expressed by clinicians and patients that failure to remove a disk herniation will likely have catastrophic neurologic consequences. The SPORT study provides evidence that this scenario is extremely unlikely.

Patients choosing surgery had more severe symptoms than those who opted for conservative management. At two-year follow-up, both surgical and nonsurgical groups showed substantial improvement; however, improvements were greater and occurred more rapidly in patients who chose surgical intervention. Patients who underwent discectomy had significantly better self-reported outcomes than those pursuing nonoperative treatment. Consistent with clinical experience, the SPORT study found that relief of leg pain was the most striking and consistent improvement with surgery.

Although this work represented a monumental effort in spine research, the data were difficult to evaluate because of limited adherence to the assigned treatment. Only 50% of patients assigned to surgery received surgery within 3 months of enrollment, while 30% of those assigned to conservative treatment received surgery in the same period. Because of this high crossover rate, data analysis on an intent-to-treat basis underestimated the true effect of surgery. As-treated analysis based on treatment received showed strong, statistically significant advantages for surgery at all follow-up times through 2 years.

This high crossover rate also indicates that, to a large extent, the study patients received the treatment of their choice regardless of how they were randomized.

Also, the study results are not applicable to patients with acute, severe sciatica of less than 6 weeks' duration. Many of those patients, especially those with significant neurologic deficits, should be considered for early surgical intervention.

In a broader context, the SPORT study demonstrated the difficulties associated with conducting randomized studies in non-life-threatening, heterogeneous conditions, in which patient preferences are a major determinant of the course of treatment selected. This study also demonstrates the limitations of using intent-to-treat analysis in situations where the patients essentially make their own treatment decisions, regardless of assignment based on randomization.

How much disk tissue should be removed?

Until recently, there was no reliable guidance on how much disk material should be removed during a lumbar discectomy. Some surgeons have advocated simply removing the herniated or extruded disk, leaving the contents of the interspace in place, while others have advocated a more aggressive removal of disk material from the interspace in order to prevent a recurrence.

Evidence is now emerging that a more aggressive discectomy does not lower the recurrence rate, and may actually be detrimental by producing more back pain and disk degeneration.

A recently presented randomized prospective study compared simple disk fragment removal (sequestrectomy) with standard microdiscectomy. The only difference between the two treatment groups was that no disk material was removed from the interspace in the sequestrectomy group, while additional disk material was removed from the interspace in the standard microdiscectomy group.

Initial clinical improvement was dramatic and identical in both groups. Improvement was maintained in the sequestrectomy group; however, the standard microdiscectomy group deteriorated somewhat over time, and, at 2-year follow-up, had more back pain and worse functional status than the sequestrectomy group. In addition, patients undergoing standard microdiscectomy had more advanced disk degeneration at the operated level on MRI at the 2-year follow-up interval. There was no difference in reherniation rates between the two groups.

In another recent study, investigators weighed the disk tissue removed during surgery, and found that a more extensive disk removal did not lead to a better outcome or lower recurrence rate.

Although this issue is not fully resolved, these recent studies support a more limited operation, with the goal of simply removing the herniated disk material causing neural compression.

Long-term spine health following microdiscectomy

Patients undergoing lumbar discectomy frequently inquire as to whether they are at increased risk for future back-related problems. A recently published report on a large series of patients with 25-year follow-up after lumbar discectomy provided a mixed answer to this important question. The encouraging finding was that this cohort of discectomy patients had generic health status measures that were comparable to those of age- and gender-matched controls; however 10% of the surgical cohort did require additional discectomy surgery at various time intervals after the index procedure.

These data suggest that patients undergoing lumbar discectomy fare just as well as the general population regarding long-term symptoms and functional status. On the other hand, the fact that 10% did require subsequent discectomy surgery does suggest that these individuals are at increased risk for future spine problems.

Illustration of microdiscectomy technique

The steps involved in lumbar microdiscectomy are outlined in Figure 11.7. Figure 11.8a depicts the MRI of an extruded disc at L5–S1 on the left, which was successfully treated with microdiscectomy. Figure 11.8b depicts an intra-operative photograph of the case, showing the extruded disk fragment and its relationship to the S1 nerve root and common dural sac.

Less invasive alternatives such as endoscopic and laser-assisted discectomy are being performed at some centers and are discussed in Chapter 12.

Lumbar spinal stenosis

Lumbar spinal stenosis is a very common disorder, which may be either congenital or degenerative in nature. Degenerative, or acquired, stenosis is the more common form and is typically seen in older adults. Congenital stenosis, which is less common, is

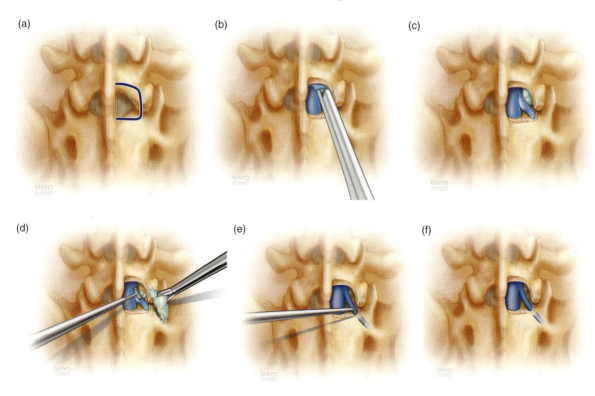

Figure 11.7. a–e. Steps involved in lumbar microdiscectomy. (a) Exposure of lamina and facet joint with outline of the anticipated partial hemilaminectomy and medial facetectomy. (b) Removal of laminar bone and ligament flavum with the Kerrison punch. (c) Extruded disk is exposed. Note medial and posterior displacement of the traversing nerve root. (d) Removal of disk fragment, while gently retracting the traversing nerve root and common dural sac. (e) Probing the foramen of the traversing nerve root to check for additional disk fragments. (f) Appearance of surgical site after discectomy. Note excellent decompression of the common dural sac and traversing nerve root. Figure reproduced with permission from Mayo Foundation for Medical Education and Research.

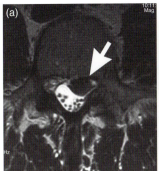 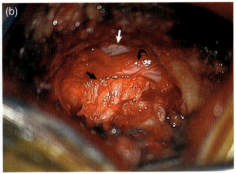

Figure 11.8. (a) Axial T$_2$-weighted lumbar spine MRI depicting a left L5–S1 disk extrusion. (b) Intra-operative photograph depicting the extruded disk (straight, black arrow) and its relationship to the traversing S1 nerve root (curved, black arrow) and common dural sac (white arrow).

associated with short pedicles and a shallow spinal canal and may be seen in young or middle-aged adults. In its more advanced forms, lumbar spinal stenosis causes neurogenic claudication, which refers to leg pain and paresthesias, precipitated by standing and walking, and relieved by sitting down. This diagnosis is being made with increasing frequency for a variety of reasons; these include a better recognition of the clinical syndrome of neurogenic claudication, the widespread availability of MRI, and an aging population.

Although patients may present with varying degrees of low back pain, intervention usually depends on whether leg symptoms are present. A careful history is essential to establish the diagnosis. Patients with neurogenic claudication give varying descriptions of their lower extremity symptoms. Some patients report true leg pain, while others describe tingling, heaviness, or a sensation that their legs are going to "give out." The leg symptoms may be unilateral or bilateral. Sphincter dysfunction due to cauda equina syndrome is uncommon.

A syndrome which may be confused with neurogenic claudication is vascular claudication due to aorto-iliac occlusive disease. Similar to neurogenic claudication, patients with vascular insufficiency develop leg pain with walking. The key point in distinguishing between these two syndromes is the fact that the patient with neurogenic claudication also develops leg pain with standing and must sit down or bend forward at the waist in order to gain relief. In contrast, the patient with vascular claudication does not develop leg pain with standing and does not have to sit down to gain relief of exercise-induced leg pain. Patients with vascular insufficiency can simply stop walking and stand briefly and experience pain relief. Pedal pulses are diminished in patients with vascular insufficiency.

The pathophysiology of lumbar spinal stenosis is not fully understood. There is increasing recognition, from both animal and human studies, that there is a direct correlation between the severity of the stenosis of the central canal, as measured by cross-sectional area, and severity of neurogenic claudication. A smaller cross-sectional area is directly related to limitations in walking distance. However, the mechanism through which this encroachment on the spinal canal produces symptoms is still uncertain. Possible explanations include obstruction of arterial blood flow to the cauda equina, impaired venous drainage of the cauda equina due to increased CSF pressure below the stenotic area, direct neural compression at the stenotic levels, or a combination of these mechanisms.

In the patient with neurogenic claudication and spinal stenosis, the neurologic examination is usually normal, or may reveal mild abnormalities. If the patient has a moderate or severe neurologic deficit, a second diagnosis may be present. For example, the patient might have lumbar spinal stenosis with a superimposed acute disk herniation. MRI or myelogram/CT should be used to establish the diagnosis of lumbar spinal stenosis. These studies may reveal stenosis of the central canal, lateral recess, or neural foramina. Figure 11.9 depicts an MRI showing severe spinal stenosis at L3–L4. A degenerative spondylolisthesis or scoliosis may also be present. Plain radiographs with flexion and extension views are useful for surgical planning.

Symptoms may fluctuate early in the course of the disease process; however, the natural history of lumbar spinal stenosis is one of gradual progression of symptoms and increasing functional limitation over time. Conservative treatment may help in selected cases. Patients with disabling neurogenic claudication, coupled with severe spinal stenosis, usually require surgical treatment.

A key factor in deciding on a surgical referral is an assessment of how much the patient is limited in his or her usual activities of daily living. If the patient has little or no functional limitation, surgery is usually not warranted, even if there is radiographic evidence

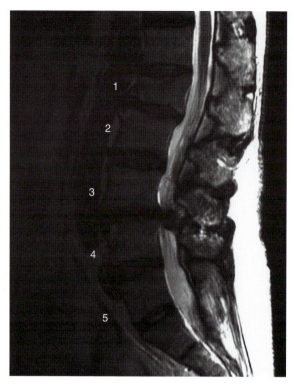

Figure 11.9. Sagittal T$_2$-weighted MRI, depicting severe spinal stenosis at L3–L4.

of stenosis. In contrast, if patient has lifestyle-limiting symptoms, surgery should be considered. For example, the author would most likely not recommend surgery for the patient who develops mild leg aching after walking 3 miles in 30 minutes. On the other hand, the patient who consistently develops severe leg pain after standing or walking for 5 minutes or less would probably be a surgical candidate.

The standard surgical treatment is a decompressive laminectomy of the stenotic spinal segments. A fusion may be required for some patients with spondylolisthesis or scoliosis. A good or excellent result can be expected in 70% to 90% of cases at 1-year follow-up. With longer follow-up, a few patients who initially do well develop recurrent symptoms and require further investigation and treatment. Despite this, surgical results are superior to those seen in patients treated nonoperatively at long-term follow-up.

Risk factors for poor outcome after decompressive laminectomy include diabetes and other co-existing medical illnesses, cigarette smoking, female gender, significant pre-operative neurologic deficit, and spinal deformity. Advanced age does not disqualify an individual from having surgery and does not appear to be a risk factor for poor outcome.

Interspinous process decompression with the X-Stop device, approved by the FDA in 2006, is an excellent minimally invasive option for patients with stenosis confined to one or two segments. This technique is described in Chapter 12.

Role of fusion in lumbar stenosis

Patients with lumbar canal stenosis often have spondylolisthesis. A common clinical question is whether this patient subgroup should undergo a fusion in addition to decompressive laminectomy. Some investigators have reported good clinical results in this patient population with decompression alone; however, several prospective studies comparing decompression and noninstrumented fusion with decompression alone have found that adding a fusion leads to better outcomes.

A related question is whether instrumentation should be added to the bone graft to enhance the success of the fusion procedure. One study found that adding instrumentation led to a higher rate of radiographic fusion but did not improve clinical outcomes at 2-year follow-up. In a separate study, the same investigators showed better clinical outcomes at 5-year follow-up among patients with a solid fusion. Synthesizing these reports, it appears that instrumentation leads to a higher rate of fusion and to better clinical results, which may not be apparent for several years. Balanced against their apparent beneficial effects, it must be recognized that instrumentation is associated with higher costs and higher complication rates. Although the issue is not fully resolved, many surgeons would recommend an instrumented fusion, in addition to decompressive laminectomy for patients with lumbar stenosis and spondylolisthesis.

A recommendation for adding instrumentation must be made in the context of the patient's age and medical co-morbidities. For example, an elderly patient with osteoporosis would be at increased risk for pedicle screw loosening and pullout. In these situations, a noninstrumented fusion may be preferable. This can be accomplished with some combination of bone morphogenetic protein, laminectomy bone chips, and allograft bone chips. Traditionally, spinal fusion has been accomplished with bone graft harvested from the iliac crest; however, in recent years, this technique has been used less frequently because of the problem of prolonged pain (donor-site morbidity) associated with bone graft harvest from the iliac crest.

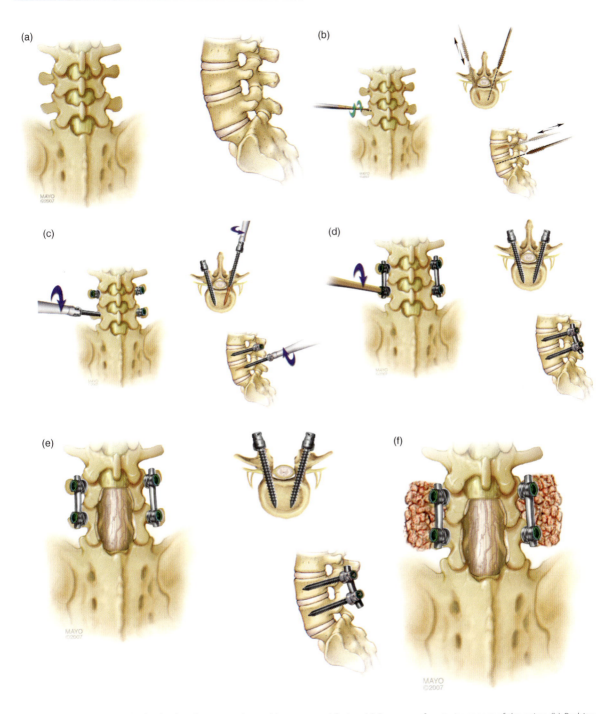

Figure 11.10. Steps involved in lumbar decompression and instrumented fusion. (a) Exposure of posterior aspect of the spine. (b) Probing and tapping of pedicles. (c) Pedicle screw placement. (d) Tightening of set screws to lock rods into position. (e) Laminectomy. (f) Posterolateral fusion. Care is taken to keep all graft material lateral to the rod and away from the exposed dura. Figure reproduced with permission from Mayo Foundation for Medical Education and Research.

Illustration of lumbar decompression and posterolateral fusion with pedicle screw fixation

The steps involved in lumbar laminectomy and instrumented posterolateral intertransverse process fusion are outlined in Figure 11.10. The illustration shows the procedure being done through a midline incision. An alternative approach is to perform the operation through bilateral paramedian incisions.

213

The laminectomy may be performed before or after placement of instrumentation. If the laminectomy is performed first, there is some risk of dropping instruments or implants on the exposed dura as the instrumentation is performed. Performing the laminectomy after placement of instrumentation, as shown, obviates this risk. At the same time, there are some situations in which the laminectomy needs to be performed first, in order to permit visualization of anatomic landmarks necessary to identify the pedicles and safely place the instrumentation.

Lumbar synovial cyst

Cysts may arise from the synovial lining of the lumbar facet joints. These are considered to be degenerative in nature and a part of the spectrum of age-related spondylotic changes that occur in the spinal column. Cysts which project posteriorly into the paraspinal soft tissues are generally not symptomatic, while cysts projecting into the spinal canal or neural foramen often produce radicular pain. Neurologic symptoms usually have a gradual onset and progression. Occasionally hemorrhage into the cyst occurs, producing abrupt, extremely intense pain.

Figure 11.11 depicts the MRI of a typical lumbar synovial cyst. Note the continuity of the cyst with the joint itself. These cysts may become quite large and obstruct the spinal canal. Figure 11.12 depicts the MRI of a very large synovial cyst, initially thought to represent an intradural tumor.

Surgical excision is the recommended treatment. Surgical outcomes are excellent, and the risk of recurrence is less than 5%.

Percutaneous cyst aspiration may be appropriate in elderly patients who are unable to tolerate surgery; however the risk of cyst recurrence is high, and repeated aspirations may be required.

Spondylolisthesis

Spondylolisthesis refers to subluxation or displacement of one vertebral body relative to the level below. The usual situation is anterior displacement of the vertebral body (anterolisthesis). Posterior displacement of the vertebral body (retrolisthesis) and lateral displacement (lateral listhesis) may also occur.

Spondylolisthesis is caused by a combination of hereditary factors, degenerative phenomena, and biomechanical stresses related to the erect posture of humans. Spondylolisthesis has never been observed

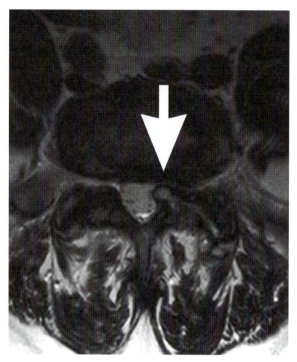

Figure 11.11. Axial T_2-weighted lumbar spine MRI depicting a synovial cyst at L4–L5, left (arrow). Note continuity between the cyst and the facet joint.

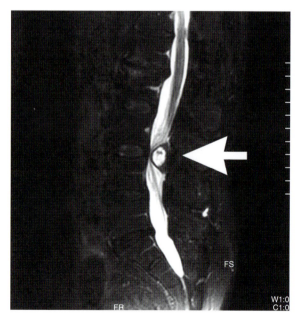

Figure 11.12. Sagittal T_2-weighted lumbar spine MRI with fat saturation, depicting a very large synovial cyst at L3–L4, initially felt to be an intradural tumor.

Table 11.2. Grading of spondylolisthesis

Grade	Degree of subluxation (%)
I	<25
II	25–50
III	50–75
IV	75–100
V	>100

in quadrupeds, nor has it been seen in humans who are chronically bedridden.

Spondylolisthesis is graded from I to V, as shown in Table 11.2. Grade V spondylolisthesis denotes complete subluxation of the vertebral body, a condition sometimes referred to as spondyloptosis. There are six basic categories of spondylolisthesis, including dysplastic, isthmic, degenerative, traumatic, pathologic, and iatrogenic forms.

Dysplastic spondylolisthesis usually occurs at L5–S1, and is caused by congenital deficiencies of the upper sacrum and arch of L5. The pars interarticularis may or may not be intact. If intact, it is poorly developed and may be elongated. These findings permit progressive anterior displacement of L5 on the sacrum. Subluxation occurs early in life and is often severe.

Isthmic spondylolisthesis is also most common at L5–S1, and is the result of a defect in the pars interarticularis (spondylolysis). This is a fairly common disorder, with an incidence of 5%–7% in the USA. Patients are born with a weak, but intact, pars interarticularis, which acutely fractures or attenuates over time with weight-bearing and stress. These patients often report a strong family history of spondylolisthesis. Female gymnasts have an incidence of isthmic spondylolisthesis four times greater than that of individuals not participating in gymnastics. The initial diagnosis is usually made in children over the age of 5, teenagers, and young adults; however, it is not unusual for the condition to remain clinically silent until patients reach middle age or advanced age. Younger patients often have high-grade slips (grade III–V), while older patients are more likely to have low-grade slips (grade I–II).

Degenerative spondylolisthesis, most commonly seen at L4–L5, is part of the cascade of degenerative lumbar spondylosis. The slippage is caused by excessive segmental mobility related to degeneration of the intervertebral disk and facet joints. The pars interarticularis remains intact, in contrast to isthmic spondylolisthesis. Most patients with degenerative spondylolisthesis have low-grade slips, most commonly grade I, and rarely higher than grade II.

Traumatic spondylolisthesis is associated with an injury which disrupts the intervertebral disk and facet joints. It may not be detected until weeks following the traumatic event, distinguishing it from an acute fracture-dislocation.

Pathologic spondylolisthesis is seen when neoplasm invades the pars, pedicle, and facet complex, destabilizing the spine and allowing for vertebral displacement.

Iatrogenic or post-surgical spondylolisthesis occurs following surgical procedures that resect or disrupt the intervertebral disk, facet complex, pars interarticularis, and/or ligamentous structures.

Clinical findings

The most common symptom is back pain. Neurologic symptoms and signs are variable. Children with dysplastic spondylolisthesis may have severe leg pain and weakness, plus incontinence of bladder and bowel due to cauda equina compression.

Isthmic spondylolisthesis at L5–S1 characteristically produces unilateral or bilateral L5 radiculopathy due to L5 nerve root compression from the associated foraminal stenosis.

Patients with degenerative spondylolisthesis initially have just intermittent back pain, without neurologic symptoms. Later in their clinical course, patients often report escalating back pain and may also develop neurogenic claudication if they have concomitant spinal canal stenosis. The neurologic examination is usually normal, even in the face of severe spinal canal stenosis. Mild distal lower extremity weakness is not uncommon; however, severe weakness and cauda equina syndrome are rare.

Patients with higher grade slips (grade III–V) often have lumbosacral kyphosis and sagittal plane imbalance. In order to compensate for this deformity and maintain an upright posture, the hamstrings tighten to rotate the pelvis into a more vertical position. If this is not sufficient, the patient must flex the hips and knees in order to stand upright.

Hamstring tightness is characteristic of symptomatic spondylolisthesis; this limits straight leg raising and forward flexion of the trunk. Originally thought to be the result of cauda equina compression, hamstring tightness is seen with all grades of spondylolisthesis and is generally not associated with neurologic deficits. It is now thought that hamstring tightness is a manifestation of the body's effort to rotate the pelvis into a more vertical position to restore sagittal plane balance.

Advanced spondylolisthesis produces foreshortening of the trunk, which has characteristic physical examination findings of absence of the waistline, flank creases, and abdominal protuberance. In severe cases, the rib cage abuts the iliac crest, further adding to the patient's discomfort.

Gait abnormalities are frequently seen. The typical spondylolisthetic gait is a wide-based waddle, with limited hip flexion, and shortened stride length.

Imaging

Radiographic evaluation of spondylolisthesis should begin with a full series of plain radiographs, including oblique and lateral flexion-extension views. Oblique radiographs provide the best view of the pars interarticularis and are often the best study for detecting spondylolysis. Flexion-extension views are important for assessing dynamic instability. Standing 92-cm or 36-in anteroposterior and lateral radiographs should be obtained for evaluation of coronal and sagittal plane deformities.

Advanced imaging with MRI or CT/myelography should be obtained in any patient with neurologic involvement, to look for stenosis of the central canal or neural foramina and abnormalities of the conus, cauda equina, and spinal nerve roots.

Radionuclide bone scanning may be helpful in patients with spondylolysis, to assess the age of the pars fracture. An acute fracture shows uptake, while a chronic fracture does not.

Treatment

Patients with mild symptoms and low grade slips can be managed conservatively. Patients with more severe symptoms and higher grade slips often require surgical intervention. The goals of surgery are neural decompression, deformity correction, and stabilization. The surgical approach must be tailored to the abnormal anatomy encountered in each case.

Decompressive procedures include laminectomy for central stenosis and foraminotomy for foraminal stenosis. In some cases, reduction of the spondylolisthesis provides additional decompression of neural elements.

Fusion is performed to stabilize the listhetic segment and prevent further slippage. In patients with high grade slips, correction of the slip and restoration of sagittal balance are often needed; however,

complete correction of the slip is not necessary and in some cases may cause further neurologic injury. For example, overly aggressive correction of a high grade L5–S1 slip may result in injury to the L5 nerve root. Deformity correction is easier in younger patients with more mobile spines, and is more difficult in older patients, who tend to have more degenerative changes and fixed deformities.

In selected patients with isthmic spondylolisthesis, repair of the pars interarticularis fracture with screw fixation has been performed with good relief of back pain.

SPORT study, Part II (degenerative spondylolisthesis)

Part II of the SPORT study, published in 2007, compared the effectiveness of surgery and nonoperative treatment for degenerative spondylolisthesis.

The study included a randomized cohort, in which patients were randomized to receive either surgery or nonoperative management, and an observational cohort, for patients who declined randomization.

The protocol surgery consisted of a standard decompressive laminectomy with or without fusion (iliac crest bone grafting with or without pedicle screw instrumentation). Decompression alone was used in 6% of cases, decompression plus fusion without instrumentation in 21%, and decompression plus fusion with instrumentation in 73%.

The nonsurgical protocol was usual care, recommended to include at least physical therapy, instruction in home exercises, and nonsteroidal anti-inflammatory medications if tolerated.

Patients were followed for two years, and outcomes were assessed using established outcomes measures, including the SF-36, Oswestry Disability Index, and stenosis bothersomeness index.

Similar to the SPORT study of lumbar disk herniation, critical analysis of the SPORT study of degenerative spondylolisthesis was limited by poor adherence to the assigned treatment. In the randomized cohort, 36% of patients in the surgical arm never had an operation, and 49% of patients in the nonoperative treatment arm crossed over to have surgery. Because of this high crossover rate, the intent-to-treat analysis showed no difference in outcome between the two groups. However, using an as-treated analysis, which reflects the treatment actually received, there was a significant advantage for surgery at all time intervals.

This report showed that patients with degenerative spondylolisthesis and spinal stenosis treated surgically, in most cases with decompression plus fusion, experienced substantially greater improvement than patients treated nonsurgically.

Discogenic back pain

The benefit of surgery for patients with the discogenic and degenerative processes just described is well established, provided the predominant symptom is radicular pain due to nerve root compression. If the primary complaint is back pain, surgery is less likely to be successful.

The main reason for this is that it can be difficult to pinpoint the source of the patient's discomfort. Imaging studies can precisely identify disk degeneration, annular fissures, facet arthritis, and other degenerative changes; however these are age-related phenomena, commonly seen in individuals without back symptoms. Thus, when imaging studies show only common degenerative changes, it is difficult to know whether these findings are the cause of the patient's back pain. MRI may be supplemented with provocative discography; however, this modality has a high rate of false positives, and results must be interpreted cautiously (see Chapter 8).

Furthermore, many studies have shown that patients with chronic low back pain are more likely to have abnormal psychological profiles, chronic pain behavior, and disability/compensation issues, all of which will limit the chance of obtaining a good surgical result.

Accepting these caveats, surgery may be an option for psychologically healthy patients with severe discogenic back pain unresponsive to conservative treatment, and confirmed with discography.

There are two goals of surgery for discogenic pain: first, to remove the pain generator consisting of the disk and posterior annulus; and, second, to perform an arthrodesis to stabilize the spine and prevent painful micromotion at the symptomatic level.

Over the years, a variety of surgical procedures have been used, including anterior, posterior, and combined approaches. The operation has traditionally been done through open techniques, although recently a host of minimally invasive approaches have been developed for this purpose.

Some form of bone grafting is used in all cases. Options include autograft harvested from the iliac crest or posterior spinal elements, allograft, and bone morphogenetic proteins (BMP). Grafts may be placed anteriorly within the interspace, posteriorly within the facet joints, and/or laterally around the transverse processes.

In some cases, instrumentation is used to enhance stability. A multitude of devices have been developed for this purpose, including pedicle screw fixation, facet joint fixation, interbody devices, and anterior plates.

When the operation is done posteriorly, one common strategy is posterolateral intertransverse process bone grafting with pedicle screw fixation. The posterior fusion may be supplemented with a posterior lumbar interbody fusion (PLIF), which consists of an interbody cage made of carbon fiber, polyether-ether-ketone (PEEK), or metal, with additional bone graft placed within and around the cage. The advantage of the PLIF procedure is that it provides additional structural support to the anterior lumbar spine. The drawbacks include the expense of the device, additional procedure time and blood loss, risk of damage to the exiting nerve root or cauda equina during device insertion, and risk of migration or subsidence of the device before fusion takes place. A PLIF is sometimes not feasible with an extremely narrowed and degenerated interspace. Scarring from previous surgery may preclude the safe placement of an interbody device. There are no definite guidelines on when to add a PLIF to a posterior lumbar fusion. The decision is based on surgeon preference and specific clinical and anatomic factors in each case.

Anterior lumbar interbody fusion (ALIF) is an alternative method of performing an interbody fusion. It is similar to the PLIF procedure in that the intervertebral disk is removed and replaced with bone graft and some form of cage device. ALIF differs from PLIF in the route of access to the spine. When performing an ALIF, the surgeon approaches the spine anteriorly through the abdomen, while the PLIF involves a posterior approach as described above.

The ALIF has the advantage of allowing for a more complete disk removal and placement of interbody devices and bone grafts with a larger footprint on the adjacent vertebrae. The surgeon is also better able to place bone grafts in compression, which increases the likelihood of a successful fusion. Another benefit of ALIF surgery is that the posterior paraspinous musculature is undisturbed and there is less dissection around the dura and exiting nerve roots.

The major risk of ALIF is great vessel injury. The approach involves exposure and retraction of the aorta, vena cava, and iliac arteries and veins. Injury to these vessels can result in catastrophic hemorrhage. The risk of this complication ranges from 1% to 15%, and can occur even when the procedure is performed by experienced surgeons. The risk of vascular injury is much greater in revision surgery as a result of scar tissue and adhesions around the vessels.

For males, another risk that is unique to the anterior approach to the lumbar spine is sexual dysfunction, most commonly retrograde ejaculation. This complication is thought to be the result of damage to very fine nerves in the presacral space. Sexual dysfunction tends to improve over time, but is permanent in about 1% of cases.

A third option for lumbar fusion is a circumferential fusion, which incorporates both ALIF and posterior fusion.

Regardless of the surgical technique used, outcomes of fusion for discogenic back pain have been somewhat disappointing. Randomized trials of lumbar fusion compared with nonoperative management have shown only modest improvement with surgery and no clear benefit over nonoperative treatment.

It is crucial for the clinician and the patient not to expect miraculous results with surgery for discogenic back pain. Under the best of circumstances, with expert surgeons operating on carefully selected patients, the expected improvement on the visual analog scale (VAS) pain scale is 3–4 points, with many patients still requiring narcotic pain medications following the procedure.

When patients fail to improve, this has often been attributed to poor patient selection or to procedure-related trauma. However, recent investigation has suggested that treatment failure may actually result from the failure of diagnostic testing, usually discography, to adequately define the source of the patient's pain.

More recently, lumbar disk arthroplasty has been promoted as a treatment alternative for discogenic back pain; however, this procedure met with limited success as well (see Chapter 13).

Trauma

Fractures may occur at any level of the lumbar spine, most frequently at the thoracolumbar junction. Assessment of fracture stability is often based on the three-column model of the spine. The anterior column includes the anterior longitudinal ligament plus the anterior half of the vertebral body and intervertebral disk. The middle column includes the posterior half of the vertebral body and intervertebral disk and the posterior longitudinal ligament. The posterior column includes the posterior bony arch and ligamentous structures, plus the facet joints.

Although it is impossible to make definite guidelines, this model has proven useful in evaluating fracture stability and guiding treatment. For example, a minimal compression fracture with an intact posterior column without neurologic compromise would be considered to be a stable injury, which could be managed conservatively with bracing, analgesics, and progressive ambulation. In contrast, a two- or three-column injury would most likely be considered unstable and surgical reconstruction would have to be considered.

Recent work has shown that CT and MRI can provide useful information regarding injury stability, beyond that provided by the three-column injury model. In addition to demonstrating fractures, neural compression, and deformities, CT and MRI can also help define the integrity of the posterior ligamentous complex. This information is particularly important in assessing stability of injuries at the thoracolumbar junction.

Diastasis of the facet joints on CT and posterior edema (high signal intensity) in the region of the posterior ligamentous complex on T_2 STIR (short TI inversion recovery) or fat saturation sagittal MRI appear to be useful predictors of instability. T_1-weighted sagittal MRI can also depict clinically important damage of the posterior ligamentous complex.

These findings suggest an expanding role for CT and MRI in the evaluation of thoracolumbar injuries.

Regardless of the type of injury being treated, if nonoperative treatment is selected, there is some risk that a significant kyphotic deformity will develop over time. If this occurs, major reconstructive surgery may be needed to correct the deformity. These patients should therefore be followed with serial radiographs to assess for late instability and progressive deformity.

An example of an unstable three-column injury is shown in Figures 11.13a–c, which demonstrate severe burst fractures at L2 and L4. Note the presence of severe spinal canal compromise at L2 and to a lesser extent at L4, due to retropulsion of bone fragments. The patient underwent circumferential reconstruction with an expandable cage anteriorly and pedicle screw fixation posteriorly. The post-operative plain radiographs are shown in Figures 11.13d and 11.13e.

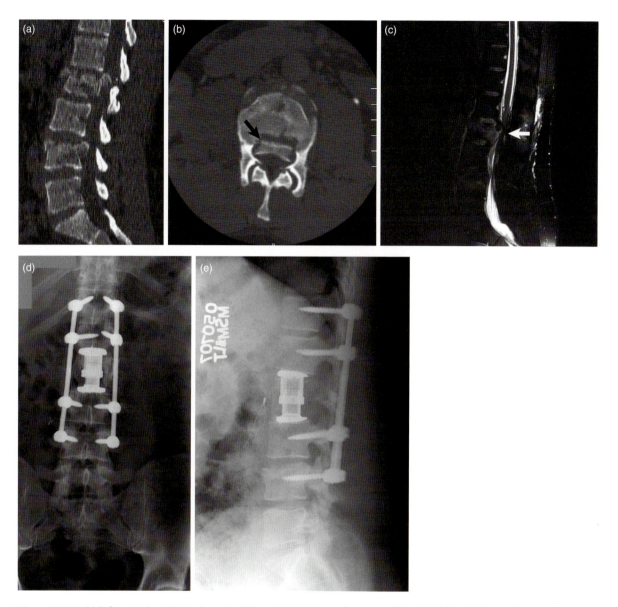

Figure 11.13. (a) Reformatted sagittal lumbar spine CT scan depicting burst fractures at L2 and L4. (b) Axial CT image depicting bony retropulsion with severe spinal canal compromise at L2 (arrow). (c) Sagittal T_2-weighted MRI further delineating the extent of the burst fracture and spinal canal compromise at L2 (arrow). (d) Anteroposterior and (e) lateral radiographs depicting circumferential reconstruction with anterior expandable cage and posterior pedicle screw fixation.

Osteoporotic vertebral compression fracture

Osteoporotic compression fractures may occur in either the thoracic or lumbar region, typically at the thoracolumbar junction. The approach to diagnosis is similar to that taken to treatment regardless of the level of the fracture, and is discussed in Chapter 10.

Sacral insufficiency fracture

Sacral insufficiency fracture is a relatively common, but sometimes unrecognized, cause of low back pain in the elderly. Osteoporosis is the leading cause, and older women are at particular risk. Other risk factors include chronic steroid use, inflammatory arthritis, radiation exposure, and previous lumbar fusion surgery. These fractures may be precipitated by minimal trauma.

Sacral insufficiency fractures are often not visualized on plain film radiography. It should also be emphasized that a standard lumbar MRI does not provide adequate imaging of the sacrum and will often miss a

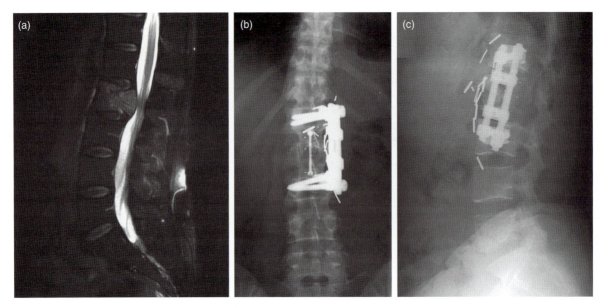

Figure 11.14. (a) Sagittal T$_2$-weighted lumbar spine MRI depicting a metastatic tumor in the L2 vertebral body with compromise of the spinal canal. (b) Anteroposterior and (c) lateral post-operative radiographs depicting anterior reconstruction with carbon fiber cage and Kaneda instrumentation.

sacral fracture. The clinician should consider the possibility of sacral insufficiency fracture in the at-risk patient with acute severe lumbosacral pain, who has a negative or unremarkable lumbar MRI. In these cases, a dedicated MRI study of the sacrum and pelvis should be obtained. CT and radionuclide bone scanning may also be useful in establishing the diagnosis. The characteristic fracture location is in the sacral ala, parallel to the sacroiliac joint. The bone scan reveals an H-shaped pattern of increased uptake.

Similar to osteoporotic fractures of the thoracic and lumbar spine, management of sacral insufficiency fractures has traditionally included periods of bed rest and narcotic analgesics. These measures often fail to provide adequate pain relief, and may lead to complications associated with prolonged bed rest in the elderly, including deep venous thrombosis, pulmonary embolus, pneumonia, and deconditioning, among others.

As vertebral augmentation with methylmethacrylate has proven to be an excellent treatment for osteoporotic vertebral body fractures, this treatment is now being extended to insufficiency fractures in the sacrum. The rationale for this approach is the concept that sacral insufficiency fractures result from transmission of weight-bearing, or axial loading, into the sacrum. Application of methylmethacrylate across the fracture provides mechanical stabilization and prevents painful micromotion.

Although there are some technical differences as compared with standard kyphoplasty or vertebroplasty, several studies have shown sacral augmentation with methylmethacrylate, or "sacroplasty," to be a safe and effective treatment for painful sacral insufficiency fractures.

Metastatic disease

Metastatic tumors may occur at any level of the spinal column, including the lumbar region. Figure 11.14a depicts the sagittal MRI of a woman with a solitary metastasis at L2 with spinal canal compromise, treated with anterior decompression and fusion with instrumentation. Post-operative radiographs are shown in Figures 11.14b and 11.14c. Diagnosis and treatment of spinal metastatic disease are discussed in more detail in Chapter 10.

Intradural tumor

The most common intradural tumors in the lumbar region are schwannoma, ependymoma, and meningioma. The typical clinical course is one of gradual onset and progression of symptoms, with varying degrees of back and radicular pain. Surgical excision is the recommended treatment for all symptomatic lesions. Figure 11.15a depicts sagittal T$_1$-weighted MRI with contrast enhancement, showing a small intradural tumor at L3. The tumor was removed and proved to be an ependymoma. Figure 11.15b depicts

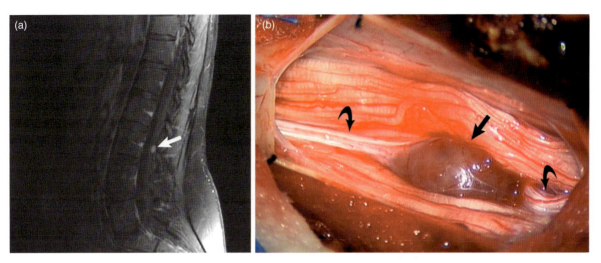

Figure 11.15. (a) Sagittal T_1-weighted lumbar spine MRI with contrast enhancement depicting an enhancing intradural tumor at L3. (b) Intra-operative photograph depicting the tumor (single straight arrow) arising from a thickened filum terminale (curved arrows). For orientation, the patient's head is to the right and feet are to the left.

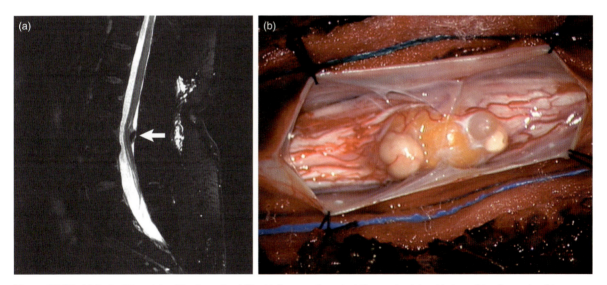

Figure 11.16. (a) Sagittal T_2-weighted lumbar spine MRI with fat saturation, depicting a mixed-signal lesion arising from a low lying conus medullaris at the L3 level (arrow). (b) Intra-operative photomicrograph of the lesion prior to excision. Pathology confirmed a teratoma. For orientation, the patient's head is to the right and feet are to the left.

an intra-operative photograph of the tumor arising from a thickened filum terminale, which is distinguished from the adjacent spinal nerve roots by its silvery, gray appearance.

Tumors of the conus medullaris may also occur. The most common tumors occurring at this location include astrocytoma, ependymoma, and lipoma. The lumbar MRI in Figure 11.16a depicts a mixed signal mass lesion arising from a low lying conus medullaris. An intra-operative photomicrograph in

Figure 11.16b shows the appearance of the lesion, which proved to be a teratoma. Complete resection was achieved.

Lumbar intradural tumors are occasionally discovered as incidental findings in patients undergoing either imaging for an unrelated problem or a "screening" CT scan. In these cases, a period of observation with serial imaging studies may be appropriate, although these lesions will usually become symptomatic over time.

Tethered cord syndrome

Tethered cord syndrome usually presents in children, but can also occur in adults of all ages. Presenting symptoms include back and radicular pain, progressive lower extremity weakness, gait impairment, bladder dysfunction, and progressive spinal deformity. Examination of the low back may reveal hypertrichosis, subcutaneous lipomas, and other cutaneous abnormalities.

Children are less likely to have significant pain at the time of diagnosis, but are more likely to have spinal deformity and cutaneous stigmata of dysraphism. Adults are more likely to present with significant pain, but less likely to have spinal deformity and cutaneous stigmata. Urological symptoms are prominent in both age groups. In children, symptoms may be aggravated by growth spurts.

Characteristic MRI findings include a low lying conus medullaris below the L2 level and a thickened filum terminale (>2 mm diameter). In some cases, the conus may be tethered by a lipoma, which can be purely intradural or combined intra- and extra-dural. MRI may also reveal other congenital abnormalities, such as diastematomyelia.

Any patient being considered for surgery should have a careful evaluation of bladder function, including formal urodynamic studies.

If the cord is tethered only by a thickened filum terminale, the patient can generally be managed by a limited lumbosacral laminectomy and division of the thickened filum. Differentiating the filum from the surrounding nerve roots of the cauda equina is aided by the observation that the filum is a midline structure, light silver in color, often with a characteristic squiggly vessel on its surface. By comparison, the nerve roots are slighter darker and more cream-colored, and located more peripherally in the spinal canal. A consistent observation during surgery is the retraction of the conus, often by a centimeter or more, after the filum is divided. This indicates the tension on the conus and upper cauda equina as a result of the tethering process.

If a lipoma is found, it may be resected if it can be dissected easily from the adjacent neural structures. However, in many cases, the lipoma is intimately involved with the conus and/or cauda equina. In these situations, complete resection of the lipoma may not be possible, as the procedure would cause an unacceptable degree of neurologic morbidity.

It is difficult to assess the benefits of surgery for tethered cord syndrome, as this is a heterogenous disorder, presenting in all age groups. Furthermore, there have been no controlled studies comparing surgery with observation. Based on available information, pain relief can usually be achieved. Milder motor deficits, urinary symptoms, and spinal deformities may improve. More severe deficits are unlikely to recover, however symptom progression can usually be arrested. Pediatric cases, especially those untethered in early childhood, are at risk for retethering. Even with its risks and limitations, surgery appears to provide a better outcome than the natural history for patients with symptomatic tethered cord.

The management of the child with asymptomatic tethered cord, discovered as an incidental finding, is more controversial. Because of the likelihood of future neurologic deterioration, especially in the younger child, prophylactic untethering is often recommended.

Spinal infection

The term spinal infection encompasses a spectrum of specific entities, including intervertebral discitis, osteomyelitis of the vertebral bodies, epidural abscess, infection of the paravertebral structures (e.g., psoas abscess), or some combination of these. Spinal infections may be pyogenic, tuberculous, or fungal.

Historically, spinal infection has historically been fairly uncommon, but is now being seen with increasing frequency. Recent spinal surgery is a known risk factor, but spinal infection frequently occurs in patients who have never had spinal surgery. Other risk factors include spinal injections, dental work, and infections elsewhere in the body, such as bacterial endocarditis. Patients with diabetes, human immunodeficiency virus (HIV) disease, chronic steroid therapy, and other causes of immunosuppression are also at increased risk.

Clinically, the patient harboring a spinal infection presents with severe localized back pain. The combination of fever and back pain strongly suggests the diagnosis of spinal infection; however, most patients harboring spinal infections are afebrile. Thus, the presence of a fever can help confirm the presence of spinal infection, but the absence of fever in no way excludes this diagnosis.

There is a spectrum of neurologic findings. The patient may be completely intact neurologically if there is no spinal canal compromise from the infection. Alternatively, the patient may have varying degrees of neurologic compromise, up to complete paraplegia, depending on the degree of epidural compression.

Magnetic resonance imaging is the imaging procedure of choice. The classic MRI findings include destructive changes in the interspace, with signal change in the adjacent vertebral bodies, sometimes associated with inflammatory changes in the epidural space. There is often a rind of enhancing tissue around the disk, extending into the psoas muscle on either side. Dural enhancement usually just represents a secondary inflammatory response, but is often overdiagnosed as representing an epidural abscess. A localized collection of pus which would be amenable to drainage, like a soft tissue abscess, is usually not seen. Thus, the MRI diagnosis of epidural abscess must be interpreted cautiously and in the context of the clinical findings. An infection usually begins in the disk space and spreads to the adjacent vertebral bodies. In contrast, a tumor usually begins in the vertebral body and is, at least initially, confined by the disk above and below.

White blood cell count (WBC), erythrocyte sedimentation rate (ESR), and C-reactive protein (CRP) should be obtained. The WBC is often normal, however the ESR and CRP are almost invariably elevated, and can be very helpful in confirming the diagnosis and in monitoring the response to antibiotic therapy. Blood cultures should be obtained at baseline and are often positive in these cases.

Fluoroscopic or CT-guided biopsy of the interspace should be carried out. The most common pathogen is staphylococcus (coagulase positive or negative); however, a wide range of pathogens, including Gram-negative and anaerobic organisms, and fungi may be seen. If the cultures are negative, options include repeating the CT-guided biopsy, open biopsy, or empiric treatment for so-called culture-negative discitis, usually with a course of anti-staphylococcal therapy.

Once a microbiologic diagnosis is established, appropriate intravenous antibiotic therapy is administered, usually over a 4- to 6-week time course. In selected cases, an additional course of oral suppressive therapy may be used. Bracing with a lightweight lumbar corset is recommended for symptomatic relief.

Spinal infections can usually be managed non-operatively; however, there are some situations where surgical management is needed. These include debridement of draining wounds, open biopsy to establish a microbiologic diagnosis (when CT-guided needle biopsies are negative), early decompressive

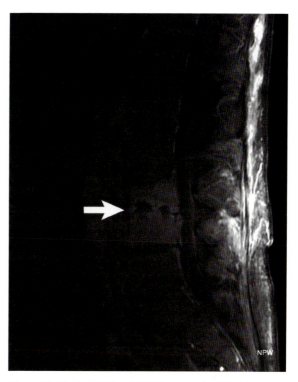

Figure 11.17. Sagittal T_1-weighted lumbar spine MRI with contrast enhancement, depicting destructive changes at the L3–L4 interspace consistent with discitis/osteomyelitis.

surgery for patients who present with acute neurologic deficits, and late reconstructive surgery for patients who develop instability or deformity as a consequence of the infection.

Figure 11.17 depicts the typical MRI findings of osteomyelitis/discitis. Cultures of the interspace grew coagulase-negative staphylococci, and the patient was managed with 6 weeks of intravenous vancomycin and bracing.

Ankylosing spondylitis

Ankylosing spondylitis is an inflammatory arthropathy, which can severely affect the spine and sacroiliac joints. Males are affected more often than females. Epidemiologic studies have shown an association between the HLA-B27 antigen and ankylosing spondylitis. This condition results in gradual fusion of the entire spinal column, giving a radiographic appearance described as a "bamboo spine." The diagnosis is based on clinical and radiological criteria. There is no serum marker to confirm the diagnosis.

Patients present with progressive rigidity and kyphosis. Chest expansion is limited. It is often possible to establish the diagnosis with plain film

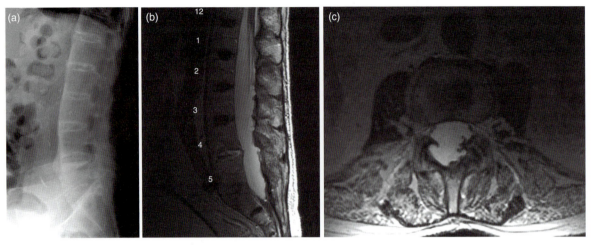

Figure 11.18. (a) Lateral radiograph of a man with ankylosing spondylitis, depicting extensive ankylosis of the entire spine and sacroiliac joints. (b) Sagittal and (c) axial T$_2$-weighted MRI, depicting severe arachnoiditis with nerve root clumping and thecal diverticula.

radiography alone. MRI may be useful in patients with neurologic findings, as some patients with this diagnosis develop arachnoiditis.

Figure 11.18a depicts the lumbar spine radiographs of a man with ankylosing spondylitis. Note the extensive ankylosis of the vertebral bodies and sacroiliac joints. Figures 11.18b and 11.18c depict the lumbar MRI of the same patient. Note the coalescence of spinal nerve roots along the lateral thecal sac margins and multiple thecal diverticula eroding the spinal lamina. These findings are hallmarks of ankylosing spondylitis.

Treatment consists of nonsteroidal anti-inflammatory medications, exercise, and avoidance of smoking.

Because of increased rigidity of the spine, these patients are at increased risk for fractures, which can be sustained after minimal trauma. More prevalent in the sixth to eighth decades of life, fractures in ankylosing spondylitis are frequently associated with a high degree of instability and neurologic deficits. Surgery is often required. Management of such patients is difficult in all respects, and high rates of morbidity and mortality are seen regardless of the treatment methods used.

Failed back syndrome

The term "failed back syndrome" refers to patients who experience persistent or new symptoms following lumbar surgery. A fairly extensive differential diagnosis must be considered and treatment must be individualized. This important issue is discussed in detail in Chapter 7.

Clinical issues
Lumbar and lumbosacral orthoses

Several orthotic devices are commonly used for immobilization of the lumbar spine after surgery or trauma. These include lightweight corsets and rigid, bi-valved thoracolumbosacral or lumbosacral orthoses.

When a fusion is extended to the sacrum, a hip spica extension may be included to enhance spinal immobilization by restricting motion of the hip joint. Patients find this very bothersome, as it significantly limits normal physical activities and activities of daily living. Patient compliance is often poor with any brace that incorporates a hip spica extension.

Few studies have addressed the role of postoperative bracing, and interpretation of the available data is further compromised by the fact that most studies have failed to control for the surgical approach (anterior or posterior) or use of instrumentation. No study has yet shown that bracing improves clinical outcomes or increases the fusion rate. Despite the lack of clear evidence that bracing improves outcomes, many surgeons use some form of bracing after fusion procedures to help with pain control and to remind patients of their activity restrictions.

Bone growth stimulators for spinal fusion

Spinal fusion surgery involves placement of bone grafts, which grow together and fuse to the spine over time. One of the risks of spinal fusion surgery is resorption of the bone grafts and failure of the fusion.

This condition has been variously described as a pseudarthrosis, failed fusion, nonfusion, or non-union. Risk factors for a failed fusion include previous failed fusion, multi-level fusion, smoking, high grade spondylolisthesis, osteoporosis, vascular disease, obesity, diabetes, renal disease, alcohol abuse, and medications that deplete calcium.

In patients with any of these risk factors, bone growth stimulation may be considered. Application of electrical stimulation has been shown to enhance the process of bone healing in difficult fractures of the extremities and spinal column, and has also been shown to enhance the healing of a spinal fusion. There are two general types of bone growth stimulators used in the spine: internal devices, which are surgically implanted, and external devices, which are worn externally.

Internal devices are implanted at the time of the fusion procedure and deliver an electrical current directly to the area where bone growth is to occur. These devices are considered very safe, but would be contraindicated in pregnant women and in patients with pacemakers and defibrillators. Patients implanted with these devices have no particular activity restrictions, and cannot feel any electrical stimulation or other sensation from the device. The stimulator can be removed at the end of its useful life, usually 6–12 months after implantation, depending on the preference of the surgeon and patient. Removal of the battery is straightforward and can be performed on an outpatient basis. The wire leads are usually left embedded in the fusion mass. Explantation is not mandatory, as there is no harm in leaving the device in place after treatment is completed.

As the name implies, external bone growth stimulators are completely external to the body, and, therefore, can be implemented without a surgical procedure. Stimulation is delivered through electrodes or coils placed on the skin over the fusion site. Coils may also be placed in a corset at the surgical site. Stimulation is carried out for varying time periods, ranging from 30 minutes to several hours per day, depending on the device. The treatment regimen typically lasts from 3 to 9 months.

These devices are considered very safe, but would have the same contraindications as internal stimulators: pregnancy and cardiac pacemakers and defibrillators. As with implanted devices, patients wearing external bone growth stimulators do not feel any electrical shocks or vibrations.

A significant advantage of the external stimulator is that the device can be employed without a surgical procedure for implantation or explantation. Another advantage is that an external system can be added later in the post-operative period, if there is a concern that the fusion mass is not maturing properly.

Effectiveness of the external stimulator will be compromised in situations where the patient is unable or unwilling to wear the device for the required amount of time each day. If it is anticipated that patient compliance may be a significant issue, an internal bone growth stimulator may be preferable.

Bone morphogenetic proteins

Historically, most spinal fusions have been performed with iliac crest autograft. This bone is harvested from the patient's iliac crest, in large slabs or in chips, and then transplanted to the recipient bed. Iliac crest autograft has proven to be an excellent substrate for spinal fusion, as it has the three fundamental factors that any graft material must possess in order to encourage new bone growth and the maturation of a spinal fusion: osteogenicity, osteoconductivity, and osteoinductivity.

Although iliac crest autograft has been used extensively and has many advantages, it has significant drawbacks as well. The bone harvesting procedure prolongs the operation, increases blood loss, slows post-operative recovery, and often results in significant and prolonged post-operative pain. There is a limited quantity of bone available for harvesting. This can be problematic in situations where a high volume of graft material is required and in patients in whom the iliac crest has already been harvested for previous spine or orthopedic procedures. In addition, this bone grafting technique does not always result in a successful fusion.

These factors have led to efforts to produce alternative materials to promote and enhance the spinal fusion process. One of the most promising strategies has been the use of bone morphogenetic proteins (BMP), a family of growth factors and cytokines, which have been shown to have significant osteoinductive capability. Seminal work on BMP dates back to the 1960s, when it was discovered that osteoinductive proteins that promote bone growth and healing are contained within the bone substance itself. As of 2007, approximately sixteen separate BMPs have been identified and genetically reproduced. BMPs have a wide range of functions. Some play a role in the

225

development of the central nervous system, heart, kidneys, and reproductive organs; however, most are involved with bone and cartilage development.

BMP-2 and BMP-7 are FDA-approved for human applications, with BMP-2 being more widely used in the USA. The specific FDA approval for BMP-2 requires the product to be used in tapered cages, implanted via an anterior open or anterior laparoscopic approach, in skeletally mature patients with single-level degenerative disk disease at either L4–L5 or L5–S1. Grade I spondylolisthesis is an approved indication, while patients with grade II or higher spondylolisthesis are excluded. BMP-2 is contraindicated in patients with known hypersensitivity to BMP-2 or bovine type I collagen, tumor, or infection, and in skeletally immature patients. Pregnancy is also a contraindication, as the potential effects of BMP on the human fetus have not been evaluated.

Building on the initial FDA approval for anterior lumbar fusion with cages, use of BMP-2 has been extended to other anterior lumbar fusion procedures, such as fusion with femoral allograft ring, and also to posterior lumbar fusion procedures, including posterior lumbar interbody fusion, posterolateral intertransverse process fusion, and facet fusion. BMP-2 has also been used in selected cervical fusion procedures. These additional uses are considered off-label. BMP-2 should be used with particular caution with procedures on the anterior cervical spine, as local swelling and swallowing difficulties have been reported with BMP usage in this location.

BMP-2 is supplied in lyophilized form. At the time of surgery, it is reconstituted with sterile water, to achieve a concentration of 1.5 mg/ml. This solution is placed on an absorbable bovine collagen sponge, which serves as a carrier. The collagen sponge is cut to the appropriate size and placed in the desired location. When BMP-2 is used for posterolateral intertransverse process fusion, the carrier sponge may be rolled around blocks or granules of calcium phosphate, or allograft bone chips. This serves to provide bulk to the sponge, which helps resist compression by the paraspinous musculature.

The biologic events of spinal fusion include two distinct but overlapping stages: an initial inflammatory response with bone resorption, followed by a bone growth phase. BMP has been shown to play a role in the regulation of both osteoclastic and osteoblastic activity. When exogenous BMP-2 is used in spinal fusion procedures, the inflammatory phase is sometimes quite pronounced, and in some cases early post-operative radiographs show significant osteolysis. It is thought that excessive doses of BMP-2 or rapid release of BMP-2 from the carrier sponge may lead to excessive bone resorption. This process is not fully understood. Further work will be needed to determine the optimal dose and carrier to minimize this complication.

In addition to concerns about the bone resorption phase, problems can potentially occur in the bone growth phase. When BMP-2 was first introduced, there was concern that the osteoblastic process could not be controlled and that exuberant local bone formation would occur, potentially leading to spinal canal compromise and neurologic complications. Ectopic bone formation was also a theoretical concern. There appears to be minimal risk of these complications, provided that the appropriate dose of BMP-2 is used and care is taken to keep the material well away from the dura.

Inflammatory fluid collections are occasionally seen after posterior interbody fusions performed with BMP-2. These fluid collections may cause nerve root compression and may require re-operation and drainage.

BMP-2 is now playing a significant role in the treatment of patients who require spinal fusion. The main advantage is that bony fusion can be achieved without harvesting bone from the iliac crest. Avoidance of "donor-site morbidity" results in a faster operation, less blood loss, a shorter hospital stay, and a faster recovery.

The main drawback of BMP-2 is its cost, which is currently $3 600 for a small kit and $5 100 for a large kit in the USA. Although BMP-2 is expensive, it may be cost-effective if its use prevents subsequent and costly revision surgery for pseudarthrosis.

When BMP-2 is used for off-label indications, such as intertransverse process fusion and facet fusion, surgeons are currently using the same dose/carrier combination that has been approved for anterior lumbar fusion. Further work is needed to determine the optimal dose and carrier for these applications.

BMP-7, also known as osteogenic protein 1 (OP-1), is approved by the FDA under a Humanitarian Device Exemption (HDE). Once implanted in the body, BMP-7 recruits stem cells from the surrounding tissues and initiates bone growth. BMP-7 is indicated for high-risk posterolateral lumbar fusion procedures, including patients with previous failed fusion, osteoporosis, smoking, and diabetes.

This product is supplied in a vial containing 3.5 mg of BMP-7 and 1 g of purified type I bone collagen. At the time of surgery, this substance in mixed with 230 mg of carboxymethylcellulose and 2.5 ml of sterile saline to yield a moist putty, which is implanted between the transverse processes of the lumbar spine to promote a fusion.

At the present time, all BMP products must be delivered to the spine by direct implantation. In the future, it may be possible to deliver BMP to the spine less invasively through the use of gene therapy.

Compensation and disability issues related to low back pain

Workers' compensation and disability issues related to low back pain have long been problematic in the workplace in the USA and in some other developed countries as well. There are several reasons for this.

1. For decades, back pain occurring in the workplace has been viewed as an injury, compensable under workers' compensation programs. Under this paradigm, the task being performed by the worker with back pain is assumed to be the proximate cause of the pain, and therefore the cause of the injury.
2. Back pain in general has been attributed to degenerative changes that are readily identified on MRI. This has been particularly true for work-related back pain.
3. Huge amounts of money have been expended in an effort to evaluate and fix the "injured" spine, and then to compensate individuals who are unable to return to work. For example, in the USA, workers' compensation insurance costs employers 2%–4% of gross earnings, a significant portion of which underwrites claims related to back-related symptoms.

Over the last decade, the injury model of work-related back pain has been called into question through several lines of investigation.

1. Multiple studies have shown little correlation between the vast array of tasks performed in the modern workplace and the incidence of disabling back pain.
2. It is now recognized that genetic factors may play a larger role in age of onset and progression of symptoms, with environmental influences playing a lesser role than previously thought.
3. Psychosocial issues often play a greater role in the genesis of back-related complaints than the physical demands of the task being performed. Workers who find their jobs boring and dissatisfying are more likely to claim disability due to back-related symptoms.
4. The degenerative changes seen on sensitive imaging studies, such as MRI, are predominantly age-related phenomena, have little to do with one's occupation or life activities, and often cannot be shown to be the cause of back discomfort. MRI obtained soon after an episode of low back pain generally does not reveal any new structural change that would explain the clinical event.

Further investigation will be needed to better define the causes of regional back pain and their relation to work and other physical activities. As the injury model for work-related back pain is refined and modified, this will undoubtedly lead to future modifications of the current system of workers' compensation for low back pain.

Emerging technology and new surgical procedures

Major recent developments in lumbar spine surgery include biological materials to facilitate spinal fusion, disk arthroplasty, disk nucleus replacement technology, and computer-assisted image guidance to assist with placement of instrumentation. In addition, there has been a trend over the past decade toward making all procedures less invasive, in an effort to avoid approach-related morbidity.

Less invasive methods of decompressing nerve roots and performing spinal fusions are now available. Further work will be needed to determine whether these new approaches will lead to improved outcomes and lower complication rates. Pharmacologic treatment aimed at local inflammatory processes is also under investigation. Further details on these topics are found in Chapter 13.

Conclusions

Low back pain is a very common symptom, which usually does not require extensive investigation or imaging studies. In most cases, symptoms resolve spontaneously. When low back pain occurs in the setting of major trauma, systemic illness, such as cancer or infection, or progressive neurologic deficit, a broad differential diagnosis must be considered and rapid investigation carried out.

Most lumbar operations are performed for discogenic and degenerative processes. Surgical outcomes are generally favorable when the predominant symptom is radicular leg pain secondary to spinal nerve root compression. Surgery is less successful, and more controversial, when the predominant symptom is axial back pain without a significant radicular component. Spinal surgery should not be viewed as the final common pathway for every patient with persistent back pain.

Emerging technology in the lumbar spine includes biological materials to enhance spinal fusion, disk arthroplasty, disk nucleus replacement, image guidance, and minimally invasive techniques.

Further reading

1. Atlas SJ, Keller RB, Wu YA, Deyo RA, Singer DE. Long-term outcomes of surgical and nonsurgical management of sciatica secondary to a lumbar disc herniation: 10 year results from the Maine lumbar spine study. *Spine* 2005; **30**:927–935.

2. Atlas SJ, Keller RB, Wu YA, Deyo RA, Singer DE. Long-term outcomes of surgical and nonsurgical management of lumbar spinal stenosis: 8 to 10 year results from the Maine lumbar spine study. *Spine* 2005; **30**:936–943.

3. Bridwell KH, Anderson PA, Boden SD, et al. What's new in spine surgery? *J Bone Joint Surg* 2006; **88**-A:1897–1907.

4. Caragee EJ. Persistent low back pain. *New Engl J Med* 2005; **352**:1891–1898.

5. Caragee E, Alamin T, Cheng I, et al. Are first-time episodes of serious LBP associated with new MRI findings? *Spine J* 2006; **6**:624–635.

6. Deyo RA, Nachemson A, Mirza SK. Spinal fusion surgery: the case for restraint. *N Engl J Med* 2004; **350**:722–726.

7. Fraser RD. Chymopapain for the treatment of intervertebral disc herniation: the final report of a double-blind study. *Spine* 1984; **9**:815–818.

8. Hadler NM, Tait RC, Chibnall JT. Back pain in the workplace. *J Amer Med Assoc* 2007; **297**:1594–1596.

9. Mariconda M, Galasso O, Secondulfo V, et al. Minimum 25-year outcome and functional assessment of lumbar discectomy. *Spine* 2006; **31**:2593–2599.

10. Sirven JI, Malamut BL (eds). *Clinical Neurology of the Older Adult*. Philadelphia: Lippincott Williams & Wilkins, 2002.

11. Waddell G, McCulloch JA, Kummel E, et al. Nonorganic physical signs in low-back pain. *Spine* 1980; **5**:117–125.

12. Weinstein JN, Tosteson TD, Lurie JD, et al. Surgical vs. nonoperative treatment for lumbar disk herniation: the spine patient outcomes research trial (SPORT): a randomized trial. *JAMA* 2006; **296**:2441–2450.

13. Weinstein JN, Lurie JD, Tosteson TD, et al. Surgical vs. nonoperative treatment for lumbar disc herniation: the spine patient outcomes research trial (SPORT): observational cohort. *JAMA* 2006; **296**:2451–2459.

14. Weinstein JN, Lurie JD, Tosteson TD, et al. Surgical versus nonsurgical treatment for lumbar degenerative spondylolisthesis. *New Engl J Med* 2007; **356**:2257–2270.

15. Weinstein JN, Tosteson TD, Lurie JD, et al. Surgical versus nonsurgical therapy for lumbar spinal stenosis. *New Engl J Med* 2008; **358**:794–810.

Chapter 12

Minimally invasive spine surgery

Philosophy of minimally invasive spine surgery

There has been an explosion of interest in minimally invasive spine surgery over the last decade, with extensive coverage in both the medical literature and media. This concept has been driven by new technology and by a desire for operations that involve smaller incisions, less operative blood loss, less post-operative pain, a shorter stay in the hospital, and a faster return to work and normal physical activities. Percutaneous discectomy and fusion, laparoscopic anterior fusion of the lumbar spine, vertebral augmentation with polymethylmethacrylate, intradiscal electrical thermal therapy (IDET), and X-Stop interspinous decompression are among the procedures that have been introduced over the last 10 years.

Some of these new procedures have proven to be valuable additions to the spine surgeon's armamentarium, while others have not. These developments are often heralded by euphoric reports of success in the media, only to be discarded after they fail to withstand the test of time.

Although there has been a great deal of recent interest in minimally invasive approaches to the spine, it is important to note that this is not a new concept. Chymopapain chemonucleolysis dates back to the early 1960s, while automated percutaneous discectomy and laser-assisted discectomy were first described in the mid 1980s. After periods of initial enthusiasm, interest in each procedure has waned, and none of the three currently enjoys widespread usage in North America or Europe.

A major source of confusion relates to terminology. Even a cursory review of the literature reveals a lack of agreement as to what constitutes a minimally invasive operation. Consider, for example, lumbar discectomy. If the surgeon removes a disk herniation through a rigid endoscope placed in the interspace through a small lateral stab incision, most would agree this is a minimally invasive technique. At the

other end of the spectrum, if the surgeon performs a discectomy through a long incision, with bilateral exposure of the posterior elements, without the benefit of magnification, most would agree this is not a minimally invasive approach. However, for all procedures falling between these two extremes, there is no consensus as to what constitutes a minimally invasive discectomy. If the surgeon makes a smaller incision, carries out a limited, unilateral bony exposure, and uses an operating microscope, some would consider that to be a minimally invasive operation, while others would consider that to be merely a refinement of traditional lumbar discectomy. If the surgeon uses a tube retractor in addition to the microscope, some would consider that to be a distinctly different and minimally invasive procedure, while others would consider it simply a modification of existing techniques.

Perhaps the best perspective is to consider minimally invasive spinal surgery as a concept, in which the surgeon attempts to achieve the goals of the operation through small incisions with less approach-related morbidity. For this reason, the term "minimal access spine surgery" may be a better term for this group of procedures.

At the same time, the length of the incision is not the sole factor in determining whether operations should be classified as minimally invasive. For example, X-Stop interspinous decompression for lumbar spinal stenosis, described later in this chapter, requires an incision the same length as that used for the standard procedure, decompressive laminectomy. However, the X-Stop procedure is faster and does not require dissection around the dura and spinal nerve roots. For this reason, X-Stop interspinous decompression is generally considered to be a minimally invasive procedure, despite the length of the incision.

Regardless of how one defines minimally invasive spine surgery, patients being considered for these operations must meet the same criteria that are required for the traditional procedure. In addition, outcomes after minimally invasive procedures should be judged by the same criteria that are used for standard procedures. For most spine operations, these would typically include the results of patient-centered outcomes instruments, such as the SF-36 and Oswestry Disability Index (ODI), plus complication and re-operation rates.

One of the concerns about some minimally invasive procedures is that proponents have highlighted parameters that are of marginal benefit to the patient, such as hospital length of stay. From the patient's perspective, whether the post-operative hospitalization lasts 2 or 3 days is irrelevant. The key factor to the patient is the outcome of treatment, not how long he or she spends in the hospital. Furthermore, it must be emphasized that minimally invasive spine surgery should not be viewed as cosmetic surgery or a marketing tool.

It is also important to note that while minimally invasive procedures may offer advantages, such as a smaller incision or less blood loss, there may be drawbacks as well, for example increased radiation exposure to the patient and surgical team from prolonged fluoroscopic imaging, which would not be necessary during a standard open procedure.

Cost is another major concern of minimally invasive spine surgery, as these procedures are technology intensive. For example, a minimally invasive spinal fusion typically requires an image guidance system, fluoro-CT, and an operating microscope, bone morphogenetic protein (BMP), pedicle screws, and interbody devices. When image guidance is used, a specialized pre-operative CT scan is required, further adding to the expense of the procedure.

It appears that a minimally invasive operation may result in a slightly shorter hospital stay than a standard open procedure; however, the cost savings related to the shorter hospital stay may not be enough to offset the greater expense of the procedure itself.

Ultimately, a new procedure, minimally invasive or otherwise, must be shown to be superior, or at least equivalent, to existing treatments before it can become the standard of care. In the case of vertebral augmentation, the procedure is generally regarded to be superior to either nonoperative treatment or major open reconstructive surgery for vertebral compression fractures. Vertebral augmentation has therefore become the procedure of choice for most patients with acute vertebral compression fracture. In contrast, several minimally invasive procedures have been introduced for lumbar disk herniation, but none has been shown to be superior to standard microdiscectomy, which at this point remains the gold standard procedure for lumbar disk herniation.

Finally, it is important to note that not all new technology is minimally invasive. To give just one example, the lumbar disk arthroplasty is sometimes presented as a minimally invasive procedure. In reality, the device must be implanted through a major open anterior approach, which is anything but minimally invasive.

Minimally invasive procedures for lumbar disk herniation

The early minimally invasive spine procedures were directed at lumbar disk herniation, perhaps because it is such a common problem. Although some of these procedures have been abandoned and are of historic interest only, a brief review will be provided, since the spine clinician routinely encounters patients having had a variety of these procedures.

Central nucleectomy procedures

The first percutaneous therapy for lumbar disk herniation was chemonucleolysis with chymopapain, a procedure that was initially reported in 1964. In many ways, this was the prototype minimally invasive spine procedure. Chemonucleolysis was followed by automated percutaneous discectomy, and later by laser-assisted percutaneous discectomy in the 1980s. Each of these procedures has the same goal: to relieve nerve root compression by removing a portion of the central nucleus pulposus. Chemonucleolysis accomplishes this by means of a chemical reaction, automated percutaneous discectomy by means of mechanical removal, and laser-assisted discectomy by means of thermal energy.

These techniques can do only a central nucleectomy; they cannot be targeted at localized areas of disk pathology. They are limited to patients with contained disk herniations with an intact annulus. Unlike microdiscectomy, these procedures cannot be used in patients with extruded disk fragments that have broken through the annulus and posterior longitudinal ligament.

Chemonucleolysis enjoyed widespread usage in North America in the 1970s, with a second resurgence in the early 1980s. Chemonucleolysis was demonstrated to be more effective than placebo injections, but was ultimately discarded because of devastating neurologic complications associated with inadvertent injection into the subarachnoid space, infrequent though sometimes life-threatening anaphylactic reactions, and because the procedure was found to be less effective than open microdiscectomy. Currently, chemonucleolysis has been essentially abandoned in North America and Europe, although there has been recent renewed interest in the procedure in Asia, in particular Korea.

As interest waned in chemonucleolysis in the mid 1980s, automated percutaneous discectomy was introduced, followed by laser-assisted percutaneous discectomy. Both procedures appear to be safe in experienced hands, but are generally regarded as being less effective than microdiscectomy. In particular, critical assessment of laser-assisted discectomy has been hampered because it has never been directly compared with standard microdiscectomy. Neither procedure has gained widespread acceptance.

Endoscopic discectomy

Endoscopic discectomy represents another minimally invasive approach to the removal of herniated lumbar disk material. This is not a new technique. Endoscopes have been used since the 1980s to inspect the intervertebral disk space and spinal canal after completion of a standard open microdiscectomy. Use of the endoscope as an adjunct to an open procedure has subsequently evolved into full endoscopic discectomy.

A variety of different endoscopic techniques have been described by different investigators. As a result, the term endoscopic discectomy actually encompasses several different, but related, procedures. This lack of procedural uniformity has made it difficult to assess the usefulness of the technique. No single endoscopic technique has emerged as being superior to the others or as superior to microdiscectomy.

The theoretical advantage of the endoscopic approach is that it produces less damage to paraspinal soft tissues and less scarring in the epidural space.

While the procedure does have the potential to reduce approach-related morbidity, there are significant drawbacks as well. First, although the endoscopic approach provides excellent access to the intervertebral disk space, it provides limited access to the spinal canal. This means the surgeon has limited ability to access and remove sequestered disk fragments which have migrated away from the interspace. Second, patients undergoing discectomy procedures often need bony decompression such as a foraminotomy or hemilaminectomy to adequately decompress the affected nerve root. This is difficult, if not impossible,

using an endoscopic technique. Third, the iliac crest may block posterolateral access to the lower lumbar region. This is especially problematic at L5–S1. Fourth, endoscopic procedures done with continuous irrigation have at least a theoretical risk of causing neurologic injury from retained irrigation fluid within the spinal canal.

Fifth, some investigators have found a higher recurrence rate, as high as 12%, with endoscopic discectomy, substantially higher than that seen with conventional microdiscectomy.

A recent study of full-endoscopic discectomy showed relief of leg pain in 84% of patients and a recurrence rate of 6.0% at 2-year follow-up. These results are similar to those for microdiscectomy; however, it must be noted that only a limited subset of patients with symptomatic disk herniations were eligible for the procedure. Patients with sequestered disk fragments, radiologic evidence that the iliac crest would block posterolateral access to the disk space, and cauda equina syndrome were excluded from the study.

From a practical standpoint, excluding patients with sequestered disk fragments and common anatomic factors that prevent posterolateral access to the disk space means that many patients with lumbar disk herniation are not eligible for the procedure. Difficulties associated with bone removal through an endoscope further limits use of the technique in individuals with significant spondylosis, who require a foraminotomy or lateral recess decompression, in addition to the discectomy.

Endoscope technology continues to evolve, and results of endoscopic discectomy have shown some improvement; however, endoscopic discectomy has not been widely adopted at this point. Perhaps the main drawback of the procedure is its limited applicability to the population of patients with symptomatic lumbar disk herniations. In order for it to be a useful technique, the endoscopic technique will have to be refined so that it can be used for the full spectrum of disk disease encountered in clinical practice.

Thermal disk decompression

Other minimally invasive procedures for lumbar disk herniation are currently under investigation, including disk ablation using thermal energy applied via heating catheters placed within the disk using percutaneous approaches. There are insufficient data on disk ablation using thermal energy to make any definite recommendations regarding this technique. The procedure should be regarded as investigational at this time.

Microdiscectomy using a tubular retractor

Tubular retractor systems are now available for microdiscectomy and other spinal procedures. Some have internal lighting systems to provide illumination of the operative site. Once the retractor is placed, the operation proceeds in the same manner as a standard microdiscectomy.

Some surgeons regard the use of a tube retractor as creating a distinctly different minimally invasive procedure, while others consider it to be simply a refinement of the standard open procedure. These retractors may be beneficial when a deep exposure is required in very large patients. One drawback is the requirement for fluoroscopic imaging, resulting in increased radiation exposure to the patient and surgical team, which is not necessary during a routine microdiscectomy. Further work will be needed to determine whether this procedure has any other benefit relative to the standard procedure.

Current status of minimally invasive procedures for lumbar disk herniation

Numerous minimally invasive procedures have been proposed for lumbar disk herniation over the last 40 years. Most are safe, and some have shown some clinical benefit, but none has been shown to be superior to open microdiscectomy. Thus at this time, microdiscectomy remains the gold standard for surgical treatment of lumbar radiculopathy secondary to disk herniation.

Minimally invasive spinal fusion

Conventional techniques for spinal fusion require lengthy midline incisions, extensive muscle dissection, with the potential for significant blood loss and post-operative incisional pain. Another major source of pain following conventional spinal fusion is "donor-site" pain at the site of iliac crest bone graft harvest.

It has long been recognized that it would be desirable to have less invasive fusion procedures, utilizing smaller incisions, which achieve equivalent or better outcomes with less approach-related morbidity. This concept is now possible as a result of the convergence of three recent technological developments.

Computer-assisted image guidance systems permit the accurate placement of pedicle screws, interbody devices, and bone grafting materials through small incisions. Vastly improved fluoroscopic units, some of which have a CT scan-like image quality, are also available. These two systems can be linked, so that an intra-operative CT-like image is transmitted to the image guidance system, further enhancing the accuracy of implant placement.

Concurrent with advances in intra-operative imaging, new instrumentation, which is designed to facilitate placement of implants and bone grafts through small incisions, has been developed.

Finally, new bone graft substitutes are also playing a role in making spinal fusion a less invasive procedure. The most prominent example is BMP, which facilitates bony fusion, while at the same time obviating the need for bone graft harvest and its associated donor-site pain. In 2004, recombinant human bone morphogenetic protein-2 (rhBMP-2) was approved by the Food and Drug Administration, for clinical use in anterior lumbar interbody fusions. BMP is now widely used for posterior lumbar fusions as well, albeit as an "off-label" indication.

To date, these less invasive fusion techniques have found their greatest application in posterior lumbar fusion procedures, including posterior lumbar interbody fusion (PLIF) and transforaminal lumbar interbody fusion (TLIF). These procedures can be done through small bilateral paramedian incisions and are gaining greater acceptance in the USA.

In contrast, there is less current interest in minimally invasive anterior lumbar fusion. In the early 2000s, there was a surge of interest in laparoscopic anterior approaches to the lumbar spine; however, significant limitations have been identified. When compared with standard open techniques, the laparoscopic approach results in longer operative times and a higher rate of sexual dysfunction in males, while the open approach provides better visualization and is technically less demanding. As a result, interest in laparoscopic anterior approaches has declined considerably over the last few years.

Recently developed minimally invasive fusion techniques include extreme lateral interbody fusion (X-LIF) and pre-sacral approaches to the L5–S1 segment (Axia-LIF). These new techniques are discussed in Chapter 13.

Minimally invasive spinal fusion techniques are in their infancy and evolving quickly. At the present time, the majority of lumbar fusion procedures are done via open approaches, with laparoscopic anterior and percutaneous posterior approaches being utilized at selected centers, based on surgeon preference. A better understanding of the role of these techniques will undoubtedly emerge over the next few years.

Vertebral augmentation procedures

Vertebral augmentation encompasses two procedures: vertebroplasty and kyphoplasty with an inflatable balloon tamp. These procedures are discussed in Chapter 10.

Spinal cord stimulation

There are three main types of neurosurgical procedures for pain: anatomic removal of the pain generator; ablative procedures, which destroy pain pathways; and augmentative procedures, which modulate pain pathways. Spinal cord stimulation is an example of the latter group. The procedure was originally known as dorsal column stimulation (DCS), as the site of action was initially thought to be in the dorsal columns of the spinal cord. Spinal cord stimulation (SCS) is now the preferred term, as it has been shown that pain relief also occurs with stimulation of ventral cord pathways.

Spinal cord stimulation is a neuromodulation procedure, which attempts to relieve pain of spinal origin through modulation (as opposed to destruction) of pain pathways. The goal of SCS is to create paresthesias that cover a painful area. If the treatment is successful, patients report that the painful sensation is replaced by a pleasant, or at least more tolerable, tingling sensation.

The primary indication for SCS is failed back surgery syndrome (FBSS), a catch-all diagnosis, which includes patients who have failed to gain relief after one or more operations on the spine. FBSS encompasses a heterogeneous group of patients, and often there is little attempt to distinguish the initial indications for surgery or the reasons for failure to relieve symptoms. Further complicating matters is the fact that patients with FBSS often have chronic pain and secondary gain issues. For these reasons, FBSS is very difficult to manage.

Spinal cord stimulation may also play a role in selected patients with complex regional pain syndromes (reflex sympathetic dystrophy), painful peripheral neuropathy, peripheral nerve injury, multiple sclerosis, bladder dysfunction, and angina.

Taking the common situation of FBSS, a specific diagnosis for the patient's pain complaints should be established based on objective clinical findings and imaging studies. Patients with a surgically correctible abnormality should be considered for re-operation, although in some of these cases, SCS may offer a higher chance of success and lower risk than re-operation. All patients with FBSS should be carefully evaluated for functional overlay and psychosocial problems. Major psychiatric issues, narcotic abuse, and secondary gain issues should be carefully addressed in a multidisciplinary fashion, and in some cases will preclude SCS.

For the patient being considered for SCS, the initial step is a screening trial, which is conducted with a percutaneously placed epidural lead, connected to an external pulse generator. In order for the treatment to help, the patient must feel stimulation in the painful area. If the trial is successful, a fully internalized stimulator system is created by connecting the epidural lead to a pulse generator placed in the subcutaneous tissues of the upper buttock or abdomen. Once inserted, the device may be turned on and off, and stimulator settings may be adjusted by either the patient or the medical team.

A paddle-type electrode placed via a laminectomy may be used if percutaneous lead placement is not technically feasible or a broader coverage pattern is needed. Two disadvantages of the paddle electrode are that it generally requires a general anesthetic for placement and that it is not maneuverable within the spinal canal to any significant degree. These factors effectively rule out a screening trial of different lead positions when using the paddle electrode.

Complications include infection, electrode migration or breakage, cerebrospinal fluid (CSF) leak from inadvertent subarachnoid lead placement, radicular pain, and interference with some cardiac pacemakers. Serious complications such as epidural hematoma or abscess are uncommon.

It was initially thought that SCS might have an undesirable effect on normal sensation, perhaps placing the patient at risk for thermal injury in the area of stimulation. This was subsequently shown not be a cause for major concern. Studies have shown that vibratory sensation is impaired; however, acute pain sensation is not affected to a degree that would increase the risk of insensible injury.

Outcomes studies of SCS often use 50% pain reduction and patient satisfaction as criteria for success. Using these parameters, success rates of

233

approximately 50% have been reported at 2-year follow-up, with a slight recurrence rate with longer follow-up. Leg pain is more likely to improve than back pain. Pulse generator replacement is required periodically, usually every 2–4 years. Lifespan of the pulse generator is based on stimulator settings and patterns of usage.

Spinal cord stimulation is less likely to relieve back pain than radicular pain for two reasons. First, it is technically more difficult to achieve paresthesia overlap of the low back than the leg. Second, low back pain is thought to have a greater component of nociceptive pain, which is less responsive to SCS, while radicular pain has a greater component of neuropathic pain, which is more responsive to SCS. For these reasons, axial back pain has proven to be particularly difficult to treat. Systems of dual or parallel electrode arrays have shown some promise in treating this difficult problem.

Although SCS is not overwhelmingly successful in the treatment of FBSS, results should be viewed as satisfactory, in the context of the very difficult patient population being treated.

The main advantage of SCS is that a screening trial is done before implantation. Thus, if the trial does not provide pain relief, the patient is not subjected to a futile intervention. Another advantage is that, like other augmentative procedures, SCS is fully reversible, meaning that if a treatment failure occurs after implantation, the device can be explanted without causing further damage. In addition, SCS is minimally invasive and involves minimal risk to the patient.

The major drawback to the use of SCS is the initial high cost of the stimulator system; however, the long-term costs of SCS have been shown to be substantially less than those associated with re-operation (e.g., repeated laminectomy and/or fusion). Another limitation is that SCS cannot be used in patients with some cardiac pacemakers or other neuromodulation devices, including deep brain stimulators and bladder stimulators. In addition, MRI is precluded after placement of an SCS system.

Since its introduction in the 1980s, SCS has become an established modality for the treatment of chronic pain of spinal origin. FBSS is the most common indication for its use. More stringent patient selection criteria and technical advances have led to better outcomes. All patients should be carefully screened using a multidisciplinary approach. SCS is a minimally invasive, reversible, neuromodulation

technique, which is useful in carefully selected patients with FBSS and other chronic pain states.

Intrathecal drug pumps

Intrathecal drug delivery systems consist of an infusion pump, which is implanted in the subcutaneous tissues of the abdomen, and an intraspinal catheter, which delivers medication from the pump into the spinal subarachnoid space. The catheter is typically inserted in the lumbar region. The pump can be programmed to deliver medication at constant or variable flow rates.

These devices were introduced in the early 1980s, and initially were used only for cancer-related pain. Indications for treatment were later expanded to include patients with pain of nonmalignant origin, including FBSS. Morphine and hydromorphone (Dilaudid) are the most commonly used analgesic agents.

One of the key mechanisms in the neurophysiology of pain is release of substance P in the dorsal horn of the spinal cord. Substance P then acts on dendrites of ascending neurons. Opioids inhibit the release of substance P and other neurotransmitters by bonding to opioid receptors, a process which serves to block pain transmission. Intrathecal delivery of opioids is particularly effective because it does not have to circulate systemically to reach the CSF and dorsal horn of the spinal cord.

Intrathecal drug therapy for intractable pain has several potential advantages, including a decreased need for oral analgesics, reduction in side-effects associated with oral analgesics (nausea, vomiting, sedation, and constipation), and improved physical functioning. Drawbacks include the high cost of the device, the development of tolerance, and the risk of device-related complications.

Selection criteria for intrathecal morphine therapy are relatively straightforward. The patient must have failed an adequate trial of oral narcotics or have had unacceptable side-effects, such as confusion or nausea. If the patient has cancer, an assessment of the patient's life expectancy should be made. The patient should be expected to live at least 3–6 months in order to justify the cost of the device. If the life expectancy is less than that, a percutaneous catheter and external pump should be considered.

Once these initial screening criteria are met, a trial of intrathecal morphine should be carried out. This step is necessary to confirm that the patient responds favorably to intrathecal morphine. The trial may be conducted with either a bolus injection or short-term continuous infusion using an external pump. The trial is important because it enables the patient and clinician to understand the degree of pain relief and improvement in function and quality of life that can be expected with an implanted system.

The use of intrathecal drug pumps in patients with nonmalignant pain, typically FBSS, is more controversial. Selection criteria are similar to those for patients with cancer-related pain; however, patients with nonmalignant pain generally have a much longer lifespan. This means that drug side-effects and tolerance and device malfunction are more likely to come into play in this patient population, because treatment is potentially required for decades. Despite these concerns, one large study of intrathecal morphine infusion showed similar outcomes for pain of malignant as for pain of nonmalignant origin.

A variety of complications may arise from placement of intrathecal drug pumps, including approach-related, device-related, and drug-related events. Serious complications are uncommon; however, even minor problems often require revision surgery, and thus prove to be bothersome to the patient and at times vexing to the clinician. Neurologists and other spine care clinicians often care for patients with intrathecal pumps, and should, therefore, have a basic understanding of problems which these patients may encounter. Once identified, most pump-related complications will be managed by the implanting physician.

Approach-related complications include infection, CSF leak, and inappropriate placement of the catheter in the subdural or epidural space.

Device-related complications include pump and catheter failure. Long-term complications related to the pump are uncommon; however, catheter breakage, disconnection, kinking, and occlusion are significant long-term risks. An unexpected reduction in pain control usually indicates a drug delivery problem, usually involving some problem with the catheter.

A rare, but serious complication is the development of an inflammatory mass at the catheter tip (catheter-tip granuloma). This diagnosis should be suspected in the patient with a history of good pain control, who experiences a sudden escalation in pain and new clinical signs of cauda equina or conus compression.

Catheter-tip granulomas have occurred only in patients receiving intrathecal opioids, usually morphine, administered alone or in combination with other medications, or rarely in patients who received agents that were not approved for intrathecal use. These masses have not been reported in patients receiving intrathecal baclofen.

This phenomenon also appears to be dose related as patients receiving higher doses of morphine are at greater risk than those on low dose regimens. Thus, the process of catheter-tip granuloma formation appears to depend on both the medication and dosage being used, although the precise pathophysiologic mechanisms have not yet been defined.

Once the diagnosis is suspected on clinical grounds, imaging should be carried out with MRI with contrast enhancement or CT/myelography. The usual MRI finding is an enhancing intradural mass, with the catheter tip embedded within it. It can be difficult at times to visualize the intraspinal catheter on MRI. In these cases, it is important to obtain biplane radiographs and correlate these studies with the MRI in order to positively identify the catheter tip and its relation to the mass.

Management of these uncommon problems must be individualized, taking into account the size of the mass and the patient's neurologic condition. Smaller masses sometimes regress after removing or repositioning the catheter or by altering the dose, concentration, or medication being infused. This may be an appropriate strategy in patients with relatively small lesions and less severe neurologic involvement. Large masses that fill the spinal canal and cause major neurologic deficits should be removed. Figure 12.1 depicts an intra-operative photograph of a catheter-tip granuloma compressing the cauda equina.

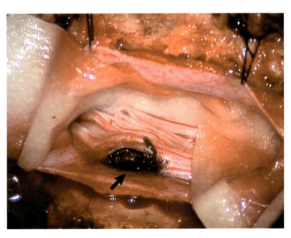

Figure 12.1. Intra-operative photograph of a catheter tip granuloma displacing and compressing the cauda equina (arrow). For orientation, the patient's head is to the right and feet are to the left.

Medication-related adverse events include tolerance and inadvertent overdose, which may occur when there are errors in dose or concentration of the analgesic agent.

Intrathecal drug pumps are also useful in the treatment of spasticity, with baclofen (Lioresal) being the medication of choice. Administration of intrathecal baclofen by continuous infusion has proven to be an effective treatment of spasticity of the lower extremities. Similar to pain patients being screened for intrathecal morphine infusion, patients with spasticity should have a successful response to a test dose of intrathecal baclofen before undergoing implantation of a pump system.

Magnetic resonance imaging is contraindicated in patients with intrathecal drug pumps.

Intradiscal electrothermal therapy

Intradiscal electrothermal therapy (IDET) was introduced in 1997 as a treatment for lumbar discogenic pain. The procedure involves the application of thermal energy to a painful disk by means of a percutaneously placed flexible electrode. The IDET catheter is analogous to the heating element in an oven, except with IDET radiofrequency energy is converted to thermal energy. The mechanism of action is not fully understood, but various theories have been advanced, including stiffening of collagen, repair of annular fissures, and destruction of nerve endings in the annulus thereby eliminating the source of nociceptive input.

Intradiscal electrothermal therapy is a controversial procedure. One of the major concerns has been patient selection. In this respect, IDET is similar to all other treatments for discogenic pain. To be a candidate for this therapy, the patient must have greater than 6 months of discogenic pain with failure of 3 months of medical and physical therapy, have pain consistent with his or her usual pain during discography, and have recent MR of CT imaging demonstrating at least 50% residual disk height and no significant compressive abnormality (i.e., disk herniation, stenosis) at the offending level(s). Exclusion criteria include significant radicular pain or motor deficits, spondylolisthesis, sequestered disk herniation, spinal canal stenosis, scoliosis. IDET may not be technically feasible if the symptomatic disk is severely narrowed; in these cases it may not be possible to navigate the intraspinal thermal catheter into proper position for treatment. IDET may be difficult at the L5–S1 level if there is a high iliac crest, which can block access for needle and catheter placement.

The IDET procedure is performed in either a surgical suite or interventional radiology suite. Biplane fluoroscopy is desirable; however, the procedure can be performed with uniplane fluoroscopy. Anesthesia consists of local anesthetic agents supplemented with small quantities of intravenous fentanyl and midazolam (Versed).

During the procedure, the patient is placed prone, and a 17-gauge needle is inserted percutaneously into the offending disk(s) from a posterolateral approach. A small catheter is then inserted through the needle into the disk and maneuvered to position a 5-cm-long heating element across the posterior annulus. Efforts are made to position the catheter over any annular tears that were identified at discography. In the typical patient with single level discogenic pain, the catheter is heated from 65°C to 90°C over 12.5 minutes and then is maintained at 90°C for an additional 4 minutes.

During treatment, the patient generally feels pain in his/her usual distribution, especially as catheter temperature is increased. The patient should be instructed to promptly report any new or unusual pain, especially pain in the rectum or genitals, as this may indicate the catheter is too close to the sacral nerve roots and should be repositioned. Intravenous narcotics and sedatives must be used sparingly. Serious complications such as a thermally induced cauda equina syndrome could occur if the patient were under heavy sedation or general anesthesia and unable to give appropriate verbal feedback during the procedure.

Once the treatment is completed, the catheter and needle are removed and the patient is observed for a few hours. The patient is then discharged into the care of a responsible adult.

Post-procedure care consists of a soft back brace for 6 weeks and a structured physical therapy program, which begins approximately 6 weeks after the procedure. Complications are rare but may include disk infection and thermal injury to a nerve root. Theoretically, a patient could sustain a traumatic disk herniation in the peri-operative period since heating of the disk causes some acute softening; however, this complication is very uncommon.

Uncontrolled clinical series have yielded conflicting results. Early data indicated that IDET-treated patients had a statistically significant improvement in their back pain when compared to their pre-procedure pain. However, later studies were unable to confirm these initial positive results. Uncertainty about the efficacy of IDET led to a randomized, blinded study in which IDET was compared with a sham procedure. In this study, mean visual analog scale (VAS) pain score in the IDET-treated cohort decreased from 6.6 to 4.2. Although this improvement was modest, it was significantly greater than that observed in the sham group. Of note, 22% of the patients receiving IDET experienced resolution of more than 75% of their pre-treatment pain.

A subsequent prospective, randomized, double-blind, placebo-controlled trial failed to show any benefit of IDET. Thus, at this point, there are two Class I studies of IDET, with one showing modest benefit of the procedure and the other showing no benefit. In the face of such conflicting data, it is difficult to make clear-cut recommendations on the use of IDET; however, the procedure may be of some benefit in highly selected patients with discogenic low back pain, whose only alternative would be a more invasive procedure, such as fusion or disk arthroplasty.

Thoracoscopic sympathectomy

Sympathectomy for treatment of hyperhidrosis and pain syndromes of the upper extremities has traditionally required an open thoracotomy or posterior paraspinal approach. With the advent of video-assisted endoscopy, sympathectomy has now evolved to a minimally invasive endoscopic technique.

The procedure is performed with standard endoscopic equipment. A double-lumen endotracheal tube is needed for ventilation of the contralateral lung, while the ipsilateral lung is deflated during the procedure. A biportal or uniportal technique may be used. The sympathectomy involves cauterization of the T2 and T3 ganglia. Denervation should not extend rostral to the T2 ganglion in order to avoid injury to the stellate ganglion. The lung is re-expanded at the conclusion of the procedure. A chest tube is usually not required. Both sides are done under the same anesthetic.

Clinical outcomes are excellent, with relief of hyperhidrosis being achieved in almost all cases. Potential complications include Horner syndrome (transient or permanent) from damage to the stellate ganglion, compensatory hyperhidrosis, gustatory sweating, hemothorax and pneumothorax, intercostal neuralgia, and wound infection. Serious complications are uncommon.

X-Stop interspinous decompression

X-Stop interspinous decompression was approved by the FDA in 2006, for treatment of symptomatic lumbar spinal stenosis, and is emerging as an effective, and less invasive, alternative to traditional laminectomy procedures.

Neurogenic claudication is a specific symptom complex, in which the patient experiences pain, paresthesias, or weakness of the lower extremities while standing or walking, and gains relief by bending forward at the waist or sitting down. The explanation for this phenomenon is that a reduction in spinal canal diameter occurs when the spine is extended during standing and walking, resulting in nerve root compression and ischemia. This process is reversed when the patient sits or bends forward; this maneuver increases the diameter of the spinal canal, thereby relieving nerve root compression.

X-Stop interspinous decompression relieves symptoms of neurogenic claudication by preventing spinal extension at the stenotic level(s). The X-Stop implant is a titanium alloy device, which is inserted between the spinous processes. In effect, the X-Stop device eliminates extension or lordosis at the treated level(s), thereby relieving neurogenic claudication symptoms. This is accomplished without impairing global sagittal balance.

The X-Stop procedure is indicated for patients with disabling neurogenic claudication, coupled with one- or two-level lumbar canal stenosis demonstrated on MRI or CT/myelography. Patients with pain at rest, significant neurologic deficits, or stenosis affecting more than two levels should not undergo an X-Stop procedure, but would be better served by a standard decompressive laminectomy. The procedure may be performed in patients with a grade 1 degenerative spondylolisthesis, but is contraindicated in patients with degenerative spondylolisthesis grade 2 or higher, and in all patients with isthmic spondylolisthesis.

The X-Stop device is implanted between the spinous processes of the two vertebrae at the stenotic level. Therefore, if the spinous processes have previously been removed during a laminectomy or other procedure, X-Stop interspinous decompression cannot be performed.

The procedure can be performed with the patient positioned either lateral or prone. The first cases were done with the patient placed in the lateral position with the low back and hips flexed to open up the interspinous space at the stenotic level. Patients operated in the lateral position are anesthetized with local agents plus small quantities of intravenous sedation. The correct level(s) are identified with fluoroscopic guidance, and the spinous processes are exposed through a vertical midline incision. Using a sizing instrument, the appropriate sized X-Stop device, measuring from 6 to 14 mm, is selected and then

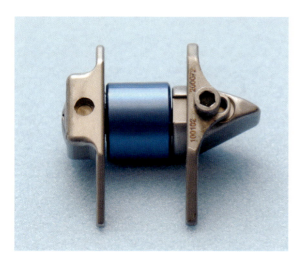

Figure 12.2. Photograph of the X-Stop interspinous decompression device.

inserted. The X-Stop device is depicted in Figure 12.2 and Figure 12.3.

The procedure may also be performed with the patient prone on a flexed spine frame. The prone position offers some technical advantages, especially in very obese patients, although a general anesthetic is required.

Post-procedure requirements are minimal. The procedure is often done on an outpatient basis. Elderly patients or those with significant medical co-morbidities may require an overnight stay in the hospital. Patients are allowed to walk immediately and resume normal physical activities once the wound has healed. Bracing is not required. Physical therapy is not required in all cases, but may be beneficial for deconditioned and sedentary patients.

Procedural complications are minimal since there is no dissection around the spinal nerve roots or dura. When the procedure was first reported, there were

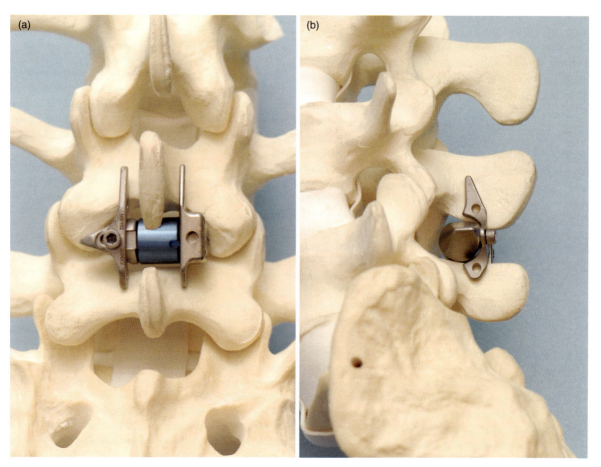

Figure 12.3. (a) Anteroposterior and (b) lateral photographs depicting the usual appearance of an X-Stop interspinous decompression device inserted between the spinous processes of L4 and L5.

concerns that the device could aggravate back pain by impairing global sagittal balance and inducing a "flat back syndrome." Another concern was that the device would fail by becoming dislodged or by fracturing the spinous processes, thereby permitting spinal extension and recurrent nerve root compression. Based on available information, both of these complications appear to be uncommon. Spinous process fracture has been reported. This complication can be minimized by avoiding both overdistraction and placement of a device that is too large. Long-term follow-up data will be needed to fully address these concerns.

Short- and mid-term outcomes of X-Stop interspinous decompression have been encouraging. Two large prospective trials with 2-year follow-up data found that the procedure yielded significantly better results than nonoperative treatment. Preliminary data suggest the outcomes with the X-Stop procedure are equivalent to those achieved with decompressive laminectomy.

Although X-Stop interspinous decompression is a new procedure, it appears to be an effective, low risk, minimally invasive alternative to decompressive laminectomy and laminectomy/fusion. If symptoms recur, the patient can be converted to laminectomy or laminectomy/fusion without any added procedural complexity or risks incurred by the X-Stop device.

The X-Stop is currently the most frequently used interspinous device; however, numerous other interspinous spacers and distraction devices are under development, with clinical trials in progress for some of them.

The Wallis device (Abbot Spine Inc., Austin, TX) is a poly-ether-ether-ketone (PEEK) spacer, which is placed between the spinous processes and held in place with Dacron retention bands. This device restricts both flexion and extension. For this reason, it may have a role for mechanical back pain with disk degeneration, in addition to lumbar spinal stenosis. An FDA IDE trial is currently in progress for this device.

The Coflex device (Paradigm Spine, LLC, New York, NY) is a U-shaped titanium implant, which is held in place through attachments to the adjacent spinous processes. Biomechanical studies indicate that Coflex restores normal flexion and extension, rather than simply holding the spine in flexion. An FDA IDE trial is currently underway to compare Coflex with instrumented fusion.

The FLEXUS Interspinous Spacer (Globus Medical Inc., Audubon, PA) is a unitary PEEK implant

which fits between the spinous processes. Proponents of the device believe the unilateral insertion technique may result in less disruption of ligamentous structures. It is also possible that a device made of PEEK, rather than metal, may result in less erosion of the spinous processes over time. An FDA IDE trial is in progress to compare FLEXUS with X-Stop.

The DIAM, or device for intervertebral assisted motion (Medtronic Sofamor Danek, Memphis, TN), is an H-shaped silicone bumper with polyester covering that is placed between the spinous processes. Two clinical trials are in progress, one in patients with lumbar spinal stenosis, and another in patients with low back pain secondary to degenerative disk disease.

The PercuDyn system (Interventional Spine, Inc., Irvine, CA) consists of a 10-mm-diameter bumper, over a cannulated titanium screw, which is inserted into the pedicle below. The PercuDyn, which can be placed through an open procedure or percutaneously, sits below the inferior facet and acts as a soft cushion to limit extension. There are limited clinical data on this device.

Interspinous implant technology represents an area of active investigation. It is anticipated that some of these newer devices will be approved for clinical use in the near future. Depending on design, interspinous implants may have a role in the treatment of mechanical low back pain and degenerative disk disease, as well as lumbar spinal stenosis. Further work will be needed to clarify the optimal design and clinical indications for these techniques.

Conclusions

Minimally invasive spinal surgery is a concept in which the surgeon attempts to achieve the goals of the operation through small incisions with reduced approach-related morbidity. The term "minimal access spine surgery" has been applied to these types of procedures. Many new minimally invasive spine procedures have been introduced over the last decade. Some have proven useful and have become part of standard surgical practice, while other have proven ineffective and have been discarded.

Patients being considered for minimally invasive procedures must meet the same criteria as those being considered for standard open procedures. Patient selection, outcomes, and cost should be considered using the same criteria as those used for evaluating standard open surgery.

Further reading

1. Anderson PA, Tribus CB, Kitchel SH. Treatment of neurogenic claudication by interspinous decompression: application of the X STOP device in patients with lumbar degenerative spondylolisthesis. *J Neurosurg Spine* 2006; **4**:464–471.

2. Freeman BJ, Fraser RD, Cain CMJ, Hall DJ, Chapple DCL. A randomized, double-blind, controlled trial: intradiscal electrothermal therapy versus placebo for the treatment of chronic discogenic low back pain. *Spine* 2005; **30**:2369–2377.

3. Hsu KY, Zucherman JF, Hartjen CA, et al. Quality of life of lumbar stenosis-treated patients in whom the X STOP interspinous device was implanted. *J Neurosurg Spine* 2006; **5**:500–507.

4. Johnson JP, Patel N. Uniportal and biportal endoscopic thoracic sympathectomy. *Neurosurgery* 2002; **51**:S79–S83.

5. North RB. Neurostimulation for pain of spinal origin. *Clin Neurosurg* 2006; **53**:272–278.

6. Pauza KJ, Howell S, Dreyfuss P, Peloza JH, Dawson K, Bogduk N. A randomized, placebo-controlled trial of intradiscal electrothermal therapy for the treatment of discogenic low back pain. *Spine J* 2004; **4**:27–35.

7. Penn RD. Intrathecal drug infusion for pain. In: *Youmans Neurological Surgery*, Fifth Edition, ed. Winn HR. Philadelphia: Saunders, 2004, pp. 3133–3142.

8. Ruetten S, Komp M, Merk H, Godolias G. Use of newly developed instruments and endoscopes: full-endoscopic resection of lumbar disc herniations via the interlaminar and lateral transforaminal approach. *J Neurosurg Spine* 2007; **6**:521–530.

Chapter

13 New technology in spine surgery

Disk arthroplasty

The artificial disk, or disk arthroplasty, was one of the most highly publicized technological developments in spine surgery in the mid 2000s. This interest has been stimulated by an effort to treat painful intervertebral disks in a way that preserves motion and decreases the risk of adjacent segment degeneration that may occur after a fusion. This general concept has come to be known as motion-sparing technology.

Historically, painful disks have been treated with spinal fusion in an effort to relieve pain by eliminating motion at the painful segment. One of the shortcomings of this approach is that segments adjacent to the fused level are under greater biomechanical stress, and are at risk for accelerated degenerative changes with disk degeneration, facet arthropathy, and spinal stenosis. This constellation of clinical and radiographic findings is known as "adjacent segment disease" or "fusion disease." This phenomenon is sometimes a source of ongoing pain and disability. When adjacent segment disease occurs, revision surgery to decompress and stabilize the adjacent level is sometimes required. Unfortunately, the new adjacent segment is then at risk for accelerated degeneration, with the end result being a series of operations marching up the spine, with progressive lengthening of the fusion construct.

Artificial spinal disks have been developed as a means of preserving motion at the affected segment, thereby minimizing biomechanical stress on adjacent levels. It should be emphasized that disk replacement is not a new concept. Investigation into these devices dates back to the 1950s, but only at the start of the twenty-first century were randomized trials conducted allowing the procedure to be critically compared with the standard operation of spinal fusion. Clinical trials have been completed or are in progress for both lumbar and cervical artificial disks.

Lumbar artificial disk

The first lumbar artificial disk to be introduced in the USA was the Charité disk (DePuy Spine, Johnson &

Johnson), approved by the FDA in 2004, after completion of a multicenter FDA-IDE trial, in which the Charité disk was compared with a stand-alone anterior lumbar interbody fusion. The device is shown in Figure 13.1.

Inclusion criteria for the trial included single-level degenerative disk disease at L4–L5 or L5–S1 confirmed by magnetic resonance imaging (MRI) and provocative discography, age 18–60 years, Oswestry Disability Index (ODI) score of 30 or greater, back pain visual analog score (VAS) score of 40 or greater, with no radicular component, and failed nonoperative treatment of at least 6 months' duration.

The primary exclusion criteria included previous lumbar or thoracic fusion, multi-level disease, facet joint arthropathy, extruded disk, osteoporosis, spondylolisthesis with slip greater than 3 mm, scoliosis greater than 11°, and mid-sagittal stenosis less than 8 mm.

The study found that disk arthroplasty with the Charité device was equivalent to fusion at 2-year follow-up.

Despite receiving FDA approval, this device has not gained widespread acceptance in the USA for several reasons.

1. Placement is technically demanding and requires a major open anterior approach to the lumbar spine. A larger surgical team is required. In addition to the spine surgeon, a general or vascular surgeon (access surgeon) is generally needed for the approach.

2. The revision strategy is complex. Once implanted, devices cannot be easily removed or repositioned. If revision surgery is undertaken anteriorly, there is a high risk of great vessel injury due to scarring around the great vessels from the index procedure. Posterior revision to fuse the level is safer and technically more straightforward, but is more prone to failure since a potentially mobile device remains in the interspace. Anterior revision is generally required for an expelled or migrated

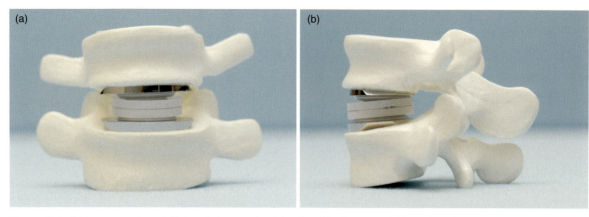

Figure 13.1. (a) Anteroposterior and (b) lateral photographs of the Charité lumbar artificial disk implanted in an anatomic model.

device, which puts vascular or neural structures at risk.

3. The clinical results have not been impressive. The FDA-IDE study showed that the clinical results with the disk arthroplasty were no better than an anterior lumbar fusion. A finding of equivalence, or noninferiority, to anterior lumbar fusion is only faint praise for the disk arthroplasty. Furthermore, 64% of the disk arthroplasty patients classified as successful outcomes were still on narcotic analgesics at 24-month follow-up.

4. The fusion procedure performed in the control group, stand-alone anterior lumbar interbody fusion with BAK (Bagby and Kuslich) cages, is of dubious efficacy and has given way to better fusion techniques, either circumferential fusion or posterior fusion with pedicle screw fixation. Thus, if the study were to be repeated today utilizing contemporary techniques, the control (fusion) group might well have better outcomes.

5. One of the goals of disk arthroplasty is to preserve motion, yet this does not occur consistently. In the FDA-IDE study, almost 40% of patients classified as successful outcomes did not have preserved motion on flexion-extension radiographs, indicating that the treated level had essentially fused.

6. It is technically difficult to achieve optimal positioning of the device, and suboptimal position correlates with worse outcomes. In the FDA-IDE study, with experienced surgeons operating on highly selected patients, 17% of devices were inserted in a suboptimal position, which speaks to the difficulty in achieving optimal implant

placement. Post-operative outcomes were worse among patients with suboptimal implant placement.

7. Some patients and clinicians are under the impression that lumbar disk arthroplasty is a minimally invasive procedure. This is not the case.

8. Many third-party payors are not providing insurance coverage for the procedure in the USA.

A second lumbar disk, the ProDisc-L (Synthes Inc.) was approved by the FDA in 2006, and is now available in the USA. The ProDisc-L is a semi-constrained implant consisting of two cobalt-chromium molybdenum alloy endplates with central keels and a polyethylene convex inlay.

The FDA-IDE study of the ProDisc-L was published in 2007. All study patients had single-level degenerative disk disease. The investigational group was implanted with the ProDisc-L device, and the control group received circumferential fusion. The study design was different from the Charité study, in that control patients in the Charité study received a stand-alone anterior lumbar interbody fusion, while the control patients in the ProDisc-L study received a combined anterior-posterior fusion. At 24-month follow-up, VAS pain scores had improved by an average of 39 points in the ProDisc-L group and 32 points in the fusion group (using a 100-point scale). This difference was not statistically significant, but trended in favor on the ProDisc-L cohort. There were no major vascular injuries or neurologic complications. Retrograde ejaculation was reported in two patients (1.2%). Six of the ProDisc-L recipients (3.7%) required re-operation, including four with device migration, one with a technical error in device insertion, and one with unresolved pain, which required conversion to a fusion. Radiographic range of motion was maintained in 93.7% of the ProDisc-L cohort and averaged 7.7°.

The ProDisc-L was found to be safe and equivalent to fusion and to preserve useful motion in most cases. Based on the clinical trial data, motion preservation with the ProDisc-L appears to be better than with the Charité device.

However, the ProDisc-L has many of the same drawbacks that have been noted with the Charité device. Placement requires an open anterior approach, and the revision strategy is complex. The clinical benefits of the procedure were no more robust than with any other treatment for discogenic back pain. The improvement in VAS pain scores was modest, and 39% of the ProDisc-L recipients were still on narcotics at the conclusion of the study.

To date, all lumbar artificial disks have required an anterior approach for placement; however, posterior lumbar disk arthroplasty systems are now under development. An example of this technology is the Triumph Lumbar Disc (previously known as the Secure-P Disc, Globus Medical, Inc., Audobon, PA). The advantage of this technique is that it can be inserted through posterior and posterolateral approaches, which are more familiar to many spine surgeons and do not require a vascular surgeon to assist with exposure.

Despite a great deal of research, the role of disk arthroplasty in the treatment of low back pain remains uncertain.

Cervical artificial disk

Anterior cervical decompression and fusion (ACDF) is commonly performed for herniated cervical disks and osteophytes causing cervical radiculopathy and/or myelopathy. The procedure allows for excellent neural decompression, and the arthrodesis effectively arrests the degenerative process at the treated level. The operation is safe, and outcomes are generally excellent.

The major concern about ACDF has been its impact on adjacent spinal segments. Biomechanical studies have documented increased motion and increased intradiscal pressure at segments adjacent to the operated segment. These factors accelerate the rate of disk degeneration at the adjacent segments, in a process that has come to be known as adjacent segment disease.

The rationale for cervical disk arthroplasty is its potential to provide the benefit of neural decompression, while preserving segmental mobility, thereby avoiding the long-term problems of adjacent segment

degeneration. This has stimulated intense interest in the development of cervical artificial disks.

Candidates for the procedure must meet the usual criteria for ACDF, including intractable radiculopathy or myelopathy due to soft disk herniation or osteophytes. In addition, imaging studies must demonstrate normal spinal alignment and mobility. The device should not be expected to restore motion at a level which has already lost motion due to advanced degenerative changes. The device should not be implanted in patients with radiographic instability, significant deformity, or significant facet degeneration. These patients should receive the standard ACDF procedure. Clinical outcomes are unknown in patients with congenital spinal canal stenosis. Recent infection or osteomyelitis represents an absolute contraindication, while rheumatoid arthritis and osteoporosis represent relative contraindications to cervical disk arthroplasty.

One significant conceptual difference between the lumbar and cervical disk arthroplasty is that the lumbar device is used to treat axial back pain, while the cervical device is used to maintain motion after a discectomy has been performed to relieve radicular pain or cord compression. Cervical disk arthroplasty is not a treatment for neck pain.

Clinical trials approved by the FDA are underway or have been completed on several different devices. Trials of three different cervical disks have shown clinical outcomes that are equivalent to standard anterior discectomy and fusion, with motion preservation and an acceptable complication profile.

The first device to enter routine clinical use in the USA was the Prestige ST Cervical Disc System (Medtronic Sofamor Danek), which gained FDA approval in 2007. This is a stainless steel device consisting of two articulating components, which are attached to the anterior vertebral bodies (Figure 13.2).

The original design incorporated a ball-in-socket articulation, which permitted flexion and extension, but not anterior-posterior movement, or translation. The ball-in-socket articulation is appropriate for a hip joint; however, subsequent biomechanical studies have shown that a normal segmental motion in the cervical spine includes an element of anterior-posterior movement, in addition to flexion and extension. This means that the superior vertebral body slides forward relative to the inferior vertebral body for a distance of 1–2 mm, as flexion occurs.

This evolving understanding of cervical motion led to the current design, featuring a ball-in-trough

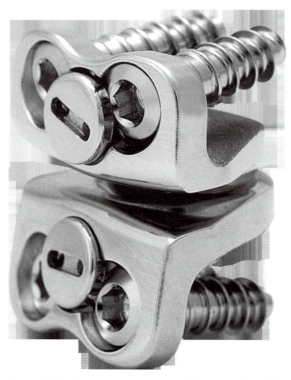

Figure 13.2. Photograph of the Prestige ST Cervical artificial disk.

articulation, which permits translation as well as angular rotation in the sagittal plane.

The Prestige ST device is available in heights ranging 6–8 mm, and lengths ranging 12–18 mm. An appropriate fit can be obtained in almost all patients; however it is possible that an occasional very small or very large individual cannot be accommodated with the available range of sizes. In these situations, a fusion should be performed.

A large, prospective, randomized trial, with 2-year follow-up data comparing the Prestige ST device with a standard allograft fusion, was recently published. All patients were adults and had single-level symptomatic cervical disk disease with intractable radiculopathy, myelopathy, or both. Patients were excluded from the study if they had multi-level disease, cervical instability or sagittal plane deformity, severe facet disease, or osteporosis. The mean age of the study participants was 43 years.

In this study, the Prestige ST device achieved outcomes that were equivalent to those of fusion in terms of SF-36 scores and relief of radicular pain. At 2-year follow-up, relief of neck pain was equivalent between the two groups, although neck pain resolved

faster in the arthroplasty group. Patients receiving the arthroplasty were able to return to work sooner.

Neurologic outcomes were equivalent at 3 and 6 months. The neurologic improvement experienced by the arthroplasty cohort was durable throughout the study period, while the fusion cohort showed a slight but statistically significant decline after the 6-month interval. As a result, the arthroplasty cohort had significantly better neurologic status than the fusion cohort at both the 12- and 24-month interval. The reasons for this are unclear. If a solid fusion has been achieved at the index level and neurologic findings relate to new pathology at an adjacent level, this may herald the early stages of adjacent segment degeneration. An alternative explanation is unrecognized pseudarthrosis in the fusion group, leading to recurrent symptoms at the index level. Longer term follow-up data will be required to resolve this issue.

Physiologic motion was maintained in all patients who received the disk arthroplasty. There were no device-related complications, and the approach-related complication rate of 6.2% was similar to that seen in patients undergoing fusion. The rate of secondary surgery was 3.3% in the arthroplasty group, compared with 8.7% in the fusion group. Re-operation for adjacent segment disease was more common in the fusion cohort.

The incidence of dysphagia and dysphonia was similar in the two groups. This is not surprising, as the profile of the Prestige ST device is similar to that of an anterior cervical plate. Some of the second generation devices in clinical trials have lower profiles, which may lower the incidence of swallowing complications.

Based on this study, it appears that disk arthroplasty with the Prestige ST device is a reasonable alternative to fusion in carefully selected patients. The inclusion/exclusion criteria should be carefully observed. Results will undoubtedly not be as good if the procedure is offered to patients with multi-level disease, deformity, loss of disk height, significant facet disease, and poor bone quality. Further study will be needed to determine whether the disk arthroplasty prevents or limits adjacent segment degeneration.

While a motion-preserving operation will likely prove to be an appropriate option for patients presenting with radiculopathy, there is less certainty regarding myelopathy. Some experts have argued that patients with myelopathy should have a fusion to protect the spinal cord, while others believe these patients will do just as well with a motion-preserving operation. It is also possible that the optimal management will not be the same in every myelopathy case. For example, the young patient with midline soft disk herniation without signal change in the cord might prove to be a good candidate for disk arthroplasty, while the older patient with a hard disk/osteophyte complex and signal change in the cord might be better served with a fusion. There were not enough myelopathy cases in the FDA-IDE study to answer this important question. The optimal management of these patients will hopefully be clarified over time as further clinical experience is accumulated with disk arthroplasty.

Whenever a disk arthroplasty procedure is planned, the surgeon should be prepared to convert to a fusion procedure if there are unanticipated intraoperative findings, such as poor bone quality or a mismatch between the size of the interspace and the arthroplasty device. This means that the surgical team must be prepared in advance for both arthroplasty and fusion. The patient should be made aware of this possibility through the oral and written informed consent process.

A second cervical disk arthroplasty, the ProDisc-C (Synthes Spine) was approved by the FDA in December 2007. Several other devices are currently under development.

The two currently available devices are approved only for single-level placement; however, it is anticipated that future devices will be designed for use at multiple levels if needed. It is known that fusion outcomes decline as more levels are treated, so disk arthroplasty may ultimately be found to be more beneficial with multi-level cases than with single-level cases. Further clinical experience will be needed to answer this question.

Another area of current investigation is a motion-sparing device for patients requiring a vertebral body resection. At the present time, the only surgical option for these patients is a fusion using structural bone graft of the appropriate length or a cage packed with bone graft materials, followed by application of an anterior plate. Motion-sparing vertebral body replacements, which incorporate a disk arthroplasty above and below the artificial vertebral body, are currently under development.

Although the early results of cervical disk arthroplasty are encouraging, the ultimate success of these devices remains to be determined. Several factors suggest that the cervical device may gain acceptance faster, and to a greater extent, than the lumbar device.

1. The approach for cervical disk arthroplasty is identical to that used for the standard anterior discectomy and fusion procedure, and is therefore familiar to all spine surgeons. This means that a spine surgeon can do the entire operation, and that an approach or access surgeon is not required.

2. Once the approach is completed, placement of the cervical disk arthroplasty is relatively straightforward. Slightly more bone removal is required than with an ACDF, but otherwise the two procedures are virtually identical.

3. The revision strategy is less complex than that associated with the lumbar disk arthroplasty. If revision is necessary, the usual approach would be to convert the arthroplasty to an ACDF.

There are several issues, however, which may limit acceptance of cervical disk arthroplasty.

1. The procedure it is designed to replace – anterior cervical discectomy and fusion – is one of the most successful spine operations available, with a long history of excellent outcomes and safety. The cervical artificial disk will have to meet a very high standard in order to gain clinical acceptance.

2. Relative to the discectomy and fusion procedure, cervical disk arthroplasty with the Prestige ST device does not lower the risk of approach-related morbidity, specifically hoarseness and dysphagia. From the patient's viewpoint, these are among the most bothersome complications of anterior operations on the cervical spine.

3. The durability of the cervical disk arthroplasty in high impact trauma situations is unknown. The biomechanical and early clinical data show good durability; however, it is unknown how well the device will withstand violent acceleration and deceleration, which may occur in high speed motor vehicle accidents and in collisions in professional sports, such as American football. In contrast, among patients undergoing anterior cervical fusion, the operated segment is stronger, and therefore less vulnerable to injury, than the remainder of the spine.

4. There are unanswered questions about the long-term durability of these devices. Based on the orthopedic experience with hip and knee arthroplasty, it could reasonably be expected that some cervical disk arthroplasties will eventually wear out and fail. There is also a risk that some of these devices will autofuse over time, with the end

result being a fused segment, with loss of physiological motion.

5. As with any new device, outcomes may not be as good in routine clinical practice as they were in the clinical trial setting with expert surgeons operating on highly selected patients. Particular concerns include the results of disk arthroplasty in patients with advanced age, poor bone quality, facet disease, and decreased lordosis.

6. A final concern relates to insurance coverage. It is unknown at this point whether third party payors will cover the device, and this will clearly have an impact on its ultimate acceptance in the USA.

New lumbar fusion techniques

Extreme lateral interbody fusion (X-LIF)

X-LIF (Nuvasive, San Diego, CA) is a new, minimally invasive fusion technique for degenerative disk disease of the lumbar spine, in which the spine is approached from a direct lateral approach through two small incisions. The approach is guided by fluoroscopy and by electrical stimulation during instrument placement to avoid damage to the lumbar plexus. The damaged disk is removed, and fusion is performed by placing an interbody device, bone graft and/or bone morphogenetic protein (BMP) into the interspace. Lateral fixation devices are available, and supplemental posterior fixation is sometimes employed.

The advantages of this technique are that it avoids muscle dissection associated with posterior approaches and avoids great vessel manipulation involved with anterior approaches. Potential drawbacks include the risk of injury to the lumbar plexus and bowel injury. This technique cannot be used at L5–S1 because the iliac crest blocks lateral access to the interspace. A high iliac crest may also limit access at L4–L5. It is also unclear when the X-LIF can be used as a stand-alone procedure and when supplemental posterior fixation should be performed.

Axia-LIF

Axia-LIF (Trans1, Wilmington, NC) is a new presacral approach to fusion at the L5–S1 segment. The procedure is done with the patient in the prone position. The incision is made just in front of the coccyx. Using fluoroscopic guidance, a guide pin is advanced through the L5–S1 disk space into the L5 vertebral body. Discectomy is performed and bone graft and/or BMP is placed into the interspace. A large screw is advanced across the interspace into the L5 vertebral

body. Distraction and height restoration of the interspace can be accomplished. In some cases supplemental posterior fixation with pedicle screws or facet screws is also performed.

The advantage of Axia-LIF is that it avoids the muscle dissection required for posterolateral fusion, and avoids great vessel manipulation required with anterior approaches. The Axia-LIF device has better purchase on the L5 vertebral body and sacrum than posterior (PLIF) and transforaminal (TLIF) lumbar fusion interbody devices, which are just tapped into position. A potential risk of the procedure is bowel injury, which could require a colostomy. Early results are encouraging; however, further work will be needed to define the long term outcomes with the device and to determine when the procedure can be done on a stand-alone basis and when supplemental posterior fixation should be performed.

Nucleus replacement

The preceding section covered disk arthroplasty, which refers to replacement of the entire intervertebral disk complex, including the nucleus, annulus, and both endplates. Lumbar disk nucleus replacement is an alternative, less invasive, concept, which involves replacing the nucleus with an artificial device or substance, while leaving the annulus and endplates intact.

Nucleus replacement has several theoretical benefits. First, the technique may be able to preserve disk height after lumbar disk herniation and discectomy, thereby preventing two potential sequelae seen in these patients: disk space collapse, leading to persistent/recurrent back pain, and recurrent disk herniation.

Second, nucleus replacement is less invasive than total disk replacement. The procedure can be performed through a small posterior incision. From a practical standpoint, this means that a nuclear replacement device can be inserted at the same time as microdiscectomy, using the same incision. In contrast, total disk replacement, or disk arthroplasty, is a much more demanding operation, which requires a separate anterior, transabdominal approach. There is some potential for disk nucleus replacement to become a strictly percutaneous procedure.

Third, there is little scarring and approach-related morbidity associated with nucleus replacement. This is helpful in cases where nucleus replacement has not provided adequate relief, and additional surgery is needed. In these situations, both disk arthroplasty and fusion are viable options, as neither of these procedures is excluded by a nuclear replacement device. In order words, nuclear replacement does not "burn any bridges" in terms of more definitive interventions.

Despite the theoretical benefits of the procedure, the role of disk nucleus replacement remains uncertain. The procedure has been studied fairly extensively, although much of the work has been done in cadavers or in small cases series without appropriate controls. In work dating back to the 1950s, investigators have placed polymethylmethacrylate, Lucite pegs, vitallium spheres (a cobalt–chromium alloy now primarily used for dentures), silicon inserts, and metal ball-bearings into the intervertebral disk space. Plastics, ceramics, polymers, injectable fluids, hydrogels, inflatable devices, and elastic coils have also been studied.

Currently, several disk nucleus replacement procedures are under investigation, including the prosthetic disk nucleus (PDN), Newcleus, and Aquarelle Hydrogel Nucleus, among others. Some are devices that are implanted through open incisions, while others are fluids that are injected percutaneously into the interspace and then harden to the appropriate consistency.

The PDN (Raymedica PDN) is perhaps the most widely studied implant. The PDN is composed of a hydrogel core, inside a flexible, inelastic woven polyethylene jacket. After insertion, the hydrogel core begins to absorb fluid and expand. Most of the expansion occurs within the first 24 hours after implantation; however, maximal expansion may require 4–5 days. Expansion of the device produces distraction and restoration of disk height. Currently, the PDN is the only nucleus replacement that is capable of distraction.

The device is implanted via an open posterior or lateral approach. After implantation and hydration, the hydrogel core deforms and re-forms in response to changes in compressive forces.

Initial clinical experience was reported to be favorable with good pain relief and increased mean disk height. Problems with device migration were encountered in the early clinical experience; however, this has become less common after modification of the surgical technique. The initial clinical studies were performed outside the USA. The recently released PDN-SOLO device is now being implanted in the USA in an FDA-IDE study.

The Aquarelle Hydrogel Nucleus (Stryker Howmedica Osteonic) is a hydrogel-based nuclear replacement. The device has performed well in biomechanical studies, and has shown no evidence of local or systemic toxicity in animal studies. Placement is carried out through a 4- to 5-mm cannula, which is inserted into the disk space. Animal studies have been conducted in the USA, and a small amount of clinical experience has been developed in Europe.

The Newcleus (Sulzer Spine-Tech) is an elongated elastic coil made of polycarbonate urethane. It is inserted through a posterolateral approach after discectomy, and then spirals around within the annulus to fill the nuclear cavity. This device has undergone laboratory and animal investigation, and has been implanted in a small number of patients in Europe.

There are at least two injectable polymers under development for disk replacement. The Prosthetic Intervertebral Nucleus is a polyurethane and the BioDisc (NanoSpine) is a protein hydrogel. Both materials are injected into the disk space and cure within minutes.

The lack of adequate clinical data and diversity of implants and methods of implantation have made it difficult to critically assess the utility of disk nucleus replacement. Currently, none of these devices is approved for clinical use in the USA. Most of the investigative work has been done in Europe. The ultimate role of disk nucleus replacement will have to be defined through prospective clinical trials, with appropriate control groups.

Facet bone dowels

Small machined allograft bone dowels have recently become available for stabilization of the facet joints after laminectomy. These small grafts are inserted into the facet joints either before or after neural decompression, and can be placed using either open or percutaneous techniques. Facet bone dowel placement is technically straightforward and takes only a few minutes to complete.

This should be considered a noninstrumented fusion technique in that it involves only placement of allograft bone, without concomitant metal implants. Decreased segmental motion is immediately apparent after dowel placement.

At this time, the technique is being used mainly in patients undergoing decompressive laminectomy for degenerative lumbar stenosis. The precise role for stabilization with facet bone dowels remains to be determined; however, preliminary experience suggests that the technique holds promise for providing added stability and reducing back pain after lumbar decompressive laminectomy.

Disk transplantation

Anterior cervical fusion is a well-established procedure with excellent outcomes, but may lead to accelerated degeneration of the adjacent segments. Disk arthroplasty has been developed as a means of maintaining motion at the treated segment and maintain integrity of the adjacent segments. Although disk arthroplasty is a promising new treatment, there are unanswered questions about the optimal choice of implant material and design, as well as uncertainty about the long-term effects of disk arthroplasty, specifically issues related to wear debris, loss of fixation, and spontaneous fusion of the device. Thus, neither interbody fusion nor disk arthroplasty may be the optimal solution for replacement of a degenerated cervical disk.

Recent advances in molecular biology may lead to a biological solution to this problem. Expanding on the success that has been achieved with transplantation of other organs, including the kidney, liver, and heart, investigators have begun to explore the possibility of transplanting the entire intervertebral disk. Reliable methods of harvesting and preserving disk material have been developed. Animal studies have shown that a transplanted intervertebral disk can survive and preserve motion.

The first report of intervertebral disk transplantation in humans was published in 2007. In this study, five patients underwent transplantation of fresh-frozen disk allograft after excision of a symptomatic cervical disk herniation. There were no procedural complications and no evidence of graft rejection. Good union of the graft endplates with the native spine was seen in all cases at 3-month follow-up. At 5-year follow-up, all five patients demonstrated improvement in neurologic symptoms. Four of the five had preserved segmental motion, and none developed instability. Two of the five patients had preservation of disk hydration on MRI. In all cases, the transplanted disk demonstrated mild degeneration, which was no more pronounced than that seen at other spinal segments.

This preliminary report suggests that intervertebral disk transplantation is safe and effective in relieving neurologic symptoms, and has the potential to preserve segmental motion and stability at long-term follow-up. For cervical disk disease, biological disk replacement may ultimately become an alternative to interbody fusion and artificial disk replacement. Extending this technique to the lumbar spine, where the biomechanics are different and the magnitude of loading is much greater, will undoubtedly be challenging. Further work will be needed to clarify the role of this new procedure.

Gene therapy for intervertebral disk degeneration

Interest in gene therapy for disk disorders has been stimulated by several observations. Disk degeneration is associated with a loss of proteoglycan content in the nucleus. Certain growth factors may stimulate proteoglycan synthesis, thereby slowing or reversing the process of disk degeneration. A chronic process such as intervertebral disk degeneration would appear to require a sustained delivery of growth factors. Management strategies are complicated by the fact that growth factors have a relatively short half-life and repeated injections of exogenous growth factors into the intervertebral disk are impractical. Therefore, there is a need for a method of continuous and sustained delivery of growth factors to the disk.

Gene therapy may be applicable to the treatment of disk degeneration by providing a mechanism through which intervertebral disk cells would be able to produce growth factors endogenously.

The general concept of gene therapy involves the use of a viral vector to transfer a nucleic acid sequence encoding a gene of interest into a population of cells that will express that gene. This concept has been explored in animal studies, in which exogenous genes encoding growth factors were delivered to the intervertebral disk by an adenoviral vector. Rabbit intervertebral disks treated in this manner have exhibited increased growth factors, thus confirming both gene transfer and gene expression. In addition, these studies have shown increased proteoglycan synthesis, thus providing evidence that gene therapy can alter the biological activity of the disk.

Further laboratory work with bone morphogenetic proteins (BMPs), tissue inhibitors of matrix metalloproteinases, the Sox9 gene, and LIM mineralization protein-1 (LMP-1) has also shown the capability of gene therapy to effect therapeutic change within the intervertebral disk.

Although gene therapy has shown significant potential as a treatment of degenerative disk disease in various animal studies, its safety will have to be studied further and confirmed before it can be used in humans. At least one death has been reported in early clinical trials of gene therapy, when an 18-year-old man with an inherited enzyme deficiency died after receiving adenovirus vector injection in the liver. This event indicates the potential for catastrophic outcomes with this form of treatment.

Various safety issues, including dosing, delivery, and regulation, will require thorough investigation. Concerns about safety are particularly important when considering elective therapy for a nonlethal condition, such as intervertebral disk degeneration. The proximity of the disk to neurologic and vascular structures underscores the need for careful examination of all possible risk factors.

Animal studies have shown that errant injection, leakage, or incorrect dosing can lead to devastating side-effects. Since the clinical application of gene therapy will most likely be accomplished through percutaneous injection into the disk, there is a small, but definite, risk of inadvertent injection into the subarachnoid space due to incorrect needle placement. This could be viewed as a "worst case scenario." There is also potential for leakage of the injectate in the epidural space, even with correct needle placement and injection technique. The potential for complications of this sort mandates a regulation system that allows transgenes to easily be turned "off" or "on." This is necessary in order to avoid toxicity to surrounding normal tissues or excessive expression.

Laboratory studies have shown that an adenoviral tetracycline-regulatable system can be developed, in which tetracycline regulates transgene expression in transduced human nucleus pulposus cells. The clinical relevance of this work is that tetracycline may have the potential to obviate the toxicity associated with errant injection, leakage of the injectate, or dosing error.

Gene therapy clearly has significant potential in the treatment of intervertebral disk degeneration; however, further work will be required before this treatment modality will be available for use in humans.

Stem cell therapy for spinal cord injury

In January 2009, the FDA approved a phase I, multi-center study of human embryonic stem cells in the treatment of spinal cord injury with paraplegia. The treatment will involve an injection of stem cells into the spinal cord at the site of injury. Patients will be followed for at least one year. The major goal of the

study is to assess the safety of the procedure; however, investigators will also monitor the neurologic function of the study patients. This study will be followed closely, as patients with spinal cord injury and their physicians and other care providers are hoping for a major breakthrough in the treatment of this very difficult problem. Regardless of its outcome, this study signals a new era in the field of spinal cord injury research.

Dynamic stabilization

Dynamic stabilization is a group of procedures for the treatment of degenerative spondylolisthesis or degenerative disk disease that represent an alternative to fusion and disk arthroplasty, which have already been discussed.

The goal of fusion is to provide rigid immobilization of a symptomatic spinal segment. In contrast, the goal of dynamic stabilization is to allow controlled motion that is more consistent with normal motion of the spine. In this sense, dynamic stabilization can be viewed as an internal brace.

Dynamic stabilization has been considered both as a stand-alone treatment and as an adjunct to spinal fusion. In the latter situation, the symptomatic level would be fused and the adjacent level would be implanted with a dynamic stabilization device, in an effort to limit motion and prevent degeneration at the level adjacent to the fusion.

Several dynamic stabilization devices have been studied and are in various stages of development. Most are pedicle screw based and use a flexible longitudinal member which permits motion. The systems differ in the type of longitudinal member used.

The system with perhaps the most extensive experience in the USA is Dynesys (Zimmer Spine), which uses pedicle screws and a longitudinal member consisting of a cord inside a plastic sleeve.

Instead of a rigid rod or plate that would be used in a fusion device, Dynesys uses a cord inside a plastic sleeve as the longitudinal member to connect the pedicle screws. This allows controlled movement of the treated spinal segment, instead of rigid immobilization.

Another potential advantage of Dynesys is that it alters spinal anatomy less than a fusion procedure. Dynesys does not disturb the intervertebral disk and does not require bone grafting.

Dynesys has received FDA clearance for use as an adjunct to spinal fusion and for prior failed fusion (pseudarthrosis). It has not been cleared for use as a stand-alone device as the initial treatment of degenerative disk disease. Experience with the device outside of clinical trials has been limited, and its role in treating back pain and degenerative disk disease remains to be determined.

Other dynamic stabilization devices are in varying stages of development. All use pedicle screws to anchor to the spine, and they differ from each other in terms of the device used to connect the screws. A partial listing of these systems and longitudinal member is as follows: Graf ligament (braided polyester cables), the IsoBar (rod with mobile joint), Dynamic Soft Stabilization System (elliptical metal coil), and Stabilimax NZ (rod with spring, plus ball-and-socket articulation with pedicle screw).

Further experience will be needed to define complications and device failure rates, and long-term clinical outcomes. Radiographic outcomes will also be important. In particular, long-term results of dynamic radiographs will be needed to confirm that these devices do indeed permit motion.

In addition, some investigators are exploring the possibility of a combination of posterior dynamic stabilization and total disk arthroplasty as another motion-preserving alternative to spinal fusion.

Facet replacement

Another motion-preserving option currently under development is facet replacement. This procedure is targeted at patients with degenerative lumbar stenosis and involves completely removing the facet joints and replacing them with motion-preserving implants, thus creating an artificial facet joint. These devices are anchored to the vertebral body by means of a screw, which is inserted into the pedicle. The technique theoretically allows for a complete decompression of the affected nerve roots and preservation of spinal motion, while avoiding the morbidity associated with fusion.

Facet replacement devices are currently in clinical trials. There are no published data on the safety and effectiveness of these implants.

Annular repair technology

Herniation of the nucleus pulposus creates an opening in the annulus, which is sometimes enlarged during the course of the microdiscectomy procedure. This annular defect does not heal well; and this persistent defect puts the patient at risk for future episodes of symptomatic disk herniation, which may be as high as 10%–15%. One of the major limitations of all microdiscectomy procedures has been the inability to reliably seal or repair the annulus, after removal of the herniated disk material.

Investigators have long sought a technique to repair the annulus, in an effort to prevent recurrent herniation. A variety of biological sealants, devices, and suture techniques have been studied; however, until recently, none proved satisfactory.

In 2007, two soft tissue repair systems, the XCLOSE Tissue Repair System and the ICLOSE Surgical Mesh System (Anulex Technologies, Minnetonka, MN), gained FDA approval for general surgery and orthopedic applications. Clinical trials of these systems as annular repair techniques following discectomy are underway, but have not yet been published. These systems may prove to be useful techniques for annular repair, although usage in the spine is considered off-label at this time.

The XCLOSE system is a suture technique, which is appropriate for a slit or narrow tear in the annulus, in which the annular tissues at the margins of the tear can be easily approximated. The XCLOSE would not be appropriate for larger defects, where the annular tissues cannot be easily brought together.

The ICLOSE system involves the placement of a mesh implant in the annular defect, and would be appropriate for a larger, gaping hole in the annulus.

There is clearly a need for safe and effective methods of annular repair. Intuitively, both of these products make sense and may prove to be valuable; however, more clinical experience will be needed to determine the ultimate benefit of these particular techniques.

Metallic bone graft substitutes

Spinal fusion procedures require the use of autograft or allograft bone. Autograft provides the highest fusion rates, but may lead to donor-site pain and, in some cases, is not available in adequate amounts due to harvesting for previous surgical procedures. Allograft bone avoids the problems associated with autograft, but is associated with somewhat lower fusion rates. Other concerns with allograft bone include limited supplies and a risk, albeit very small, of disease transmission.

Metallic grafting materials have been developed in an effort to deal with the shortcomings of autograft and allograft bone. Highly porous tantalum implants, which closely approximate the physical structure of normal bone, have recently been developed. These implants have greater compressive strength and similar flexibility (elastic modulus) as compared with cancellous bone. Permeability is similar to that of cancellous bone, which permits rapid ingrowth of bone and maturation of the fusion. Another benefit of tantalum is that it is very biocompatible, with a very low risk of allergic reaction.

To date, the available published data on spinal tantalum implants have been confined to cadaveric and animal studies. No human clinical studies have been published.

Absorbable spinal implants

In contemporary practice, rigid titanium plates are used in most anterior cervical fusion procedures. Titanium plating has proven to be a safe and effective technique, which improves the fusion rate. Although representing a significant advance over previous methods (stainless steel plates or no plate at all), titanium plate-screw fixation does have some drawbacks. First, titanium devices produce susceptibility artifact, which compromises future MRI studies. Second, titanium implants create a rigid construct, which may predispose to adjacent segment degeneration. Third, despite a low profile design, metal implants can impinge on the esophagus and cause long-term problems with swallowing.

Resorbable polylactide polymers have been used for several human clinical applications, in particular craniofacial fixation. Fixation devices made from these materials would have several theoretical advantages in the cervical spine. Nonmetallic implants create less artifact on MRI, thereby facilitating subsequent spinal imaging. These implants have less stiffness than titanium, possibly decreasing adjacent segment degeneration. Once the fusion is solid, the stabilizing function of the implant is no longer needed. Resorption of the implant would not compromise spinal stability and would eliminate the possibility of late hardware-related complications.

These potential benefits of resorbable plate technology must be balanced against the fact that these devices provide less secure immediate fixation and diminishing long-term fixation as the implant is resorbed. Resorbable plates may have their greatest utility in straightforward one- or two-level procedures, in which deformity correction is not needed. They would not provide adequate structural support for longer constructs or those in which deformity correction is performed. Further clinical experience will be needed to define the specific clinical advantages and disadvantages of the property of implant resorbability.

"Hybrid" techniques of spinal stabilization

The term "hybrid" technique of spinal stabilization is now starting to appear in the spine literature. Two points require emphasis. First, the hybrid technique is not a single procedure, but rather a term which has been loosely applied to a collection of spine procedures. Second, this term does not refer to a new implant, but rather to new methods of combining existing anterior and posterior instrumentation techniques.

One procedure, which has been labeled a hybrid technique, involves the placement of a lumbar disk arthroplasty at one level and a fusion of one or more adjacent levels. This procedure is being developed for the treatment of degenerative disk disease, with the goal being to provide motion preservation at the level of the disk arthroplasty, while eliminating motion at the fused levels.

Another hybrid technique involves the use of anterior instrumentation extending down to the low lumbar spine, coupled with partially overlapping posterior instrumentation extending down to the sacrum. This technique has been described for use in thoracolumbar and lumbar scoliosis.

Surgical management of thoracolumbar and lumbar scoliosis in the adult often involves anterior mobilization of the spine followed by long posterior thoracolumbosacral constructs anchored to the pelvis. The theoretical benefit of the hybrid procedure is that it provides adequate deformity correction, while avoiding long posterior fusion constructs extending from the thoracic spine down to the pelvis. This design may limit the proximal extent of the construct thereby sparing some proximal motion segments, and may also avoid the requirement for fixation of the distal end of the posterior construct to the pelvis.

There are insufficient clinical data on any hybrid technique of spinal stabilization to make any recommendations regarding their use.

Biological vertebral augmentation

Vertebral augmentation with polymethylmethylacrylate (PMMA) is a well established technique for the treatment of vertebral compression fracture (VCF) due to osteoporosis and osteolytic tumors.

This procedure yields significant pain relief in most cases; however, there have been ongoing concerns that PMMA is not the optimal material for the procedure. First, PMMA is an inert, nonbiologic material, which is neither incorporated nor remodeled. Second, PMMA cures through an exothermic reaction, which may impair fracture healing. Third, PMMA may actually prevent fracture healing by preventing contact between fractured bone fragments. Fourth, PMMA is harder than normal cancellous bone, which may predispose the adjacent spinal segments to fracture.

In an effort to overcome the concerns related to PMMA, investigators have developed biological substances which more closely mimic the characteristics of normal bone. An example is Norian SRS (Synthes), an injectable, fast-setting biocompatible calcium phosphate, which hardens in vivo to form carbonated apatite, a substance closely resembling bone. Curing takes place with an isothermic reaction, thereby preventing thermal injury to the surrounding tissue. Norian SRS remodels gradually and is incorporated into the skeleton. At this time, Norian SRS is approved for use only in the extremities and pelvis. Usage in the spine is considered off label, and experience with spinal applications has been limited.

Another risk of PMMA vertebral augmentation relates to the fact that the PMMA is not contained after injection. Thus, the potential exists for PMMA extravasation into the spinal canal and embolus to the lung. These complications are rare, but potentially serious. This has led to a search for alternative methods of delivery that would offer better containment of the PMMA or other material after injection.

The OptiMesh System (Spineology) is a new technology, in which morcellized allograft is placed inside a porous mesh pouch, inside the fractured vertebral body. The pouch serves to prevent extravasation of the injected bone material and allows in growth of native bone to promote actual healing of the fracture. The procedure is done percutaneously, similar to conventional vertebral augmentation. The OptiMesh System is designed for use in the vertebral body, although there has also been some limited experience using the system as an interbody fusion device.

Image guidance and spinal stereotactic surgery

Sophisticated, computer-assisted image guidance systems have been available for intracranial procedures for more than 20 years, and now play an essential role in a variety of neurosurgical procedures, including those for brain tumors and movement disorders.

These techniques have more recently have been modified for spinal applications. The rationale behind image guidance and stereotactic surgery is to provide a level of precision with lesion localization and device placement that cannot be achieved with free hand techniques based on the surgeon's visualization of anatomic landmarks.

The basic steps of spinal stereotactic surgery are as follows:

1. The patient undergoes a thin-cut, "planning" CT or MRI examination. This scan may be done immediately prior to the surgical procedure or several days in advance.
2. The scan is imported into the computer software of the image guidance system.
3. Treatment planning is carried out. In spinal applications, this may involve planning entry points and trajectories for pedicle screws.
4. At the time of surgery, the initial exposure of the area of interest is carried out and a digitizing camera is brought into position. Registration is carried out, which "marries" the position of the spine and various surgical instruments in space with the CT or MRI images, which had been acquired prior to surgery.
5. The surgeon is then able to "navigate" off the imaging study and precisely place instruments and implants in the spine. In practical terms, if the surgeon touches the spine with an instrument, he/she can see exactly where the instrument is on the CT or MRI scan on the monitor. Figure 13.3 depicts a typical screen of information available to the surgeon during image guidance with the BrainLab system. In this example, the system nicely shows the anatomy of the T2 vertebra and assists the surgeon in precisely placing a cannula in the right T2 pedicle. This would be very difficult to accomplish with free hand techniques.

Advantages

The main advantage of image guidance in spinal surgery is that it allows for more accurate placement of pedicle screws and other implanted devices. Image guidance may be used at any level of the spinal column, but is especially helpful during screw placement in the lateral mass of C1, which is a very small

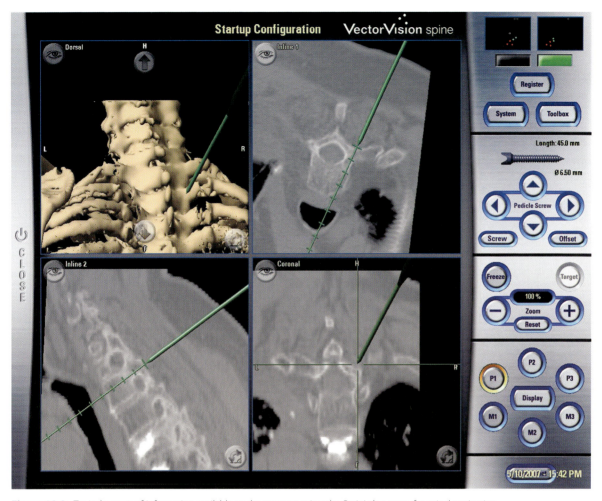

Figure 13.3. Typical screen of information available to the surgeon using the BrainLab system for spinal navigation.

target in close proximity to the spinal cord and vertebral artery, and in the upper thoracic region, where the pedicles are quite small. Image guidance is also useful in the post-surgical spine, where normal anatomic landmarks have been obscured, for example by a large fusion mass. Image guidance allows for more limited surgical approaches and can permit percutaneous placement of pedicle screws and intradiscal devices.

There are two significant limitations of image guidance of the spine. First, the technique is cumbersome, and there is a significant degree of "fiddle factor," even for an experienced surgeon. Second, image guidance in the spine is somewhat less accurate than cranial applications. The inherent mobility of the spine, coupled with the fact that the pre-operative imaging study is generally done with the patient supine while the operation is generally done with the patient prone, tends to degrade the accuracy of

the technique. If major changes in spinal alignment occur during the operation, intentional or otherwise, the pre-operative imaging study is further compromised in terms of being a viable tool for navigation.

These problems may be obviated to some extent by obtaining new planning data during the operation. This may be accomplished in one of two ways.

First, new sophisticated portable fluoroscopic systems, which can produce "CT-like" images, are now becoming available. The main benefit of this technique is that repeated scans can be obtained during the operation to account for changes in spinal alignment and to check implant position as the operation progresses. This technique also eliminates the need for a pre-operative planning scan and a post-operative CT to confirm implant placement.

A second option is intra-operative CT scanning, now available in a small number of centers, which can be used for intra-operative planning of pedicle screws and other implants.

Another advantage of intra-operative scanning, with either the fluoroscopic CT or regular CT scanner, is the ability to assess the adequacy of surgical decompression and spinal alignment during the procedure.

At present, both of these devices are expensive and somewhat difficult to use. Neither technique has been widely adopted at this point, although the future will undoubtedly see further advances in intra-operative spinal imaging.

Assessment of new devices and procedures

As with any medical field, new spinal devices and procedures are often studied first in appropriate animal models, followed by Phase I and II clinical trials to assess safety and efficacy in humans. Phase III trials are then conducted to compare the new technology with some sort of control group.

In the evaluation of new medications, placebo-controlled trials are often carried out, in which the investigational medication is compared with a placebo. For reasons that will be discussed below, placebo- or sham-controlled trials have rarely been conducted for surgical procedures, in particular those used for spinal disorders.

A common approach in clinical spine research is to trial a new device or procedure against a benchmark, or gold standard, treatment. This can be an effective methodology; however, one drawback is that there is sometimes no consensus as to which treatment represents the gold standard treatment.

This uncertainty is reflected by a review of the clinical trials of lumbar disk arthroplasty, in which the artificial disk has been trialed against lumbar fusion. A major problem with design and interpretation of these trials has been the lack of agreement about what procedure should be done in the control group: stand-alone anterior lumbar interbody fusion (ALIF) or 360° circumferential fusion.

The advantage of using a stand-alone ALIF is that it more closely approximates the approach-related morbidity of disk arthroplasty, as both procedures are performed using anterior approaches to the spine. The drawback is that stand-alone ALIF is not currently the procedure of choice for lumbar fusion. Most surgeons now supplement the interbody fusion with pedicle screw fixation, which involves a separate posterior incision.

A 360° circumferential fusion with interbody fusion plus pedicle screw fixation more closely represents the current standard of care in lumbar fusion techniques, but the drawback is that this procedure exposes the patient to morbidity related to a posterior approach to the spinal column, which is not an issue with the disk arthroplasty procedure.

Both procedures have been used in the control group of various trials of disk arthroplasty, and the lack of agreement regarding the optimal control procedure has led to controversy and has hampered critical assessment of the study results.

Trialing a new procedure against an existing procedure may also be problematic if the new procedure is minimally invasive and the existing procedure is done "open." Since the minimally invasive procedure is expected to be safer, with more rapid recuperation, it may be offered to patients earlier in their clinical course. This introduces a bias for patients in the minimally invasive cohort to be less impaired prior to treatment, which in turn would potentially bias study results in favor of the control group.

In these situations, a commonly used strategy is to trial a new device or procedure against nonoperative treatment. A limitation of this strategy is that patients have often failed nonoperative management prior to enrolling in the study. Thus, the patient randomized to nonoperative management would be expected to pursue a course of treatment that has already proven unsuccessful. Furthermore, clinical symptoms may be sufficiently bothersome that the patient may wish to proceed with definitive treatment.

These concerns are partially addressed in some studies by providing 2:1 (instead of 1:1) randomization between the surgical intervention and nonoperative management, thus increasing the odds of the patient being randomized to surgery. In addition, patients randomized to nonoperative treatment are usually given the opportunity to crossover to the surgical arm of the study after an appropriate time interval.

Another difficulty with randomized trials of surgical procedures against nonoperative treatment is that high rates of crossover can greatly compromise study results. Excessive rates of crossover nullify the effects of randomization and invalidate an intent-to-treat analysis. This was seen in the recently published SPORT study, discussed in Chapter 11.

In studies of this type, any delays between randomization and surgery will promote crossover out of the surgical cohort. The study design and logistics should facilitate immediate surgery in patients randomized to receive the surgical procedure. This will minimize crossover out of the surgical cohort, but does not address the problem of early crossover from the nonoperative cohort to surgery.

Sham trials in spine surgery

For some surgical procedures, objective outcome measures are readily available. A good example of this is coronary artery bypass grafting, where surgical mortality is a good estimate of the success of the procedure.

In contrast, with spine procedures, objective outcome measures are harder to come by. Patients rarely die after spine surgery, so mortality rates are not helpful in assessing the benefit of the intervention. Instead, more qualitative measures of outcome, such as pain, function, and patient satisfaction, are generally used. In these situations, it is necessary to distinguish between the effects of the intervention and the effect of the patient's expectation on the intervention, which is known as the placebo effect. Distinguishing between the two requires a trial, in which the patient is blinded as to the type of treatment to be received and then randomized to receive either the intervention of interest or a sham intervention (placebo).

The use of sham controls is well established in studies of new medications. In trials of this type, the patient is blinded and randomized to receive either the study medication or an inactive pill (placebo). There is no risk associated with the placebo, and patient acceptance is generally reasonable.

For a variety of reasons, sham controls have not been widely used in surgical trials. The major concern is that, unlike a placebo medication, a sham surgical procedure does involve some risk to the patient. For example, if the surgical procedure under evaluation requires a general anesthetic, patients receiving the placebo would be exposed to the risk of death, albeit small, from general anesthesia. If an incision is made, the patient is also exposed to a small risk of bleeding and infection. There are additional challenges related to the blinding process in the case of implanted devices, as it is difficult to maintain blinding if the placebo group does not have a device implanted. Finally, patients often have definite expectations of receiving a certain course of treatment, and would be reluctant to accept randomization to a sham procedure. This is particularly true of patients with spinal disorders.

Despite these concerns and limitations, a few surgical trials involving a sham control group have been published. Studies of internal mammary artery ligation for coronary artery disease, arthroscopy for osteoarthritis of the knee, and surgical treatment of Parkinson disease have been conducted with sham controls. Interestingly, in each of these studies, there was no difference in outcome between the active treatment group and the group receiving the sham procedure.

Two spine studies have been conducted with a sham control group. The first was a trial of chymopapain chemonucleolysis for the treatment of symptomatic lumbar disk herniation. In this study, chymopapain injection into the intervertebral disk was compared to placebo injection in a blinded, randomized fashion. The intervention in question, chymopapain, was shown to be superior to placebo injection. These findings gave further support to the use of chymopapain for treatment of lumbar disk herniation. Chemonucleolysis was later abandoned because it was shown to be less effective than microdiscectomy and because of occasional serious neurologic complications and anaphylactic reactions.

The second was a recent study of intradiscal electrothermal therapy (IDET) for discogenic back pain. In this study, patients were randomized to receive thermal treatment of a symptomatic lumbar disk using a heating catheter placed in the disk, or a sham treatment, in which the catheter was placed, but thermal treatment was not applied. The active treatment was found to be superior to sham treatment.

It could be argued that the chymopapain trial was more a study of a medication than a surgical procedure. Nevertheless, this work showed that it is possible to do randomized, placebo-controlled studies of interventions for spinal disorders.

More sham-controlled trials would be useful in spine surgery because the most relevant endpoints (pain, function, and patient satisfaction) are inherently subjective. The potential benefits of sham-controlled trials must be balanced against the potential risks, e.g., death from general anesthesia, the logistical difficulties associated with randomization, and an overall reluctance of patients to participate in such a study.

Government regulation of new devices

In the USA, marketing and distribution of any new medical device requires approval of the Food and Drug Administration (FDA). This is accomplished by one of three pathways. First, the device may be considered to be exempt. Second, the device may require 510(k) approval (premarket notification). Third, the device may require premarket approval (PMA), the most stringent form of review.

Most spine devices are approved via a 510(k) submission, the purpose of which is to demonstrate that the new device is safe and effective, and substantially equivalent to an existing device. One to two years of clinical data are often required for 510(k) approval. Increasingly, the FDA is requiring an additional period of after-market surveillance by the manufacturer. For example, following approval of a new device via the 510(k) process, the FDA may require that all patients implanted with the device be followed for five additional years, with those follow-up data being provided to the FDA.

Conclusions

There have been numerous technological advances in spine surgery over the last decade, including lumbar and cervical disk arthroplasty, biological materials to promote spinal fusion, and computer-assisted spinal stereotactic surgery. Disk nucleus replacement is in the development stage, and annular repair appears to be a promising new technique. Spine technology is changing rapidly, and there will undoubtedly be more advances in the near future.

Further reading

1. Ames CP, Chamberlain RH, Cornwall GB, et al. Feasibility of a resorbable anterior cervical graft containment plate. *BNI Q* 2003; **19**:1–8.

2. Bindal RK, Ghosh S, Foldi B. Resorbable anterior cervical plates for single-level degenerative disc disease. *Neurosurgery* 2007; **61** (Suppl 2):ONS 305–ONS 310.

3. Boachie-Adjei O, Charles G, Cunningham ME. Partially overlapping limited anterior and posterior instrumentation for adult thoracolumbar and lumbar scoliosis: a description of novel spinal instrumentation, "the hybrid technique." *HSS J* 2007; **3**:93–98.

4. Bridwell KH, Anderson PA, Boden SD, et al. What's new in spine surgery? *J Bone Joint Surg* 2006; **88-A**:1897–1907.

5. Mummaneni PV, Burkus JK, Haid RW, Traynelis VC, Zdeblick TA. Clinical and radiographic analysis of cervical disc arthroplasty compared with allograft fusion: a randomized controlled clinical trial. *J Neurosurg Spine* 2007; **6**:198–209.

6. Nishida K, Kang JD, Gilbertson LG, et al. 1999 Volvo award winner in basic science studies: modulation of the biologic activity of the rabbit intervertebral disc by gene therapy: an *in vivo* study of adenovirus-transforming growth factor [beta]1 encoding gene. *Spine* 1999; **24**:2419–2425.

7. Ruan D, He Q, Ding Y, Hou L, Li J, Luk KDK. Intervertebral disc transplantation in the treatment of degenerative spine disease: a preliminary study. *Lancet* 2007; **369**:993–999.

8. Shapiro MD. MR imaging of the spine at 3T. *Magn Reson Imaging Clin N Am* 2006; **14**:97–108.

9. Traynelis VC. Cervical arthroplasty. *Clin Neurosurg* 2006; **53**:203–207.

10. Vadala G, Sowa GA, Smith L, et al. Regulation of transgene expression using an inducible system for improved safety of intervertebral disc gene therapy. *Spine* 2007; **32**:1381–1387.

11. Yuan PS, Day TF, Albert TJ, Morrison WB, Pimenta L, Cragg A, Weinstein M. Anatomy of the percutaneous space for a novel fusion technique. *J Spinal Disord Tech* 2006; **19**:237–241.

12. Zigler J, Delamarter R, Spivak JM, et al. Results of the prospective, randomized, multicenter Food and Drug Administration Investigational Device Exemption study of the ProDisc-L total disc replacement versus circumferential fusion for the treatment of 1-level degenerative disc disease. *Spine* 2007; **32**:1155–1162.

Medical management of the spine surgery patient: pre-operative, intra-operative, and post-operative considerations

Pre-operative medical evaluation

Any patient undergoing elective spinal surgery should have a pre-operative medical evaluation, to ensure that the patient is in optimal medical condition to undergo the planned surgical procedure. Currently, there is a trend toward "same day" admissions and outpatient surgical procedures, which increases the risk of a hurried and inadequate evaluation. However, this does not obviate the need for pre-operative medical clearance. Furthermore, with more complex operations being offered to older patients with more medical co-morbidities, a careful medical assessment is more important than ever.

The pre-operative medical evaluation is a surgically oriented process concerned with identifying and treating any significant medical illnesses which would make the surgical procedure unsafe. For many patients, this evaluation represents their first assessment of cardiovascular risk factors and other health concerns. Thus, the pre-operative medical evaluation often provides the initial diagnosis of significant, chronic illnesses, such as diabetes mellitus, hypertension, and hyperlipidemia, which require life-long treatment. In these situations, the pre-operative medical evaluation provides long-term benefits for the patient, well beyond enhancing the safety of the surgical procedure.

The extent of the evaluation is determined by the patient's age, general health, and type of surgery. Healthy patients do not require an extensive workup. Minimal testing is needed (Table 14.1). In contrast, patients with unstable cardiovascular disease, bleeding disorders, significant pulmonary disease, uncontrolled diabetes mellitus, uncontrolled hypertension, renal disease, or liver disease require more extensive evaluation. In these situations, consultation with a cardiologist or other medical specialist may be needed.

Depending on the clinical context, identification of a significant new medical problem may result in postponing the spine procedure until the medical issue is fully addressed. An example of this would be a 70-year-old man scheduled for elective lumbar laminectomy for spinal stenosis, who is found to have unstable angina with severe coronary artery disease during his pre-operative medical evaluation. A likely scenario for this patient would be to proceed directly to coronary stenting or bypass surgery, with spinal surgery being deferred until his cardiac status is stabilized.

Another role of the pre-operative medical evaluation is to review all chronic medical problems to ensure that they are stable and being optimally managed.

The American Society of Anesthesiologists (ASA) has developed a classification system, which stratifies risks according to physical status (Table 14.2). This system does not take into account the surgical procedure and is not designed to predict outcome. Nevertheless, it has been shown to correlate well with peri-operative morbidity and mortality.

Management of anti-coagulant and anti-platelet medications

A wide range of medications and herbal supplements affect blood clotting and can cause potentially serious surgical site bleeding. At the pre-operative visit, an accurate listing of anti-coagulant and anti-platelet medications must be obtained. These include both prescription medications, such as warfarin (Coumadin) and clopidogrel (Plavix), and nonprescription medications, such as aspirin, ibuprofen and other nonsteroidal anti-inflammatory medications, and vitamin E. Clopidogrel, which is being used with increasing frequency in the USA for cardiac and cerebrovascular disease, is especially dangerous, because it is a platelet inhibitory agent, which cannot be effectively reversed.

Patients should also be asked about herbal supplements, as many of these substances have anti-coagulant properties or potentiate the effects of other anti-coagulant medications, notably ginkgo biloba and ginger.

All anti-coagulant and anti-platelet medications must be stopped prior to elective spinal surgery. The

Table 14.1. Suggested laboratory tests for healthy patients undergoing elective spinal surgery

Age	Tests suggested
Under 50	None
50–59	ECG
60 and over	CBC, ECG, creatinine, glucose

Notes:
A CBC is indicated for all patients who are typed and screened.
A potassium is indicated for all patients taking diuretics.
A chest X-ray is indicated for patients with a history of cardiac or pulmonary disease or recent respiratory symptoms.
CBC, complete blood count; ECG, electrocardiogram.

Table 14.2. ASA classification of physical status

Disease state	ASA class
No organic, physiologic, biochemical, or psychiatric disturbance	1
Mild to moderate systemic disturbance	2
Severe systemic disturbance	3
Severe systemic disturbance that is a constant threat to life	4
Moribund patient, likely to die with or without surgery	5
Brain dead organ donor	6

duration of action of clopidogrel and other anti-platelet medications is 10–14 days, which is the lifespan of the platelet. Therefore anti-platelet medications should be stopped 2 weeks in advance of surgery.

Warfarin should be stopped long enough for the international normalized ratio (INR) to normalize. This typically takes 5–7 days, but can vary significantly from one patient to the next, depending on the baseline INR and other factors. If the patient is at high risk of an embolic event while off warfarin, heparin or enoxaparin sodium (Lovenox) can be used on a short-term basis prior to surgery. Consultation with a cardiologist may be necessary to stratify the risk of stopping warfarin and determine whether heparin or enoxaparin should be used.

If a patient on warfarin requires urgent or emergent spine surgery, warfarin can be reversed in several ways. If immediate surgery is not needed, warfarin can be reversed by administering vitamin K and fresh frozen plasma (FFP), with close monitoring of the INR. This process may take hours to days. Fluid balance should be monitored closely. If FFP is administered too rapidly, fluid overload and congestive heart failure may ensue. This is a particular concern in the elderly and in those with pre-existing cardiac disease.

If surgery must be performed emergently, warfarin can be immediately reversed with recombinant factor VII (Novo-7). The recommended dose ranges from 15 to 90 µg/kg. Administration results in immediate normalization of the INR. Coagulation studies must be followed closely, as the half-life of Novo-7 is only 2.6 hours. This means that the patient will often require additional doses of Novo-7 and/or FFP during and after the surgical procedure.

Novo-7 is an expensive medication; its cost is approximately $1100 per 1.2-mg vial in the USA. However, it is the only medication that can immediately reverse the effects of warfarin and facilitate emergency surgery on fully anti-coagulated patients. For this reason, the benefits of Novo-7 justify the costs in these situations.

Following percutaneous procedures, anti-coagulant and anti-platelet medications may be resumed within 1–2 days after surgery. When open spinal surgery has been performed, these medications should be withheld for 5–7 days post-operatively. The reason for the additional time in the latter group is the presence of dead space in the wound, which could promote the development of a hematoma at the surgical site. This is potentially a greater concern in patients with spinal instrumentation, as the implanted devices create even more dead space at the surgical site.

Beta-blockers

Beta-blockers have been shown to decrease cardiovascular risks in patients undergoing noncardiac surgical procedures. Beta-blocker therapy should be considered for patients with cardiac risk factors, including history of coronary artery disease, previous myocardial infarction, stable angina, symptomatic arrhythmia, compensated heart failure, positive cardiac stress test, age >65 years, hypertension, current smoker, hyperlipidemia, diabetes mellitus, poor functional status, chronic renal disease, peripheral vascular disease, and previous stroke.

Recommended agents include atenolol, bisoprolol, or metoprolol, taken orally whenever possible. Intravenous beta-blockers can be used for patients not able to take tablets orally and for those requiring urgent or emergent surgery.

Beta-blocker therapy should be started within 7 days of surgery and continued for 30 days post-operatively. At that point, follow-up should be obtained with the patient's primary care physician or cardiologist, to determine the advisability of continuing treatment on a long-term basis.

Contraindications include severe bradycardia (heart rate <50 beats per minute), second- or third-degree heart block, severe chronic obstructive pulmonary disease, decompensated heart failure, and allergy to beta-blockers. Beta-blockers should be used cautiously in patients taking calcium channel blockers, and in those with reactive airway disease, mild heart failure, and mild to moderate chronic obstructive pulmonary disease.

Prophylactic antibiotics

Prophylactic antibiotics are routinely used in patients undergoing spinal surgery. The optimal antibiotic regimen would have the following characteristics:

1. active against the most common wound pathogens
2. safe
3. inexpensive
4. adequate tissue levels present during the entire time the wound is open
5. smallest impact possible on the patient's normal bacterial flora

The organisms of greatest concern are aerobic Gram-positive cocci, including *Staphylococcus aureus* (coagulase-positive staphylococcus) and *Staphylococcus epidermidis* (coagulase-negative staphylococcus).

The choice of antibiotic must take into account local susceptibility patterns, which vary widely among communities and individual hospitals. In many hospitals, a cephalosporin, such as cefazolin, is the agent of choice, with clindamycin or vancomycin being alternative choices if the patient has a beta-lactam allergy. In some facilities, vancomycin is the agent of choice, based on local susceptibility patterns.

The timing of administration is very important, in order to ensure that adequate tissue levels are present during the procedure. Infusion of cefazolin or clindamycin should begin within 1 h of the incision and should be completed before the skin incision is made. Vancomycin requires a longer infusion time in order to avoid hypotension and flushing of the face, neck, and upper torso (red man syndrome), which can occur if the medication is infused too rapidly. Therefore it is recommended that vancomycin infusion begin 2 h prior to the incision, with completion of the infusion before the incision is made.

Typical dosing for cefazolin is 1 g IV prior to surgery, with re-dosing every 6 h during the procedure.

The usual dosing of vancomycin is 1 g IV prior to surgery, with re-dosing every 12 h during the procedure.

There is no consensus on how long to continue antibiotics following the operation. Acceptable strategies include:

1. No further antibiotics after the operation is completed
2. One additional dose after the operation
3. Continuing antibiotics for 24 h post-operatively
4. Continuing antibiotics until all surgical drains are removed

There is general agreement that prophylactic antibiotics should not be continued after removal of surgical drains.

Deep venous thrombosis/pulmonary embolism – prophylaxis

Deep venous thrombosis (DVT) with its potential for life-threatening pulmonary embolus (PE) is a risk in patients undergoing spinal surgery. This risk is increased in obese, immobile patients undergoing lengthy operations and in those with significant neurologic deficits.

In an effort to prevent this complication, several measures are recommended. Thigh-high TED hose and pneumatic compression stockings should be applied prior to surgery. These devices should be used intra-operatively and continued post-operatively until the time of discharge. Another key factor is to mobilize the patient as soon as possible after surgery.

Prophylactic anti-coagulation, for example with subcutaneous heparin, is frequently used in hospitalized patients, but is contraindicated in spine surgery patients due to the risk of surgical site bleeding.

Deep venous thrombosis/pulmonary embolism – treatment

Despite preventive measures, DVT can occur in the early post-operative period. The clinical hallmark of DVT is a red, warm, swollen, tender extremity. When DVT is suspected clinically, diagnostic ultrasound should be performed. If DVT is confirmed, treatment should be instituted promptly in order to prevent pulmonary embolism (PE).

Pulmonary embolism can occur in the post-operative spine patient, and its presence should be suspected in the patient with acute shortness of breath, chest pain, tachycardia, and hypoxemia. The diagnosis is confirmed with CT scanning.

Anti-coagulation is the recommended treatment for acute DVT and PE; however, these medications must be used cautiously in patients with recent spinal surgery. It is not possible to provide any precise guidelines on when it is safe to institute anti-coagulation following spine surgery. These decisions have to be individualized, taking into account the type of surgery, extent of dissection, amount of dead space, surgical drains, and medical condition of the patient.

Deep venous thrombosis or PE in the very early post-operative period represents a very high-risk situation, as the risk of surgical site bleeding from anti-coagulation is substantial. If DVT or PE occurs within 5 days of surgery, one possible strategy is to place an inferior vena cava (IVC) filter and defer anti-coagulation until the risk of surgical site bleeding is diminished.

If DVT or PE occurs beyond the fifth post-operative day, the decision making process is more straight-forward. By that point, the risk of surgical site bleeding is generally lower, and full anti-coagulation may be instituted.

Blood products and intra-operative transfusion

Because of limitations in the supply of banked blood and the costs involved, blood should be typed and crossmatched in advance only if there is a high likelihood that transfusion will be required. An example of this would be a multi-level thoracolumbar fusion with instrumentation, anticipated to last for several hours. Another situation in which crossmatched blood should be available is when there is a risk of sudden, high volume blood loss, for example during the surgical approach to a vascular tumor or a tumor encasing the vertebral artery.

For cases where significant blood loss may occur, but rapid blood loss is not anticipated, an order to type and screen the blood is often appropriate. An example of this would be lumbar decompressive laminectomy for spinal stenosis or a short segment lumbar fusion. If transfusion is required, the blood bank should be able to supply crossmatched blood within 30 minutes. If the patient has significant anemia at baseline, it may be appropriate to have crossmatched blood available, even if significant blood loss is not expected.

For percutaneous and minimally invasive procedures, where significant blood loss is not anticipated, it is not necessary to type and screen the patient in advance.

If emergency transfusion is needed and cross-matched blood is not available, Type O, Rh-negative blood can be administered.

If rapid or high-volume blood loss is anticipated, a Cell Saver system (Haemonetics, Braintree, MA) can be employed. These systems retrieve blood shed from the surgical site and prepare it for re-infusion into the patient. It is not cost-effective to use these systems routinely, especially when significant blood loss is not expected. The Cell Saver system should not be used in cases of spinal tumor or infection.

Informed consent

Before any spine surgery is performed, informed consent must be obtained from the patient. Informed consent is a process through which the patient is informed about the diagnosis and planned surgical procedure, including potential benefits, risks, limitations, and alternatives to surgery. Many hospitals have a written consent form, which is to be signed by the patient and the surgeon; however, the key element of the process is the discussion that takes place between the surgeon and the patient, and the documentation of this discussion in the patient's medical record.

It is essential that the surgeon discuss the procedure in simple terms that can be understood by the patient. The use of anatomic models is often helpful in this process. It is also important to inform the patient of any specific factors which would increase his/her risks, relative to the general population of patients undergoing the same procedure. Examples include diabetes mellitus, smoking, prior surgery, osteoporosis, severe baseline neurologic deficit, and significant medical illnesses. If possible, family members or close friends should also be present for this discussion.

For a straightforward problem, informed consent can often be obtained at the first visit, and the patient can proceed immediately to surgery. For more complex situations, several visits may be required. In some cases, a second opinion consultation with another neurosurgeon may be helpful.

Jehovah's Witnesses represent a special circumstance, and the informed consent process for these patients must be considered very carefully. Individuals practicing this religion do not accept transfusion of blood products, including whole blood, packed red blood cells, plasma, and platelets; however, some of these individuals will accept albumin and clotting factors. Jehovah's Witnesses do not accept transfusion of predeposited autologous blood. Some accept blood retrieved and re-infused through a Cell Saver system, while others do not. Pre-operative administration of erythropoietin (EPO), a medication used to treat anemia associated with chronic renal disease, may be an option in some cases. There is some evidence of an increased risk of thrombotic events in patients receiving EPO, therefore the decision to use this medication should be considered carefully.

Hypotensive anesthesia should also be considered, as there is some evidence that controlled hypotension during the surgical procedure decreases surgical blood loss by as much as 40%. Hypotensive anesthesia may also result in shorter operative times.

Enthusiasm for hypotensive anesthesia should be tempered by the observation in one study of lumbar fusion that most of the blood loss occurred during decortication of bony surfaces prior to placement of bone grafts. Bone bleeding is venous in origin and would not be altered by manipulations of arterial blood pressure.

As a part of the pre-operative discussion and informed consent process, it is imperative that the surgeon have a detailed discussion with the patient about the risks of declining transfusion, the situations (if any) in which the patient would consider transfusion as a life-saving measure, and whether the patient would accept the use of a Cell Saver system during the procedure.

The surgeon and patient must carefully weigh the benefits and risks of surgery performed without access to blood products. If risks outweigh benefits, the procedure may have to be deferred.

Intra-operative management
Surgical site bleeding and hemostasis

The surgeon can generally anticipate the volume of intra-operative blood loss fairly accurately, based on the spinal disorder being treated, the type of procedure being performed, and the medical status of the patient.

For surgery in the prone position, especially thoracic and lumbar procedures, the patient should be carefully positioned to allow the abdomen to hang freely. This is important because if the abdomen is resting on the operating table, intra-abdominal pressure is increased, leading to increased epidural venous pressure and sometimes copious epidural bleeding. All frames and operating tables used in spinal surgery are designed to prevent pressure on the abdomen.

It is extremely important to carefully monitor blood loss as the operation progresses. Several members of the surgical team have a role to play in this process. The surgeon is in the best position to observe bleeding at the surgical site, while the anesthesiologist should be alert for changes in hemodynamic status, which may indicate significant blood loss. The anesthesiologist and circulating nurse should closely monitor blood volumes accumulating in drainage canisters in the operating room. Depending on the estimated blood loss, hemoglobin and hematocrit levels are measured as needed. As a general guideline, an estimated blood loss exceeding 500 ml should prompt measurement of hemoglobin and hematocrit.

Venous bleeding from the paraspinous musculature is usually easily controlled with bipolar and unipolar coagulation. Epidural venous bleeding is managed with bipolar coagulation and gentle application of topical hemostatic agents such as Gelfoam (absorbable gelatin compressed sponge, Pfizer, New York, NY) or Avitene (microfibrillar collagen hemostat, multiple companies). Bone bleeding is controlled with bone wax. If it not excessive, bone bleeding can be controlled with the high speed drill using the fine diamond drill bit. This technique generates heat and stops bleeding by coagulating bleeding bone surfaces.

The incision should be no longer than necessary to perform the operation. Exposure and dissection of the paraspinal soft tissues should be limited as much as possible in order to minimize bleeding from these structures.

Unexpected blood loss should prompt an immediate response by the surgical team. For surgery in the prone position, the patient should be checked to ensure that the abdomen is hanging freely. Any pressure on the abdomen should be corrected by repositioning the patient as needed. If arterial bleeding is identified, the source should be immediately identified and controlled.

A source of potentially catastrophic hemorrhage rarely seen during lumbar microdiscectomy is great vessel injury. Overly aggressive use of pituitary rongeurs and other instruments deep within the interspace can breach the anterior longitudinal ligament and cause injury to the aorta, vena cava, and iliac vessels. Brisk arterial bleeding arising from the interspace may herald this complication. If this is suspected, the lumbar wound should be immediately closed or packed open, and the patient should be positioned supine for laparotomy. A general or vascular surgeon should be requested for immediate abdominal exploration.

It should also be emphasized that a great vessel injury, which occurs during a posterior approach, may produce little or no bleeding into the surgical field if the blood is contained in the retroperitoneal space. Thus, the finding of unexplained hypotension and hypovolemia should prompt consideration of great vessel injury, even if there is no significant bleeding in the surgical field.

Patients requiring transfusion are almost always given packed red blood cells, as whole blood is now rarely used in the USA. Transfusion of multiple units of blood can lead to a coagulopathy secondary to thrombocytopenia and a deficiency of clotting factors, as packed red blood cells are devoid of platelets and clotting factors. Thus, patients requiring more than 5 units of packed red blood cells should also receive platelets and FFP. If surgical site bleeding persists, desmopressin (DDAVP), cryoprecipitate, and recombinant factor 7 (Novo-7) may also be helpful.

Threshold for transfusion

Historically, patients undergoing spine surgery were not transfused until the hemoglobin had fallen to a level of 7–8 g/dl. In the absence of significant ischemic heart disease, hemoglobin levels in this range are generally well tolerated.

Transfusion practice is now evolving with the recent recognition of the syndrome of post-operative blindness, which appears to be related, in part, to inadequate blood replacement (see Chapter 11). As a result, there is a trend toward earlier transfusion of the spine surgery patient. For example, some surgeons and anesthesiologists now recommend that the patient be transfused to maintain the hemoglobin level above 10 g/dl during the surgical procedure.

Post-operative management
Post-operative analgesia

Post-operative analgesia requirements vary widely depending on the type of surgery being performed, and the patient's psychological makeup and pre-operative analgesic usage. Patients undergoing minimally invasive procedures, who have taken little or no narcotic analgesics prior to surgery, may not need any narcotics at all following their surgical procedures. In contrast, patients on chronic high-dose opioids often have greatly magnified pain, with

Table 14.3. Typical post-operative analgesia regimen

Parenteral narcotic	Hydromorphone (Dilaudid) 1–2 mg IV every 4 h or morphine sulfate 2–4 mg IV every 4 h as needed for pain.
Oral narcotic	Oxycodone/acetaminophen 5/325 (Percocet) 1–2 tablets by mouth every 4 h or hydrocodone/acetaminophen 5/500 (Lortab) 1–2 tablets by mouth every 4 h as needed for pain.
Non-narcotic analgesic	Acetaminophen 325 mg 1–2 tablets by mouth every 4 h as needed for pain.
Muscle relaxant	Cyclobenzaprine (Flexeril) 10 mg 1 tablet by mouth every 8 h or methocarbamol (Robaxin) 500 mg 1 tablet every 6 hours as needed for muscle spasm.

correspondingly high narcotic analgesic requirements, regardless of the surgical procedure.

Post-operative analgesia orders should include a parenteral narcotic, an oral narcotic, a non-narcotic analgesic, and a muscle relaxant, all to be used on an as-needed basis. A typical parenteral narcotic regimen is shown in Table 14.3.

A short course of parenteral or oral steroids is often helpful for acute post-operative radicular pain. Steroids should be used cautiously in diabetic patients, as these medications aggravate hyperglycemia.

Intravenous ketorolac (Toradol) is a potent non-steroidal anti-inflammatory agent, which may also be useful for acute post-operative pain. Ketorolac is contraindicated in patients with renal failure and may also precipitate surgical site bleeding.

Patient controlled analgesia (PCA) is a protocol by which the patient administers his or her own analgesia. PCA utilizes an electronically controlled infusion pump, which delivers an intravenous bolus of a narcotic analgesic, usually hydromorphone, morphine, or fentanyl, when the patient activates a button. The PCA pump can be programmed for bolus doses of narcotic, a continuous infusion of narcotics, or a combination of bolus doses and continuous infusion.

The main advantage of the PCA system is that the patient controls his or her analgesic regimen and can administer a dose of medication as soon as pain is noted. The amount of narcotic used is precisely measured and is a useful tool for the surgical team and nursing staff to gauge the patient's pain level from one day to the next.

The physician prescribes the amount of each bolus dose and time interval between doses (lockout interval). This lockout time is a safety measure, which prevents the patient from receiving an overdose of narcotics as a result of attempting to self-medicate too often. Patients using a PCA pump should be monitored with continuous pulse oximetry.

The major risk of the PCA pump is narcotic overdose due to dosing error, pump malfunction, or excessive use of the pump. This is a potentially fatal complication. The potential risks and benefits of using a PCA pump should be carefully considered on a case-by-case basis.

Activity

One of the keys to a successful outcome after spine surgery is rapid mobilization of the patient. Historically, spine surgery patients were maintained on bedrest for several days post-operatively; however, the current approach is to encourage ambulation as soon as possible.

Young, healthy patients undergoing limited procedures, such as single-level lumbar microdiscectomy, should be able to ambulate within a few hours of surgery, and will likely have very limited needs for formal post-operative rehabilitation.

Elderly patients undergoing lumbar laminectomy for spinal stenosis would be expected to progress more slowly, but are frequently able to ambulate the day of surgery. Physical therapy should be instituted immediately following surgery, and continued after dismissal from the hospital. Home physical therapy is often appropriate, and a short course of inpatient rehabilitation may be useful in selected cases.

For more complex procedures with extensive muscle dissection and blood loss, such as lumbar fusion with instrumentation, it may be appropriate to keep the patient on bedrest overnight, and begin ambulation on the first post-operative day.

Patients undergoing intradural surgery and those in whom an inadvertent cerebrospinal fluid (CSF) leak is encountered during the procedure may need a short period of bedrest. These patients were traditionally maintained on strict bedrest for several days. However, with new tissue sealants and other techniques for dural repair, there is a trend toward shorter periods of bedrest. In some cases, bedrest may not be necessary at all, if the surgeon is confident that a good dural closure was obtained.

When straightforward anterior and posterior cervical decompressions for radiculopathy are performed, the patient may ambulate immediately following the procedure.

Patients undergoing surgery for cervical spondylotic myelopathy require particular attention. This disorder can result in impaired autoregulation of spinal cord blood flow; and there is some risk of cord ischemia and quadriparesis due to postural hypotension when the patient assumes the upright position. This can be exacerbated if the patient is anemic and/or dehydrated. These patients should be mobilized very cautiously, and, in many cases, should be kept on bedrest until the first post-operative day. Anemia should be corrected and appropriate fluid replacement should be carried out before permitting ambulation. If the patient becomes quadriparetic while ambulating, he or she should immediately be placed flat in bed.

Rehabilitation

Post-operative rehabilitation is an important component of recovery from spinal surgery. Rehabilitation needs are dictated by pre-operative neurologic and functional status, medical co-morbidities, age, and extent of surgery. The physical therapist should do a "needs assessment" at the first post-operative visit to determine functional goals, evaluate the need for a walker or other assistive device, and outline a rehabilitation program. The occupational therapist should be involved if the upper extremities are affected, as in the case of cervical spondylotic myelopathy. The occupational therapist can also help with dressing and other activities of daily living. Patients with traumatic spinal cord injury should be transferred to a spinal cord injury rehabilitation facility as soon as their acute management is completed.

Return to work following spinal surgery

Decisions about return to work are based on the patient's occupation, pre-operative neurologic deficit, and type of surgery. A young healthy patient with minimal baseline neurologic deficit, undergoing lumbar microdiscectomy should be able to return to work within 2–4 weeks. Physically demanding occupations may require a longer recovery time. Patients undergoing lumbar fusion will need to be off work for 4–6 months.

For patients undergoing anterior cervical discectomy and fusion for radiculopathy, return to work is dictated, to a large extent, by how long they have to wear a hard cervical collar, typically 4–8 weeks. Because there is no need to wear a hard collar post-operatively, patients receiving a cervical disk arthroplasty can return to work sooner, often within 2–3 weeks.

Further reading

1. Berg C, Berger DH, Makia A, et al. Perioperative beta-blocker therapy and heart rate control during noncardiac surgery. *Am J Surg* 2007; **194**:189–191.

2. Fletcher S, Lam AM. Anesthesia: preoperative evaluation. In: *Youmans Neurological Surgery*, Winn HR ed. Philadelphia: Saunders, 2004, pp. 547–560.

3. Gause PR, Siska PA, Westrick ER, et al. Efficacy of intraoperative Cell Saver in decreasing postoperative blood transfusions in instrumented posterior lumbar fusion patients. *Spine* 2008; **33**:571–575.

4. Greenberg MS. *Handbook of Neurosurgery*, Sixth Edition. New York: Thieme, 2006.

5. Hines RL, Marschall KE, eds. *Stoelting's Anesthesia and Co-existing Disease*, Fifth Edition. Philadelphia: Churchill Livingstone, 2008.

6. Lubin MF, ed. *Medical Management of the Surgical Patient: A Textbook of Perioperative Medicine.* Cambridge: Cambridge University Press, 2006.

7. Mayer SA, Brun NC, Begtrup K, et al. Recombinant activated factor VII for acute intracerebral hemorrhage. *New Engl J Med* 2005; **352**:777–785.

8. O'Leary JP, Tabuenca A, eds. *The Physiologic Basis of Surgery*, Fourth Edition. Philadelphia: Lippincott Williams & Wilkins, 2008.

9. Sachs B, Delacy D, Green J, et al. Recombinant activated factor VII in spinal surgery: a multicenter, randomized, double-blind, placebo-controlled, dose-escalation trial. *Spine* 2007; **32**:2285–2293.

10. Shamji MF, Cook C, Tackett S, et al. Impact of preoperative neurological status on perioperative morbidity associated with anterior and posterior cervical fusion. *J Neurosurg Spine* 2008; **9**:10–16.

Appendix: Please don't make my mistakes

Introduction

No one in any line of work wants to make mistakes. We hate to make mistakes and do our utmost to avoid them. This is especially true in healthcare where mistakes can lead to serious adverse health consequences including death, to sanctions by our peers and state medical board, and to lawsuits with resulting deep personal anguish and substantial financial consequences. After more than 35 years of seeing patients, I have made my share of mistakes. Despite my best efforts, I am sure that I will continue to make errors. I have learned something from my experience and would like to share my observations with you in this chapter. Our editor does not like us to use the first person in our writing. Since this chapter is based on personal experience, I have convinced her that it is appropriate and necessary for me to use the first person. The potential errors will be presented in the order in which they are made in patient care: the history, the examination, patient preferences, diagnostic testing, and treatment (see Table A1).

Mistakes I have made in taking a history

Not listening to the patient or asking the right questions

The patient's history is the key to diagnosis in all of medicine and even more so in spine care. Failure to listen to the patient and their family and truly understand the patient's symptoms and their evolution is a sure path to the wrong diagnosis. The history consists of more than just what the patient and their family tell us. We must ask the right questions. For example, the patient may be embarrassed to tell us about bowel or bladder control problems or they may not think that sphincter disturbance could be related to their spine problem. Unfortunately, taking a good history requires time, and there are many pressures on providers to shorten rather than lengthen the time they spend with patients and their families.

Not getting the straight story

There are instances when the patient gives us insufficient information, exaggerated information, the wrong information, or false information. These situations increase the degree of difficulty of taking a history. They are not the patient's fault, except in those rare circumstances of malingering where the patient is overtly lying to us. Some patients are vague in their answers or tangential in their replies. Some patients are not very aware of their symptoms. Other patients think that we are more interested in the results of tests or treatments or advice from other providers. These elements are important, but not as important as the patient's symptoms. Some patients report what they believe to be the mechanism of their symptoms ("I've got a pinched nerve in my neck") instead of the symptoms that have led them to their conclusion. Usually we can tease out the patient's own symptoms, but it can be difficult and time consuming to do so.

Too many symptoms

Some patients overwhelm us with too many symptoms. These patients can be frustrating, and I personally find that I tend to get angry with patients who have what I feel are too many complaints. In this setting, we need to hear out the patient and try to separate the "wheat from the chaff" and rely more on our examination and perhaps on diagnostic testing. Many patients with multiple complaints are symptom-prone and may have a somatoform disorder. Doctors talk about these patients as being "functional" by which we mean that they do not have organic disease accounting for their symptoms. Unfortunately, patients who are symptom prone, who have somatoform disorders, or who are "functional" also get real disease affecting their spine and other organs. These patients need to be seen frequently to make sure that they are not developing serious problems and to protect them from too many tests and risky tests and interventions. Symptom-prone patients typically continue to report multiple evolving symptoms over time and are rarely cured. Caring for these patients is necessary but not gratifying.

265

Table A1. Mistakes made in patient care

In the history
  Not listening to the patient or asking the right questions
  Not getting the straight story
  Too many symptoms
On examination
  Taking shortcuts
  Over-interpreting and under-interpreting uncertain findings
    Give way weakness
    Sensory loss
  Peripheral tenderness
Patient and provider biases
  "We have to do something"
  "I just want an answer"
  "It's only a disk"
  "I'm not interested in surgery on my spine"
  "Doctor, I'm not one who likes to take a lot of pills"
In diagnostic testing
  Premature investigation
  Over-reliance on diagnostic test results
In diagnosis and treatment
  Rush to judgment
  The need to make a diagnosis
  Influenced by experience
  Jumping to conclusions
  Clinging to a diagnosis
  Attributing a peripheral process to a spine disorder
  Attributing spine-related symptoms to a peripheral process
  Going against and going along with the previous diagnosis
  Considering the possibility of more than one "lesion" or disease
  Failure to remember the natural history of the disease
  Failure to recognize the limits of treatment
  Failure to consider all available treatment options
Interacting with patients
  Failure to obtain and incorporate patient and family preferences
  Telling the patient what they want to hear
  Blaming the patient

I put so much reliance on the patient's history that there is one additional circumstance where I have made major mistakes. While infrequent, some patients report that they are getting better, when, in fact, they are getting worse. These patients are very

sincere when they report that they are improving. I suspect that their perception of improvement is based on hope and wishful thinking rather than on any objective observation. These patients want to get better, but they are not. To my regret, I have taken them at their word and often I have not re-examined them, and my mistake has only become apparent when the patient's deterioration is painfully obvious or is brought to my attention by their family or my colleagues. Corroborating history from family members and re-examination can help to prevent this kind of mistake.

Mistakes I have made in the examination of a patient
Taking shortcuts

I have gotten into trouble when I have taken shortcuts, conscious or subconscious, and failed to conduct a pertinent physical and/or neurologic examination. This can occur in the setting where the patient reports that they have no weakness or numbness, and I take them at their word, only to later find out that they did have significant weakness or sensory loss that they had not noticed. Conversely, the patient may report significant weakness or sensory loss, but on examination none is found. Patients often report that their limb is weak as well as painful when their perceived weakness is entirely due to the pain provoked by attempted use. I offer the example of the person with a broken leg who will not bear any weight on the limb, but whose strength is intact because there has been no damage to the nerves or muscles.

Sometimes in my sloppiness and hurry, I have not fully examined patients because I thought I knew what was wrong. Recently, I saw a patient with standing- and walking-induced proximal greater than distal pain from the hip down in the front and back of one lower limb. She brought with her an outside MRI scan that showed severe lumbar spinal stenosis, and I assumed that her asymmetrically narrowed lumbar spinal canal was responsible for her apparent pseudoclaudication. I did not check hip range of motion, which was severely limited and painful on her symptomatic side. Fortunately, the plain X-rays of her lumbar spine that I ordered and the spine surgeon to whom I referred her both noted bone-on-bone osteoarthritis of her right hip, which was contributing to her symptoms, and, in fact, probably the main source of her pain.

Over-interpreting and under-interpreting uncertain findings

Fortunately, the neurologic and musculoskeletal examinations provide us with some objective information to help determine if there is genuine weakness, reflex change, muscle spasm, altered range of motion, or provocative signs (such as straight leg raise testing) that help determine the presence or absence of significant spine disease. The patient who gives way on muscle strength testing presents us with a dilemma: are they truly weak or is their muscle strength really normal and they are just giving way because of pain, lack of understanding, an underlying functional disorder, or even malingering? In the past, I used to make a judgment whether or not the give way weakness was genuine or false. My guesswork was sometimes wrong, and I made mistakes. As mentioned in an earlier chapter, I think it is better to interpret give way weakness as being equal to or better than whatever the strength was before the muscle gave way. I accept the uncertainty of not knowing whether the muscle is really mildly or moderately or severely weak (when it gave way) or is normal in strength.

This is similar to the sensory examination. All partial and complete loss of sensation is subjective; we rely on the patient's report that their sensation is less than normal or absent. We use our knowledge of normal sensory innervation patterns to help determine if the patient's demonstrated sensory findings are likely to be genuine or not, but we cannot be certain that their perception is truly impaired, nor can we be sure that the sensory loss is "functional." Patients do not understand how their body is innervated, and they may try to help us find the sensory loss they have experienced. A "nonanatomic" sensory loss could well have an underlying organic basis which has been embellished by the patient in an effort to help the examiner.

Peripheral tenderness with radiculopathy

Finally, I used to think that if the patient was tender out in their limb in the muscles or ligaments or joints, their pain could not be radicular in origin and referred from the spine. For reasons that are not clear to me, patients with nerve root compression can have soft tissue tenderness in their limb. I am not referring to tenderness in a peripheral nerve that could be related to compression of a nerve root near the spine, but rather soft tissue tenderness. I can't explain it, but don't make my mistake of presuming that limb tenderness eliminates the possibility of nerve root compression.

Patient and provider biases that have led to mistakes

"We have to do something"

Desperation on the part of the patient, their family, or their providers can lead to big trouble. Pain and disability are often poorly tolerated. "Doctor, I just want my life back" puts pressure on us to figure out what is wrong and fix it now. Desperation is greater with more symptoms, more severe symptoms, and longer duration of symptoms. Desperation is also greater in patients with a low tolerance for symptoms. Such desperation should not lead to premature or inappropriate investigation or treatment, but it does and I have done it. Please don't. We must know our limitations as providers and follow established evidenced-based recommendations for care. To do otherwise will subject our patients to unnecessary tests and treatment with attendant harm and actually lessen their chances for good outcomes.

"I just want an answer"

I have heard this request from patients and their families, and the question is often tinged with desperation. The need to have an answer also frequently leads to premature or inappropriate investigation. I admit that sometimes my curiosity about a patient's symptoms has led me to want a definite answer, and, in turn, led me to order premature and unnecessary tests and consultations. In my experience, patients who "just want an answer" are not satisfied with the answer alone; all of us want effective treatment if not a cure for what we hope is a benign condition.

"It's only a disk"

I see lots of patients with back and limb pain. Most of them have disk-related pain, and others have non-discogenic musculoskeletal pain. In both instances, the natural history is favorable, and the vast majority of patients do well with conservative treatment. As has been noted, the majority of patients will have evidence of degenerative disk disease on imaging studies. Whether or not the patient has had an imaging study which confirms the presence of degenerative disk disease, I sometimes conclude that the patient's symptoms are, at worst, due to a herniated disk. I may forget to keep in mind the possibility that something else could be going on. If the patient worsens or new symptoms develop, always be open to the possibility that the patient could have something else entirely or in addition to a disk.

"I'm not interested in surgery on my spine"

On occasion, I have had patients express a strong preference, if not a mandate, that they not have surgery on their spine. This can be based on familiarity with someone else's experience with back surgery or based on their own experience. Sometimes, it is based on advice they were given by a close relative or friend. This restriction is usually predicated on the presumption that their spine problem is "only a disk," and in that sense, they are guilty of the mistake described in the preceding section. I recall one patient whose mother told him on her deathbed never to have an operation on his spine. Just because the patient is unwilling to undergo surgery on their spine for degenerative disk and joint disease should not prevent us from finding out the cause of their symptoms. Sometimes, the cause is not a disk but rather a tumor or an infection. Sometimes, it is a disk but a very large one causing spinal cord or cauda equina compression. Sometimes, if all of the facts are known, the patient and their mother might be willing to accept surgery. Don't let a patient unnecessarily restrict your recommendations for diagnostic testing based on treatment that they think they are unwilling to accept. The diagnostic test does not commit you or the patient to surgery.

"Doctor, I'm not one who likes to take a lot of pills"

No one likes to take a lot of pills! I very rarely see patients who want to take more medications. Patients who tell us that they do not want to take a lot of pills are well-intentioned, but, depending on the strength of their conviction not to take medication, may be ruling out a form of treatment that could be very helpful to them. I respect patients who do not want to take medications for their symptoms. I do point out to them that medications are one of just four treatment options that we as healthcare providers have for any medical problem. The four treatment options are medications, surgery, physical therapies, and help coping with a problem or loss. While I respect the patient's wishes and do not suggest that they take prescription or over-the-counter analgesics or other drugs, I point out the potential role that medications could play in controlling symptoms.

I also point out that an injection is the administration of a medication at the end of a needle. I have observed that patients who "don't like to take a lot of pills" are usually more than happy to receive an injection (as are most patients I see with spine and limb pain).

Mistakes I have made in diagnostic testing

Premature investigation

The indications for appropriate investigation of spine and limb complaints have been presented. These evidence-based guidelines tell us when and what studies we should order. Premature investigation is prompted by good intentions and by some of the pitfalls outlined in this chapter (see "We have to do something" and "I just want an answer"). However, premature investigation carries with it significant risks that should curb our enthusiasm for obtaining them. What could be wrong with getting the MRI scan now instead of waiting until the stable patient has had symptoms for 4–6 weeks? Well, we could find nothing in their spine which might be reassuring but might lead us to worry that we are missing something more sinister outside of the spine and prompt us to obtain more testing. Second, we might see a lot of degenerative changes in the spine which could worry the patient, their family, and their employer, and us too. Now, the patient believes that they have a "degenerated spine." Perhaps they have "spinal stenosis." They are now afraid to lift their children and grandchildren, afraid to do yard work, afraid to go back to work, and sure that they are headed for spine surgery in the future. We have shaken their confidence. The findings may prompt us to obtain additional tests now, recommend treatment based solely on the test results, or lead us to recommend follow-up studies to track the initial findings. Third, we could see something inside the spine that we were not expecting. For example, we might see an abnormality in the bone that turns out to be a benign hemangioma but requires additional investigation. Fourth, we could see something outside the spine that raises concern and prompts additional testing now and follow-up in the future. For example, we may see a renal cyst that requires additional investigation or a thyroid nodule or an enlarged aorta. The additional tests that are prompted can be associated with risk. These additional abnormalities further rock the confidence of the patient and their family and can suggest that the patient has serious health problems. I confess my sins – I have often obtained premature testing. I don't recommend it.

Over-reliance on diagnostic test results

Wonderful imaging and electrophysiologic tests are available for evaluating patients with spine disease. They have transformed our ability to diagnose and thus treat patients. Be aware that sometimes the test results are wrong or, if not wrong, they are misleading because the findings do not correlate with the patient's clinical picture.

"I saw it with my own eyes" so how can the imaging study be wrong? As has been noted, MRI can show multiple findings in asymptomatic individuals. The patient with symptoms will have the same asymptomatic findings on MRI and possibly one or two symptomatic abnormalities. Which finding, if any, is symptomatic? The most prominent finding on the imaging study may not be causing the patient's symptoms. In fact, there are some patients with clear-cut radiculopathy or myelopathy who have normal imaging studies. It is natural to attribute the patient's symptoms to their imaging findings unless, of course, they are on the wrong side of the body. The radiologist will often list abnormalities by level or by radiographic significance. I am often guilty of concluding that a prominent imaging finding explains the patient's symptoms. To help reduce this bias, my preference is to evaluate the patient before I look at their MRI or CT scan. If patients ask me if I have looked at their imaging study when I first meet with them, I tell them, "No, I don't know where to look yet."

Electrophysiologic studies are very helpful in the diagnosis of spine disease, but they, too, can be misleading. In some institutions, including my own, there is a widely held belief that electromyography (EMG) is infallible. It is not. EMG can show no abnormalities when there is a radiculopathy; it can show radiculopathy that is not related to the patient's current symptoms; it can show incidental findings such as a carpal tunnel syndrome; and it can be flat out wrong. I recently saw a 65-year-old man with diffuse and persistent lower limb pains with occasional standing-induced severe pain. His examination showed no weakness and absence of the ankle reflexes. He had already had an EMG which was reported to show myopathic changes. An MRI of his legs showed "patchy atrophy" consistent with a chronic myopathy. I referred him to our neuromuscular clinic, where my colleague obtained a peroneus longus muscle biopsy which showed denervation with reinnervation. The neuromuscular specialist who is also head of the EMG laboratory repeated the EMG and found evidence of chronic denervation mostly affecting the S1 myotomes bilaterally. An MRI of his lumbar spine showed severe central and foraminal stenosis which probably explains the EMG findings but does not explain his chronic muscle pain. I and my colleagues were fooled by the first EMG report.

One should also maintain a healthy degree of skepticism about drawing conclusions from the benefit or lack of benefit that follows injections. Injections can be performed on spine patients for purely diagnostic purposes (e.g., local anesthetic into a facet joint or a hip joint), chiefly for a therapeutic benefit (e.g., transforaminal and other epidural steroid injections), or for both purposes. Even if performed as a treatment, we often draw diagnostic conclusions from the patient's response or lack of response to these injections. However, there are many variables that affect the patient's response and make it difficult to draw firm conclusions. These include a placebo response, a genuine response which results from spread of the injectant to a location different than was intended, a response that occurs at a greater distance from the injectant than one would expect, intravascular injection such that the injectant does not stay put, and lack of benefit because the local injection is not effective for the pathology that is causing the patient's symptoms. Tests which are meant to provoke the patient's pain, chiefly discography, are infamous for false-positive results. Do not put undue weight on the results of diagnostic/therapeutic injections. Response to injection does not necessarily establish the structure injected as a pain generator, nor does lack of response exclude the injected structure as a pain generator.

Mistakes I have made in diagnosis and treatment

Rush to judgment

The pace of medical practice seems to be ever increasing. Time constraints put pressure on us to diagnose and treat quickly and efficiently. Rushing to provide care often leads to wrong diagnoses and improper or ineffective treatment. If only we had more time for each patient.

The need to make a diagnosis

Patients, families, employers, referring providers, colleagues, and we expect us as providers to have an answer for every patient's problem. I wish it were so. Recall that it has been estimated that only 15% of patients with acute low back pain can be given an accurate diagnosis that explains their symptoms. As a neurologist seeing general neurology or spine patients, I consider myself lucky to truly know what is going on in half of my patients. We can't be wrong if we tell a patient we aren't sure about their diagnosis. Of course, we can't be right either. I have often gotten into trouble because I thought I knew what was wrong with a patient when the diagnosis was far from certain. There is no harm in quoting Mark Twain's reply when you are in doubt, "I was gratified to be able to answer promptly. I said I didn't know."

While patients want to know what is wrong with them, we cannot always tell them. Rather than fool them (and perhaps ourselves) by offering a definite answer, if we are unsure it is better to tell them either that we don't know what is wrong or describe our tentative diagnosis and explain why we cannot be sure at this time. I have become comfortable living with uncertainty when it comes to my patients' diagnoses. It can be helpful to leave a little room for doubt in your mind even when you are confident that you know what is wrong with a patient. By doing so, you never completely close the door on a possible, alternative diagnosis.

Influenced by experience

Experience greatly influences our decisions. Most patients with spine problems have degenerative disk and facet joint disease, compressive radiculopathy, spondylotic myelopathy, or lumbar spinal stenosis. Given a steady diet of the same symptoms and the same diagnoses, our bias is to conclude that the next patient has a similar condition. In summary, we are stuck in a diagnostic rut. Conversely, if we have recently seen an unusual case, we may start looking for that rare disease in all of the patients we see in the next several months. It is hard to keep a truly open mind for each new patient we see.

Jumping to conclusions

Several of the mistakes listed above such as "it's only a disk," "over-reliance on diagnostic test results," "rush to judgment," and "the need to make a diagnosis" can lead us to jump to a diagnostic conclusion or a therapeutic decision which is wrong or inappropriate respectively. Even if we are not pushed for time, we sometimes "shoot from the hip" and reach a conclusion prematurely and with insufficient basis or

thought. Other factors such as overconfidence can contribute to this error. Patients sometimes jump to conclusions as well. Jumping to conclusions is almost always a bad idea in medicine. A degree of humility and a modicum of uncertainty can help to prevent this mistake.

Clinging to a diagnosis

Whether we have come to a diagnostic conclusion quickly or after much thought, we are sometimes very reluctant to give it up when evidence mounts that we might be wrong. This mistake is likely related to hubris and our distaste for being wrong. I recall a woman who told me about the young doctor at the hospital who would not let go of his wrong diagnosis. She said that he held on to his conclusion "like a puppy clenching a rag." I have made this mistake. I think that we are all guilty at one time or another of being reluctant to admit we were wrong.

Attributing a peripheral process to a spine disorder

Neck pain is common. So is carpal tunnel syndrome. When the two occur together, it is easy to mistake the numb hand of carpal tunnel syndrome for cervical radiculopathy or myelopathy. Peripheral musculoskeletal pain or deep vein thrombophlebitis can be mistaken for a radiculopathy.

Attributing spine-related symptoms to a peripheral process

This is the converse of the preceding section. For example, I have mistaken the symptoms of a cervical radiculopathy or myelopathy for the more common carpal tunnel syndrome. I have also attributed an L5 radiculopathy to a peroneal nerve palsy. Please keep in mind that a spine disorder can simulate a peripheral process and vice versa.

Going against and going along with the previous diagnosis

Doctors are a funny lot. We sometimes do our best to prove the last doctor's diagnosis wrong. On the other hand, especially if the referring provider is a colleague, there is a tendency for us to go along with the previous diagnosis. For people like me who trained before the advent of CT and MRI, I am not very good at reading spine images and often accept the radiologist's interpretation. I sometimes forget to keep an open mind, review all of the data myself, and come to an independent diagnosis and recommendation for treatment. This is especially true if I am short on time or if the previous provider is someone I hold in high esteem.

Considering the possibility of more than one "lesion" or disease

We are taught in medicine to be parsimonious and to explain everything with a single diagnosis. Patients do not always co-operate and can have more than one problem at a time. While it may true that the patient does have a carpal tunnel syndrome, they could have a concomitant cervical myelopathy. Many patients with spine disease are older and entitled to have more than one problem. Patients with spine disease will often have problems at more than one level of the spine, especially a combination of cervical and lumbar spinal stenosis or cervical and lumbar radiculopathy. They can also have spine disease and peripheral musculoskeletal disease (e.g., radiculopathy and trochanteric bursitis). I have made mistakes when I settled on a single diagnosis and I have should have been more vigilant and considered the possibility that the patient had an additional problem within or outside the spine.

Failure to remember the natural history of the disease

Acute cervical and lumbar radiculopathies typically improve on their own. If the patient is seen early in their course, we may recommend tests and interventions that are unnecessary because the patient will recover spontaneously if we give them time. Lumbar spinal stenosis and cervical spondylotic myelopathy tend to progress but only gradually over time, and there is usually no need to rush the patient into surgery before they are convinced of its need in their situation.

Failure to recognize the limits of treatment

We also need to remember the efficacy of the treatments we recommend. I recently saw a patient with a lumbar radiculopathy due to a herniated lumbar disk who had undergone surgery after having been told that there was a "99.9%" chance that the surgery would cure them. This patient did not have a good outcome from their surgery, and their disappointment was heightened by the inflated odds that surgery would relieve them of their symptoms. Surgery for acute cervical and lumbar radiculopathy is probably 90% effective in relieving patients of their pain, but neither operation is 100% effective. Surgery for lumbar

spinal stenosis is beneficial in about 75%–80% of patients. Surgery for cervical spondylotic myelopathy often keeps people where they are, although some patients do improve post-operatively. As much as we would like patients to improve with the treatment we recommend, what we tell them should be realistic and evidenced-based. I know I have overstated the potential benefit of surgery in the past. I have done so in an effort to convince the patient to have an operation I thought would help them. I should have been more honest and let the patient decide.

Failure to consider all available treatment options

I often forget to consider all of the four treatment options we can provide (medications, surgery, physical therapies, and help with coping). One can also add activity modification and lifestyle changes that are under the patient's control. Treatments can and should be used in combination rather than in isolation. Even if you and the patient decide against one or another form of treatment, it can be useful to at least mention all potential treatment options.

Mistakes I have made interacting with patients

Failure to obtain and incorporate patient and family preferences

Patients and their families are better informed than ever about their medical conditions. For most spine conditions, multiple treatments are available, and surgical intervention is often elective rather than necessary. In fact, data from the Spine Patient Outcomes Research Trials show that for many operations on the spine, patients do better if they have input into the decision whether or not to have surgery. We should find out if our patients are interested in manipulation therapy or complementary and alternative medicine and advise them about these treatment options rather than to be blind to their preferences and have them seek out such treatments on their own and without our knowledge. I need to remind myself continually to seek out the patient's and family's perspective and incorporate their preferences into the plan to evaluate and treat their symptoms.

Telling the patient what they want to hear

Healthcare providers sometimes behave like politicians; we tell patients and their families what they

271

want to hear rather than the truth. I remember an older woman who had undergone surgery for lumbar radiculopathy. Her pain was better, but her weakness was worse. Imaging showed no new nerve root compression. Her EMG showed chronic radiculopathy. I could not explain why her leg was weaker. She asked me to reassure her that she did not have amyotrophic lateral sclerosis (ALS). I thought this was unlikely and did not see any harm in telling her that she did not have this dreadful condition. She and her family were bitter when it turned out that her weakness spread and she did have ALS. Follow Mark Twain's advice, "When in doubt, tell the truth." We can tell patients and their families that "we don't think they have . . ." or "there is no evidence that they have . . ." or "the risks of surgery are low . . ." but we should not make hard and fast statements without basis even though the patient and their family crave reassurance or "an answer."

Blaming the patient

Please don't blame the patient or get angry with them. It is unprofessional and counterproductive to patient care. I am very embarrassed to say that it happens to me, and it may happen to you as well. These feelings against the patient occur in several circumstances. It can occur when the patient has too many symptoms, and I don't have the time to listen to all of them. It sometimes happens to me when I can't explain the patient's symptoms. While I may be crazed, the patient is not crazy, and I should not blame them for my inability to reach a diagnosis. Sometimes these feelings happen when there are medicolegal or workers' compensation entanglements. Sometimes I blame the patient and get angry when they have functional, apparent nonorganic findings. Sometimes it happens when I believe the patient is drug-seeking or malingering. Sometimes it occurs because I blame the patient for their bad habits (smoking, drinking alcohol to excess), their lifestyle choices (sedentary and being overweight), their personality traits (vague responses, argumentative, angry, or overly passive), or sometimes just because we don't hit it off for

reasons that I can't explain. Of course, we shouldn't blame the patient and or get angry with them. However, this is our emotional reaction, and not something we can simply turn off. We should be aware of our emotional response to patients and strive to be more accepting of their symptoms, habits, situations, and personalities. If I recognize that I have negative feelings toward a patient, I try to understand why, do my best to hide my feelings, and attempt to be objective. In the very rare instances where my interpersonal reaction with the patient is impeding care, I will ask a colleague to see them in my stead.

Further reading

Croskerry P. The importance of cognitive errors in diagnosis and strategies to minimize them. *Acad Med* 2003; **78**:775–780.

Elstein A, Dowie J, eds. *Professional Judgment: A Reader in Clinical Decision Making.* Cambridge: Cambridge University Press, 1988.

Ericsson KA. An expert-performance perspective of research on medical expertise: the study of clinical performance. *Med Educ* 2007; **41**:1124–1130.

Ericsson KA, Charness N, Feltovich P, Hoffman RR, eds. *The Cambridge Handbook of Expertise and Expert Performance.* Cambridge: Cambridge University Press, 2006.

Graber ML, Franklin N, Gordon R. Diagnostic error in internal medicine. *Arch Intern Med* 2005; **165**:1493–1499.

Groopman J. *How Doctors Think.* New York: Houghton Mifflin Company, 2007.

Hall J, Roter D. *Doctors Talking With Patients/Patients Talking With Doctors: Improving Communication in Medical Visits*, Second Edition. Westport, CN: Praeger Publishers, 2006.

Higgs J, Jones MA. *Clinical Reasoning in the Health Professions.* Woburn, Mass.: Butterworth-Heinemann, 1995.

Kassirer JP, Kopelman RI. Cognitive errors in diagnosis: instantiation, classification, and consequences. *Am J Med* 1989; **86**(4):433–441.

Redelmeier DA. The cognitive psychology of missed diagnoses. *Ann Intern Med* 2005; **142**:115–120.

Glossary

Adamkiewicz, great radicular artery of. The largest segmental radicular artery supplying the lower end of the spinal cord. In two-thirds of individuals, the vessel arises on the left side and accompanies the spinal nerve root through the intervertebral foramen, usually from T9 through L1, but ranging from T5 to L3.

Adjacent segment degeneration. Accelerated degenerative changes occurring at segments adjacent to a spinal fusion as a result of increased biomechanical stress. Other terms include adjacent segment disease and fusion disease.

Allodynia. Pain caused by a nonpainful stimulus such as a light touch which may extend beyond the area stimulated. The presence of allodynia suggests a neuropathic process and sensitization of the central nervous system.

Allograft. Bone graft obtained from another human. Allograft bone is harvested from cadavers, prepared in a variety of sizes and shapes, and stored until needed. Also known as homograft.

Annular repair. Technique used to repair the annulus after lumbar microdiscectomy in an effort to prevent recurrent herniation.

Autograft. Bone graft taken from the patient's body. Autograft bone is usually harvested from the iliac crest, although grafts may also be harvested from rib or fibula.

Baastrup disease. Adjacent spinous processes, usually in the lumbar spine, abut against one another and produce local reactive change with midline back pain.

Bent spine syndrome. This is basically a synonym for camptocormia (see Camptocormia).

Bertolotti syndrome. Anomalous enlargement of the transverse process on one or both sides of the caudal-most lumbar vertebra which may then articulate with or fuse with the sacrum or ilium.

Degenerative change in this joint or the disk immediately above can cause back pain which is termed Bertolotti syndrome.

Bone growth stimulator. Device which applies a weak electrical current to the spine to enhance the maturation of a spinal fusion. The device may be implanted at the time of surgery or worn externally after the procedure.

Bone morphogenetic proteins (BMP). Recombinant human bone morphogenetic proteins, commonly known as BMP, represent a group of growth factors and cytokines with significant bone-forming ability. BMP is often used to enhance a spinal fusion.

Brown–Séquard syndrome. A spinal cord syndrome resulting from damage to one lateral half of the spinal cord which results in ipsilateral motor weakness and loss of vibration and joint position sense and contralateral loss of pain and temperature sensation below the lesion.

Cage. Device placed into the anterior spinal column to provide structural support after discectomy or corpectomy. Cages are made of metal, carbon fiber, or poly-ether-ether-ketone (PEEK), and are filled with bone graft material prior to insertion.

Camptocormia ("bent tree trunk"). Forward flexion at the waist when standing or walking which is relieved when supine; inability to stand erect. Often accompanied by pain, camptocormia can be seen in hysteria, parkinsonian syndromes, dystonia, and severe paraspinal muscle weakness.

Cauda equina ("horse's tail"). The collection of lumbosacral nerve roots that run together from the end of the spinal cord (usually from the level of the first lumbar vertebra) down to the bottom of the sacrum within the vertebral (spinal) canal.

Cauda equina syndrome. Damage to the lumbosacral nerve roots which constitute the cauda equina. Commonly caused by a large herniated disk, trauma, tumors, inflammatory conditions, and iatrogenic causes. Manifestations include low back and lower limb pain, numbness in the perineum and lower extremities, difficulty controlling bowel and bladder function, lower limb weakness, and reduced or absent lower limb reflexes.

Central cord syndrome. A common incomplete spinal cord injury syndrome typically caused by hyperextension of the neck. Damage is greatest in the central cervical spinal cord and causes motor impairment greater in the upper than lower limbs, variable sensory loss below the level of injury, and frequent bladder dysfunction.

Chemonucleolysis. A procedure for lumbar disk herniation which involves percutaneous injection of chymopapain into the disk nucleus pulposus to shrink the protruded disk and relieve nerve root compression. After being widely used in the 1970s, chemonucleolysis has been largely abandoned in North America and Europe. However, there is currently a resurgence of interest in the technique in Asia.

Chiari (or Arnold Chiari) malformation. A spectrum of structural defects affecting the hindbrain (cerebellum and brain stem) and sometimes other parts of the central nervous system. The inferior aspect of the cerebellum, especially the cerebellar tonsils, protrudes through the foramen magnum with resulting compression of neural tissue. Valsalva-induced headache is a common presenting complaint. This is type I. A more severe Chiari malformation, type II, is usually accompanied by a myelomeningocele. Chiari malformation can be associated with hydrocephalus, spina bifida, syringomyelia, tethered cord syndrome, and scoliosis. Low CSF pressure can cause the hindbrain to sag into the foramen magnum which is sometimes termed acquired or secondary Chiari malformation.

Circumferential fusion. Combined anterior and posterior spinal fusion; may be done as a single operation or in separate stages. Other terms include "front-back," anterior-posterior, and 360° fusion.

Clearing the cervical spine. A process, which includes clinical and radiographic assessment, by which significant cervical spine injury is excluded in trauma patients.

Complex regional pain syndrome (CRPS). CRPS is a chronic pain condition that usually affects one limb

and is accompanied by changes in skin color and temperature, swelling, abnormal sweating, and hypersensitivity of the affected area. CRPS commonly follows injury, but the pain that develops, which is often burning in character, is far out of proportion to the severity of the injury. Type I, previously known as reflex sympathetic dystrophy, typically follows an injury that did not directly injure nerve tissue. Type II, once referred to as causalgia, typically follows a peripheral nerve injury.

Conus medullaris. The lower end of the spinal cord which normally ends at the level of the first vertebral body. The conus medullaris has some upper motor neuron fibers as well as anterior horn cells which supply the lower lumbar and sacral level motor nerves.

Corpectomy. Removal of a vertebral body; can be performed at a single or multiple levels as needed. Also known as vertebrectomy.

Dermatome. The area of skin supplied by a single spinal sensory nerve root and its dorsal ganglion.

Discectomy. Partial or complete removal of an intervertebral disk. Can be accomplished via an anterior or posterior surgical approach.

Disk arthroplasty. A mechanical device, available for use in the cervical and lumbar spine, which replaces the entire intervertebral disk complex, including the nucleus, annulus, and both endplates. Other terms include total disk replacement and artificial disk.

Disk extrusion. An extruded disk is where the distance between the edges of the disk beyond the disk space is greater than the distance between the edges of the base of the herniated disk when measured in the same plane or when there is a loss of continuity between the herniated disk material and the disk material within the disk space.

Disk migration. Disk herniation in which part of the disk material is displaced away from the interspace so that it lies behind the vertebral body above or below.

Disk protrusion. A protruded disk is one in which the distance between the edges of the herniated disk material beyond the interspace is less than the distance between the edges of the disk at its base when measured in the same plane.

Disk sequestration. Refers to a herniated disk in which the disk material is no longer in continuity with the parent disk and is no longer contained by annulus fibrosus tissue. By definition, a sequestrated disk is also an extruded disk.

Donor-site pain. Pain occurring at the site of bone graft harvest for a fusion procedure.

Double crush syndrome. Simultaneous compression at the peripheral nerve and nerve root level, resulting in additive signs and symptoms. For example, carpal tunnel syndrome combined with C6 radiculopathy from a disk herniation at C5–C6.

Dropped head syndrome. Inability to hold the head erect, typically due to neck extensor muscle weakness. The condition may or may not be painful and is usually secondary to a localized myopathy, a generalized myopathic process, motor neuron disease, myasthenia gravis, parkinsonian syndromes, or dystonia.

Dynamic stabilization surgery. A group of lumbar stabilization operations, allowing controlled motion, which is more consistent with normal movement of the spine. In contrast, fusion operations result in rigid immobilization of the treated segments. This term should not to be confused with dynamic lumbar stabilization, a specific exercise program for patients with low back pain.

Facet bone dowel. Small allograft bone dowel implanted into the facet joint to stabilize the spine. Usually done bilaterally, facet bone dowels may be inserted using either open or percutaneous techniques.

Failed back surgery syndrome. Not so much a well-defined syndrome as a poor outcome from lumbar spine surgery with chronic low back and/or lower limb pain that is difficult to treat.

Foraminotomy. Opening of a neural foramen to decompress the exiting nerve root. Foraminotomy may be done through an anterior or posterior surgical approach.

Fusion. A surgical procedure designed to permanently join together, or fuse, two or more segments of the spinal column. A variety of bone grafting materials and fixation devices, made of metal and other materials, are used in fusion procedures.

Hybrid construct. A loosely defined term, which applies to a collection of spine operations, incorporating new methods which combine existing surgical techniques. An example would be performing a lumbar fusion at one level and a disk arthroplasty at an adjacent level.

Image guidance. Refers to the use of CT or MRI images, acquired pre-operatively or intra-operatively, to assist with placement of instruments and implants in the spine. See Stereotactic spinal surgery.

Instrumentation. Metal rods, screws, and cages used as internal fixation devices in the spine. Instrumentation is available for use in all levels of the spinal column.

Interbody fusion, lumbar. A commonly performed procedure, which involves removal of the intervertebral disk and placement of a cage and/or bone graft. Interbody fusion may be performed via anterior, posterior, lateral, and combined approaches. At L5–S1, interbody fusion may also be performed via a presacral route.

Internal disk disruption. Degeneration and reactive change within intervertebral disks and adjacent vertebrae which cause axial spine pain without nerve impingement. The exact pathophysiology of symptoms associated with internal disk disruption is not clear.

Intervertebral (neural) foramen. Between adjoining vertebrae are paired openings, the intervertebral (neural) foramina, which contain the spinal nerves and nerve roots, dorsal root ganglia, segmental blood vessels, and sinuvertebral nerves. The intervertebral foramina are bounded by the pedicles above and below, the intervertebral disk and vertebral body anteriorly, and the zygapophyseal joints posteriorly.

Intradiscal electrothermal therapy (IDET). A procedure for treating discogenic back pain, which involves application of thermal energy to the disk annulus by means of a percutaneously placed flexible electrode.

Intrathecal drug pump. An infusion system, consisting of an infusion pump, implanted in the subcutaneous tissues of the abdomen, and an intraspinal catheter, which delivers medication from the pump into the spinal subarachnoid space.

Klippel–Feil syndrome. Congenital fusion of any two of the seven cervical vertebrae which can be associated with a short neck, low hairline posteriorly, and reduced neck range of motion.

Kyphoplasty. A percutaneous technique of repair of vertebral compression fractures, which involves inflation of a balloon tamp within the fractured vertebral body, followed by a low-pressure injection of polymethylmethacrylate (PMMA) to stabilize the fracture. See Vertebroplasty.

Kyphosis. A general term which refers to abnormal forward curvature of the spine usually affecting the thoracic spine. Also used to describe reversal of the normal backward curve of the cervical or lumbar spine. Also known as sagittal plane deformity.

Lag screw effect. This phenomenon occurs in posterior cervical lateral mass fusion procedures when there is a gap along the screw between the lateral mass and the rod or plate. As the surgeon tightens the screw to close the gap, the lateral mass can be displaced posteriorly which can in turn deform the neural foramen and compress the nerve root.

Laminectomy. Partial or complete removal of the lamina at one or more levels. Used to treat spinal stenosis or provide access to the spinal canal for removal of disks, tumors, and other lesions.

Laminoplasty. A procedure for cervical spinal stenosis, which expands the spinal canal by splitting open the laminae, removing the ligamentum flavum, and repositioning the laminae posteriorly.

Lateral mass fixation. A posterior cervical fusion procedure, which involves placement of bilateral vertically oriented rods or plates, which are secured to the spine by means of screws placed into the lateral masses.

Lhermitte sign. Tingling down the spine and/or extremities with neck flexion more commonly than with neck extension is termed Lhermitte sign and indicates inflammation or irritation of the cervical spinal cord from conditions such as multiple sclerosis, pernicious anemia, cervical spondylosis, and tumors.

Medial branch. The medial branches of the dorsal rami of the spinal nerves supply paraspinal muscles, cutaneous sensation near the midline posteriorly, and the ipsilateral facet joints. The medial branches are often targeted in attempts to relieve pain of suspected facet joint origin.

Meralgia paresthetica. Injury to or irritation of the lateral femoral cutaneous nerve resulting in tingling, numbness, and sometimes burning pain in the lateral thigh. Meralgia paresthetica is a benign syndrome but can be confused with lumbar radiculopathy.

Microdiscectomy. Removal of the intervertebral disk with the assistance of an operating microscope.

Minimally invasive spinal surgery. A concept in which the surgeon attempts to achieve the goals of the operation through small incisions with less approach-related morbidity. Another term is "minimal access spine surgery."

Modic changes on MRI. There are three types of Modic changes which describe various reactive changes in vertebral body bone marrow adjacent to and associated with degenerative disk disease. Named after the neuroradiologist who described them.

Myelopathy. Disease of the spinal cord.

Myotome. The muscles supplied by a single spinal segment.

Nephrogenic systemic fibrosis (initially termed nephrogenic fibrosing dermopathy). An illness that develops following the administration of gadolinium to patients with reduced renal function who undergo MRI. The condition is characterized by fibrosis of the skin, joints, and internal organs. There is no effective treatment.

Neuropathic pain. Caused by damage to or dysfunction of peripheral sensory nerves, the spinal ganglia, or their central connections, neuropathic pain often has a burning, prickling, lancinating, or electric quality. Allodynia (see above) and hyperalgesia (exaggerated pain with a normally painful stimulus) are frequent accompaniments.

Nociceptive pain. Caused by activation of primary sensory nerve endings, nociceptive pain can be aching, throbbing, or sharp. Nociceptive pain can be further divided into superficial somatic, deep somatic, and visceral pain, depending on where the sensory nerve stimulation occurs.

Noninstrumented fusion. Spinal fusion performed with various bone grafting materials, without concomitant metal fixation devices.

Notalgia paresthetica. Itching, tingling, and pain, sometimes accompanied by increased skin pigmentation, affecting a local thoracic paraspinal area, usually on one side. While it is thought that the symptoms may be due to a "sensory neuropathy," the condition is benign and not associated with significant nerve root or spinal cord impingement.

Nucleus replacement. A group of procedures, currently in the development stage, which involve replacing the disk nucleus with an artificial device or substance, while leaving the annulus and endplates intact. Nucleus replacement is a less invasive procedure than disk arthroplasty.

Orthosis. One of a variety of braces worn externally to immobilize the spine after fusion surgery or trauma. Orthoses are available for all levels of the spinal column. Most are made of plastic or other lightweight materials.

Osteophyte. Focal hypertrophy of bone surface and/or calcification of soft tissue attachments to bone.

Pedicle screw. Bone screw inserted via a posterior approach through the pedicle, into the vertebral body, and attached to a longitudinal member, either rod or plate, to connect two or more segments of the spinal column. Pedicle screws are available in varying lengths and diameters and can be used in the thoracic and lumbar spine and sacrum.

Perineural (Tarlov) cysts. Cerebrospinal fluid-filled nerve root sleeve diverticula. They are more common in the lumbosacral spinal canal than at higher levels. While impressive on MRI, they are usually incidental, asymptomatic findings.

Piriformis syndrome. Compression of the sciatic nerve by the piriformis muscle can cause pain, tingling, and numbness in the ipsilateral buttock and lower extremity. Piriformis syndrome is considered when sciatica occurs without an apparent spinal cause.

Plate, anterior. Metal fixation device applied to the anterior spine for stabilization. Anterior plates are anchored to the spine by means of screws in the vertebral bodies, and are available for use at all levels of the spinal column.

Plate, posterior. Metal fixation device applied to the posterior spine for stabilization. Plates are anchored to the spine with pedicle screws. Plates have largely been replaced by rods in the posterior spine.

Pseudarthrosis. Failed spinal fusion, often heralded clinically by persistent or recurrent pain. Radiographic findings include resorption of bone grafts and loosening or breakage of spinal instrumentation.

Pseudomeningocele. An abnormal extradural collection of CSF that occurs after a breach in the dura-arachnoid layer of the meninges, usually following surgery or, occasionally, trauma. They are most common in the lumbar spine and may be symptomatic. Low back pain, a local soft mass, radiculopathy, and intracranial CSF hypotension can occur.

Radiculopathy. Disease of the spinal nerves or nerve roots.

Referred pain. Used to describe pain that is perceived at a site distant from the site of injury or pain origin.

Rod. Metal fixation device applied to the posterior spine for stabilization. Rods are anchored to the spine with pedicle screws.

Sciatica. Pain in the distribution of the sciatic nerve which receives contributions from the L4, L5, S1, S2, and S3 nerve roots.

Sclerotome. Areas of bone supplied by a single spinal segment.

Scoliosis. Any lateral curvature of the spine measuring more than 11°, sometimes associated with rotation. Also known as coronal plane deformity.

Sham trial. A prospective clinical trial in which the patient is randomized to receive either the intervention of interest or a sham intervention (placebo). Sham trials are often performed using medications and less commonly with surgical procedures.

Sinuvertebral (recurrent meningeal) nerves. Arise at each spinal level from branches of the spinal nerve or its ventral ramus and a gray ramus communicans. These nerves innervate the posterior longitudinal ligament, superficial posterior and lateral intervertebral disk and periosteum, the anterior dura mater, and blood vessels, and are thought to play a role in transmitting axial spine pain related to degenerative disk disease.

Spinal cord stimulation. A treatment which attempts to relieve chronic spine and limb pain through stimulation (as opposed to destruction) of sensory pathways. Spinal cord stimulation is used primarily for patients with failed back surgery syndrome.

Spinal nerves and nerve roots. The term spinal nerve applies to the short segment of nerve after the

Index

Note: Page numbers in *italic* indicate Glossary entries

281